AF380665

Innovation of Diagnosis and Treatment for Pancreatic Cancer

Hiroki Yamaue

Editor

Innovation of Diagnosis and Treatment for Pancreatic Cancer

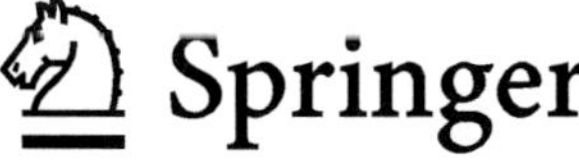 Springer

Editor
Hiroki Yamaue
Second Department of Surgery
Wakyama Medical University
Wakayama
Japan

ISBN 978-981-10-2485-6   ISBN 978-981-10-2486-3   (eBook)
DOI 10.1007/978-981-10-2486-3

Library of Congress Control Number: 2017946486

This Springer imprint is published by Springer Nature
The registered company is Springer Nature Singapore Pte Ltd.
The registered company address is: 152 Beach Road, #21-01/04 Gateway East, Singapore 189721, Singapore

Contents

Part I

Diagnosis of Pancreatic Cancer

Early Diagnosis of Pancreatic Cancer Using Endoscopic Ultrasound

1

Susumu Hijioka, Kenji Yamao, Nobumasa Mizuno, Hiroshi Imaoka, Vikram Bhatia, and Kazuo Hara

1.1 Introduction

Pancreatic cancer (PC) is the deadliest of all solid malignancies. The prognosis of patients with PC is extremely poor, as vast majority of PC is diagnosed only at an advanced stage. Over 30,000 patients died of PC in Japan during 2013, and this number is expected to rise. It is projected that PC will surpass breast, prostate and colorectal cancer to become the second leading cause of cancer-related death in the USA by 2030 [1]. Therefore, PC remains one of the greatest challenges in the fight against cancer in the twenty-first century [2]. Since the poor prognosis is attributed to difficulties with diagnosis at an early stage, early detection might offer the best hope for a cure. Therefore, detecting PC at the earliest possible stage at which it is potentially curable and identifying precursor lesions have received considerable focus. PC is usually detected by computed tomography (CT) and/or magnetic resonance imaging (MRI) with magnetic resonance cholangiopancreatography (MRCP), or endoscopic ultrasound (EUS). Although multi-detector (MD) row CT is almost universally utilized in PC evaluation, its rate of detecting small pancreatic masses is low. On the other hand, EUS can detect small pancreatic masses with high sensitivity. This chapter reviews early PC diagnosis using EUS (Table 1.1).

S. Hijioka (✉) • K. Yamao • N. Mizuno • H. Imaoka • K. Hara
Department of Gastroenterology, Aichi Cancer Center Hospital,
1-1 Kanokoden, Chikusa-ku, Nagoya, Aichi 464-8681, Japan
e-mail: rizasusu@aichi-cc.jp

V. Bhatia
Department of Gastroenterology, Fortis Escorts Hospital, New Delhi, India

© Springer Science+Business Media Singapore 2017

H. Yamaue (ed.), *Innovation of Diagnosis and Treatment for Pancreatic Cancer*,
DOI 10.1007/978-981-10-2486-3_1

Table 1.1 The characteristics of convex and radial scope

	Radial scope	Convex scope
Advantage	• Scanning range is 360° • Pancreas is easily seen as a longitudinal and continuous image	• Histological diagnosis is possible • Junction between the pancreatic head and body can be seen from the stomach
Disadvantage	• Histological diagnosis is impossible • Operator dependent	• Scanning range is 180° • Images of the body and tail of the pancreas become cross-sectional images

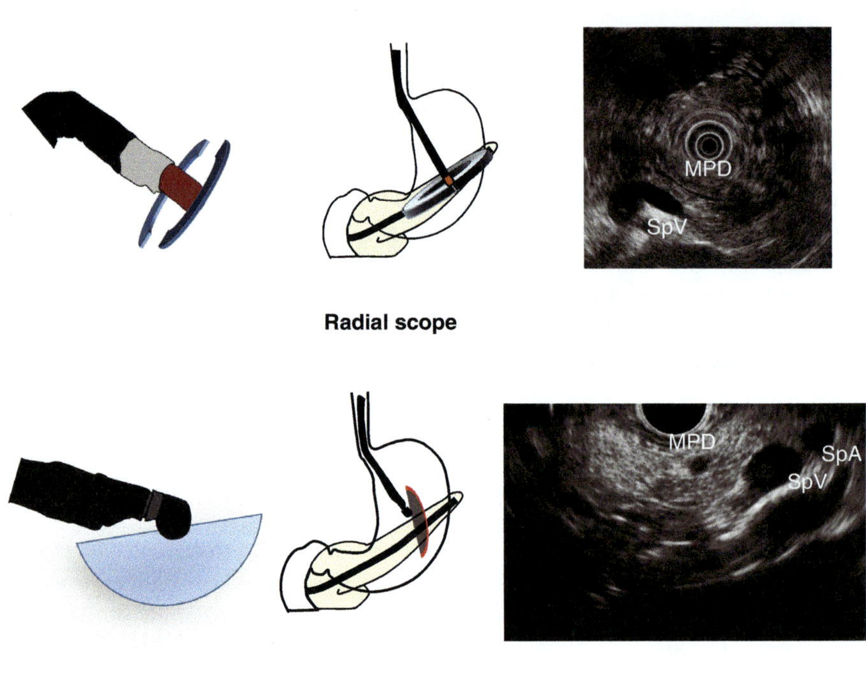

Fig. 1.1 Scheme of radial EUS and convex EUS. Radial EUS has 360° imaging perpendicular to the long axis. MPD is depicted longitudinally in pancreas body. Convex EUS has imaging along a plane parallel to the long axis of the instrument. MPD is depicted short axis view in pancreas body

1.2 **EUS** (Fig. 1.1)

The EUS equipment includes probes with different imaging methods: radial probes allow 360° imaging perpendicular to the long axis, and convex probes allow imaging along a plane parallel to the long axis of the instrument. The former only allows diagnostic imaging, whereas the latter was developed for fine-needle aspiration (FNA) [3, 4]. EUS uses high ultrasound frequencies, with imaging from the stomach or duodenum providing high resolution, real-time images of the pancreas. This modality therefore plays an important role in evaluating pancreatic diseases.

1.3 Early Diagnosis of PC Using EUS

MDCT evaluation of patients with suspected PC is the standard preoperative assessment at most medical institutions. This is because MDCT has good spatial and temporal resolution with wide anatomical coverage, and thus permits both comprehensive local and distant disease assessment during a single session [5, 6].

Among cross-sectional imaging modalities, the performance of MDCT is optimal for evaluating vascular involvement, which is the most important predictor of tumor resectability [7–9]. However, about 10% of PCs are iso-attenuating relative to the background pancreatic parenchyma (Fig. 1.2) [10]. CT enhancement of the PC and of pancreatic parenchyma surrounding a tumor is correlated with the degree of fibrosis. Contrast material is retained in PC with a predominant fibrous component. A similar degree of fibrosis in a tumor and surrounding pancreatic parenchyma might lead to overlapping enhancement on MDCT that could prevent the detection of PC, especially when tumors are ≤2 cm [11–13].

On the other hand, PC appears on EUS images as heterogeneous hypoechoic masses with irregular margins, which allows very high sensitivity for detecting PC [14, 15].

It is considered one of the most accurate means of detecting pancreatic focal lesions, especially when tumors are ≤2 cm [16–19].

Recent reports indicate that EUS can detect tumors <10 mm [20–22]. The sensitivity of EUS for detection of 25 small PC with size <10 mm was 84%, among eight Japanese high-volume centers [23]. Therefore, all patients with obstructive jaundice

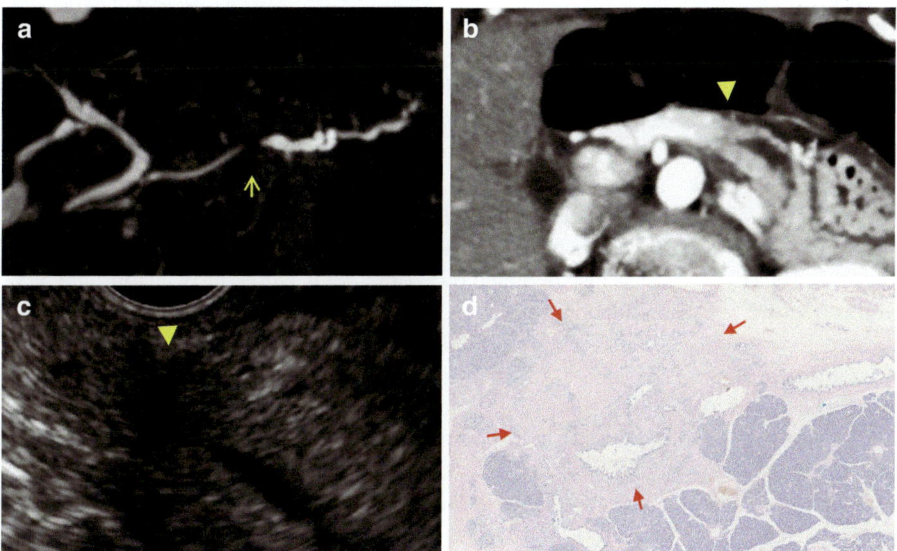

Fig. 1.2 Case: a 8 mm pancreatic cancer with invasion. MRCP (**a**) showed short duct stenosis in pancreatic body (*arrow*). Contrast-enhanced CT (**b**) could not detect the mass in pancreatic body (*arrow ahead*) though main pancreatic duct (MPD) was dilated and disrupted in the body. (**c**) EUS could detect the low echoic mass with unclear margin. (**d**) Microscopic findings revealed an 8 mm tumor with invasion accompanied with 20 mm fibrosis

or unexplained pancreatic duct dilation, in whom CT or MRI do not definitively identify pancreatic lesions should be assessed using EUS [24].

However, EUS can miss a true pancreatic mass in patients with chronic pancreatitis, a diffusely infiltrating carcinoma, a prominent ventral/dorsal split, or a recent episode (<4 weeks) of acute pancreatitis [25]. The potential for suboptimal visualization of the pancreatic gland for detection of PC by EUS and other imaging modalities should be acknowledged in the setting of acute or chronic pancreatitis. Acoustic shadowing caused by an indwelling biliary or pancreatic stents, or pancreatic stones can also interfere with the visualization of small pancreatic masses.

1.4 Pancreatic Intraepithelial Neoplasia (PanIN)

PC develops through stepwise progression from precursor lesions comprising pancreatic intraepithelial neoplasia (PanIN), mucinous cystic neoplasm (MCN), and intraductal papillary mucinous neoplasm (IPMN). Among these, PanIN is the most common precursor of PC [26]. PanIN are noninvasive epithelial proliferations within smaller pancreatic ducts (<0.5 mm) that can be flat or papillary and classified into low (PanIN-1), intermediate (PanIN-2), and high (PanIN-3) grades according to the degree of architectural and cellular atypia [26]. Based on mutations associated with each grade, normal ductal epithelium seems to progress through low-grade PanIN, high-grade PanIN, localized adenocarcinoma, and metastatic adenocarcinoma in that order. Detection of high-grade PanIN-3 would provide an optimal opportunity to reduce mortality from PC. It has been believed that PanIN cannot be reliably visualized using clinical imaging [27] as they typically arise in the small-caliber pancreatic ducts [26].

However, it has been recently suggested that PanIN is associated with localized parenchymal changes that may be detected by EUS [28, 29]. These parenchymal changes are characterized by acinar cell loss, proliferation of small ductular structures, and fibrosis referred to as lobulocentric atrophy (LCA) [30]. Localized fibrosis and/or LCA has been pathologically identified in parenchyma around PanIN-3 [21, 25, 28, 29, 31, 32]. A slightly low echoic lesion on EUS images might suggest localized fibrosis around PanIN-3 [28]. Maire et al. [29] reported that EUS changes corresponded to PanIN lesions in 83%. EUS also detected 69% of patients with PanIN lesions and 57% of those with PanIN3 lesions. However, EUS findings for PanIN lesion were not uniformed. For instance, Maire et al. [29] defined EUS findings of PanIN lesion were microcysts or hyper-echogenic foci resulting in a heterogeneous pattern. On the other hand, Hanada et al. [28] reported slightly low echoic lesion on EUS images were the findings of PanIN. However, it should be noted that these abnormalities on EUS are not specific to PanIN or early PC, and conversely, PanIN may well occur in the absence of LCA [30, 33]. Further studies are warranted to confirm these findings.

1.5 Surveillance of High-Risk Individuals

Familial pancreatic cancer (FPC) kindreds are defined as families with two or more first-degree relatives (FDR) affected with PC, in the absence of other cancers or familial diseases. Klein et al. found that the risk of developing PC was 4.5- vs.

32-fold depending on whether one or at least three FDR were affected, respectively [34, 35].

A multicenter prospective cohort study (CAPS 3) implemented by Canto et al. [36] included 216 high-risk individuals (HRI) (Peutz-Jeghers syndrome, $n = 2$; familial breast-ovarian cancer with at least one affected first- or second-degree relative with PC, $n = 19$; relatives of patients with FPC with at least two FDR, $n = 195$). All persons were evaluated by CT, MRI, and EUS, and 92 (42%) of 216 had at least one pancreatic mass (84 cystic and 3 solid) or a dilated pancreatic duct ($n = 5$) according to the findings of at least one of the imaging modalities. The prevalence of these lesions increased with age of the screened persons. Pancreatic abnormalities were detected by CT, MRI, and EUS in 11%, 33.3%, and 42.6% of the patients, respectively. Among the pancreatic lesions, 82 were IPMN, and three were neuroendocrine tumors. Five patients who were surgically treated had high-grade dysplasia in IPMN <3 cm and multiple intraepithelial neoplasms. Canto et al. concluded that screening asymptomatic HRI could detect curable noninvasive high-grade and multiple cystic lesions. Both EUS and MRI were more effective diagnostic screens for HRI than CT [37]. These findings showed that screening of high-risk families can detect early precancerous changes in the pancreas [35].

1.6 New Screening Modality Comprising Contrast EUS and Elastography

Conventional EUS sometimes cannot detect pancreatic tumors in patients with chronic pancreatitis, diffusely infiltrating carcinoma, or a recent episode of acute pancreatitis [25]. Contrast-enhanced (CH)-EUS and EUS elastography might help to improve the diagnostic accuracy of EUS.

Parenchymal perfusion and the pancreatic microvasculature can be visualized without artifacts by CH-EUS [38], and it is useful in the differential diagnosis of PC, especially small tumors [39, 40]. Fusaroli et al. [41] reported that pancreatic tumor visualization by CH-EUS is better than that of conventional EUS. A recent meta-analysis of 1139 patients found that the sensitivity and specificity of CE-EUS for a differential diagnosis of PC were 94% and 89%, respectively [39]. That study found that hypoenhancing lesions on CE-EUS images were a sensitive and accurate predictor of PC.

Because CH-EUS is more sensitive, it can be used to identify targets of EUS-FNA [41–43] and might also help to avoid puncturing necrotic and inflammatory areas of malignant masses or hard and scirrhous areas of inflammatory masses, thus reducing the need for repeated FNA assessments.

Another emerging technology is EUS elastography, which provides real-time visualization of tissue stiffness. It is based on the premise that compression causes less strain in hard, rather than in soft tissues [44]. The results of recent investigations using EUS elastography for diagnosing pancreatic focal lesions are promising [45–47]. As malignant lesions are generally harder than normal adjacent tissue, measuring strain might help to classify pancreatic masses. Two meta-analyses recently found high pooled sensitivity (95–97%) and low pooled specificity (67–76%), for a differential diagnosis of solid pancreatic masses [48, 49].

However, CH-EUS and EUS elastography are not widely available and have yet to be widely tested as screening tools for PC [37, 50].

1.7 Early Diagnosis of PC Using EUS-FNA (Fig. 1.3)

Although EUS has high overall sensitivity, differentiating PC from other solid lesions based only on endosonographic features remains challenging. Specimens for histopathological diagnosis can be collected using EUS-guided FNA. Since its introduction in the early 1990s, EUS-FNA has emerged as a safe and accurate means of tissue diagnosis in patients with pancreaticobiliary disorders, particularly confirmed PC. The sensitivity and specificity of EUS-FNA for diagnosing pancreatic masses is 80–95% and 75–100%, respectively [51–55].

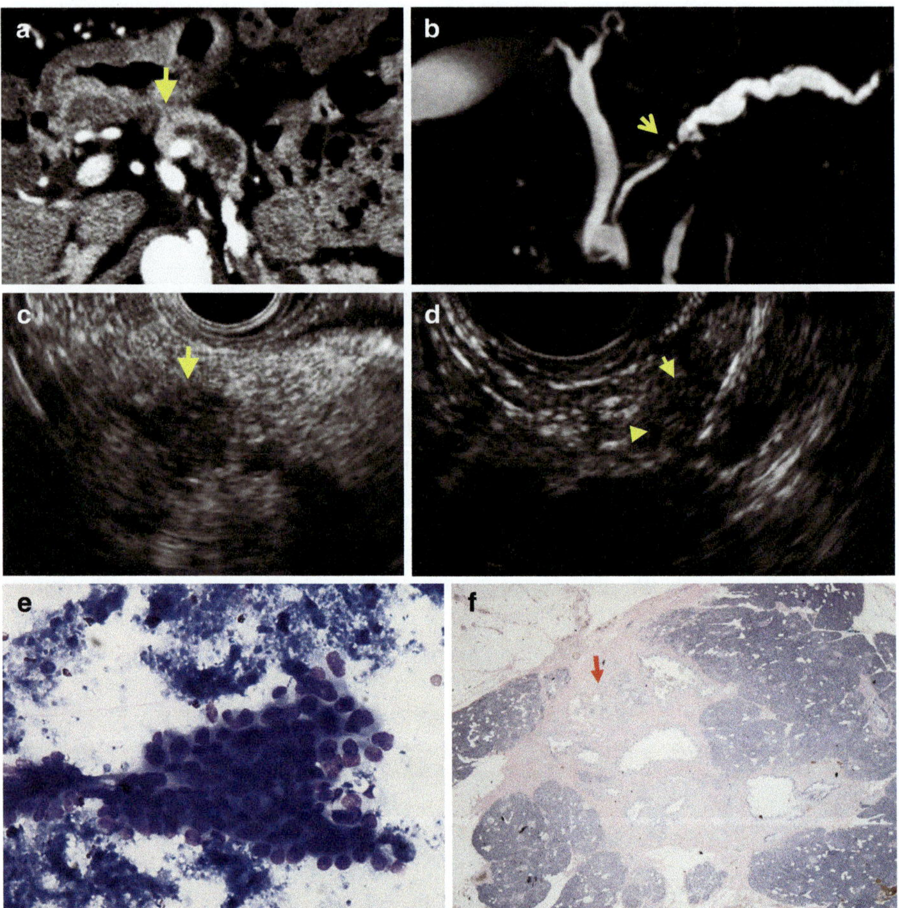

Fig. 1.3 Case: a 3 mm pancreatic cancer with invasion. Contrast-enhanced CT (**a**) could not detect the mass in pancreatic head (*arrow ahead*) although main pancreatic duct (MPD) was dilated. MRCP (**b**) showed short duct stenosis in pancreatic body (*arrow*). (**c**) EUS showed an 7 mm low echoic mass (*arrow*). (**d**) EUS-FNA was performed from the 7 mm low echoic mass using 22G FNA needle. (**e**) Cytology with Papanicolaou stain showed atypical cells consistent with adenocarcinoma. (**f**) Macroscopic findings revealed pancreatic adenocarcinoma with invasive components of 3 mm (*arrow*) with 8 mm surrounding fibrosis

Uehara et al. [56] recently reported that EUS-FNA was 96% accurate for identifying pancreatic masses <10 mm in 23 patients. Thus, EUS-FNA is useful for confirming pancreatic tumors <10 mm.

References

1. Rahib L, Smith BD, Aizenberg R, et al. Projecting cancer incidence and deaths to 2030: the unexpected burden of thyroid, liver, and pancreas cancers in the United States. Cancer Res. 2014;74:2913–21.
2. Gungor C, Hofmann BT, Wolters-Eisfeld G, et al. Pancreatic cancer. Br J Pharmacol. 2014;171:849–58.
3. Inui K, Kida M, Fujita N, et al. Standard imaging techniques in the pancreatobiliary region using radial scanning endoscopic ultrasonography. Dig Endosc. 2004;16:S118–S33.
4. Yamao K, Irisawa A, Inoue H, et al. Standard imaging techniques of endoscopic ultrasound-guided fine-needle aspiration using a curved linear array echoendoscope. Dig Endosc. 2007;19:S180–205.
5. Brennan DD, Zamboni GA, Raptopoulos VD, et al. Comprehensive preoperative assessment of pancreatic adenocarcinoma with 64-section volumetric CT 1. Radiographics. 2007;27:1653–66.
6. Lee ES, Lee JM. Imaging diagnosis of pancreatic cancer: a state-of-the-art review. World J Gastroenterol. 2014;20:7864–77.
7. Li H, Zeng MS, Zhou KR, et al. Pancreatic adenocarcinoma: signs of vascular invasion determined by multi-detector row CT. Br J Radiol. 2006;79:880–7.
8. Manak E, Merkel S, Klein P, et al. Resectability of pancreatic adenocarcinoma: assessment using multidetector-row computed tomography with multiplanar reformations. Abdom Imaging. 2009;34:75–80.
9. Gusmini S, Nicoletti R, Martinenghi C, et al. Vascular involvement in periampullary tumors: MDCT, EUS, and CDU. Abdom Imaging. 2009;34:514–22.
10. Prokesch RW, Chow LC, Beaulieu CF, et al. Isoattenuating pancreatic adenocarcinoma at multi-detector row CT: secondary signs. Radiology. 2002;224:764–8.
11. Yoon SH, Lee JM, Cho JY, et al. Small (</= 20 mm) pancreatic adenocarcinomas: analysis of enhancement patterns and secondary signs with multiphasic multidetector CT. Radiology. 2011;259:442–52.
12. Blouhos K, Boulas KA, Tsalis K, et al. The isoattenuating pancreatic adenocarcinoma: review of the literature and critical analysis. Surg Oncol. 2015;24:322–8.
13. Scialpi M, Cagini L, Pierotti L, et al. Detection of small (</= 2 cm) pancreatic adenocarcinoma and surrounding parenchyma: correlations between enhancement patterns at triphasic MDCT and histologic features. BMC Gastroenterol. 2014;14:16.
14. Ainsworth AP, Rafaelsen SR, Wamberg PA, et al. Is there a difference in diagnostic accuracy and clinical impact between endoscopic ultrasonography and magnetic resonance cholangio-pancreatography? Endoscopy. 2003;35:1029–32.
15. Mertz HR, Sechopoulos P, Delbeke D. EUS, PET, and CT scanning for evaluation of pancreatic adenocarcinoma. Gastrointest Endosc. 2000;52:367–71.
16. Tamm E, Charnsangavej C. Pancreatic cancer: current concepts in imaging for diagnosis and staging. Cancer J. 2001;7:298–311.
17. Dewitt J, Devereaux BM, Lehman GA, et al. Comparison of endoscopic ultrasound and computed tomography for the preoperative evaluation of pancreatic cancer: a systematic review. Clin Gastroenterol Hepatol. 2006;4:717–25. quiz 664
18. Agarwal B, Abu-Hamda E, Molke KL, et al. Endoscopic ultrasound-guided fine needle aspiration and multidetector spiral CT in the diagnosis of pancreatic cancer. Am J Gastroenterol. 2004;99:844–50.
19. Volmar KE, Vollmer RT, Jowell PS, et al. Pancreatic FNA in 1000 cases: a comparison of imaging modalities. Gastrointest Endosc. 2005;61:854–61.

20. Hanada K, Okazaki A, Hirano N, et al. Effective screening for early diagnosis of pancreatic cancer. Best Pract Res Clin Gastroenterol. 2015;29:929–39.
21. Hanada K, Okazaki A, Hirano N, et al. Diagnostic strategies for early pancreatic cancer. J Gastroenterol. 2015;50:147–54.
22. Greenhalf W, Neoptolemos JP. Increasing survival rates of patients with pancreatic cancer by earlier identification. Nat Clin Pract Oncol. 2006;3:346–7.
23. Hanada KIT, Hirano N. Role of EUS for small pancreatic cancer less than 1 cm. Tan Sui. 2009;30:343–8.
24. Luz LP, Al-Haddad MA, Sey MS, et al. Applications of endoscopic ultrasound in pancreatic cancer. World J Gastroenterol. 2014;20:7808–18.
25. Bhutani MS, Gress FG, Giovannini M, et al. The no endosonographic detection of tumor (NEST) study: a case series of pancreatic cancers missed on endoscopic ultrasonography. Endoscopy. 2004;36:385–9.
26. Hruban RH, Adsay NV, Albores-Saavedra J, et al. Pancreatic intraepithelial neoplasia: a new nomenclature and classification system for pancreatic duct lesions. Am J Surg Pathol. 2001;25:579–86.
27. Shin EJ, Canto MI. Pancreatic cancer screening. Gastroenterol Clin N Am. 2012;41:143–57.
28. Hanada KIT, Yamao K. Diagnostic strategies for the early diagnosis of pancreatic cancer. Gastroenterol Endosc. 2012;54:3773–82.
29. Maire F, Couvelard A, Palazzo L, et al. Pancreatic intraepithelial neoplasia in patients with intraductal papillary mucinous neoplasms: the interest of endoscopic ultrasonography. Pancreas. 2013;42:1262–6.
30. Del Chiaro M, Segersvärd R, Lohr M, et al. Early detection and prevention of pancreatic cancer: is it really possible today. World J Gastroenterol. 2014;20:12118–31.
31. Takaori K, Matsusue S, Fujikawa T, et al. Carcinoma in situ of the pancreas associated with localized fibrosis: a clue to early detection of neoplastic lesions arising from pancreatic ducts. Pancreas. 1998;17:102–5.
32. Iiboshi T, Hanada K, Fukuda T, et al. Value of cytodiagnosis using endoscopic nasopancreatic drainage for early diagnosis of pancreatic cancer: establishing a new method for the early detection of pancreatic carcinoma in situ. Pancreas. 2012;41:523–9.
33. Petrone MC, Arcidiacono PG. New strategies for the early detection of pancreatic cancer. Expert Rev Gastroenterol Hepatol. 2016;10:157–9.
34. Klein AP, Brune KA, Petersen GM, et al. Prospective risk of pancreatic cancer in familial pancreatic cancer kindreds. Cancer Res. 2004;64:2634–8.
35. Klein AP. Identifying people at a high risk of developing pancreatic cancer. Nat Rev Cancer. 2013;13:66–74.
36. Canto MI, Hruban RH, Fishman EK, et al. Frequent detection of pancreatic lesions in asymptomatic high-risk individuals. Gastroenterology. 2012;142:796–804. quiz e14–5
37. Bhutani MS, Koduru P, Joshi V, et al. The role of endoscopic ultrasound in pancreatic cancer screening. Endosc Ultrasound. 2016;5:8–16.
38. Hou X, Jin Z, Xu C, et al. Contrast-enhanced harmonic endoscopic ultrasound-guided fine-needle aspiration in the diagnosis of solid pancreatic lesions: a retrospective study. PLoS One. 2015;10:e0121236.
39. Gong TT, Hu DM, Zhu Q. Contrast-enhanced EUS for differential diagnosis of pancreatic mass lesions: a meta-analysis. Gastrointest Endosc. 2012;76:301–9.
40. Sakamoto H, Kitano M, Suetomi Y, et al. Utility of contrast-enhanced endoscopic ultrasonography for diagnosis of small pancreatic carcinomas. Ultrasound Med Biol. 2008;34:525–32.
41. Fusaroli P, Spada A, Mancino MG, et al. Contrast harmonic echo-endoscopic ultrasound improves accuracy in diagnosis of solid pancreatic masses. Clin Gastroenterol Hepatol. 2010;8:629–34.e1–2.
42. Romagnuolo J, Hoffman B, Vela S, et al. Accuracy of contrast-enhanced harmonic EUS with a second-generation perflutren lipid microsphere contrast agent (with video). Gastrointest Endosc. 2011;73:52–63.

43. Kitano M, Kudo M, Yamao K, et al. Characterization of small solid tumors in the pancreas: the value of contrast-enhanced harmonic endoscopic ultrasonography. Am J Gastroenterol. 2012;107:303–10.
44. Ophir J, Cespedes I, Ponnekanti H, et al. Elastography: a quantitative method for imaging the elasticity of biological tissues. Ultrason Imaging. 1991;13:111–34.
45. Giovannini M, Thomas B, Erwan B, et al. Endoscopic ultrasound elastography for evaluation of lymph nodes and pancreatic masses: a multicenter study. World J Gastroenterol. 2009;15:1587–93.
46. Li X, Xu W, Shi J, et al. Endoscopic ultrasound elastography for differentiating between pancreatic adenocarcinoma and inflammatory masses: a meta-analysis. World J Gastroenterol. 2013;19:6284–91.
47. Opacic D, Rustemovic N, Kalauz M, et al. Endoscopic ultrasound elastography strain histograms in the evaluation of patients with pancreatic masses. World J Gastroenterol. 2015;21:4014–9.
48. Hu DM, Gong TT, Zhu Q. Endoscopic ultrasound elastography for differential diagnosis of pancreatic masses: a meta-analysis. Dig Dis Sci. 2013;58:1125–31.
49. Mei M, Ni J, Liu D, et al. EUS elastography for diagnosis of solid pancreatic masses: a meta-analysis. Gastrointest Endosc. 2013;77:578–89.
50. Nelsen EM, Buehler D, Soni AV, et al. Endoscopic ultrasound in the evaluation of pancreatic neoplasms-solid and cystic: a review. World J Gastrointest Endosc. 2015;7:318–27.
51. Eloubeidi MA, Varadarajulu S, Desai S, et al. A prospective evaluation of an algorithm incorporating routine preoperative endoscopic ultrasound-guided fine needle aspiration in suspected pancreatic cancer. J Gastrointest Surg. 2007;11:813–9.
52. Yoshinaga S, Suzuki H, Oda I, et al. Role of endoscopic ultrasound-guided fine needle aspiration (EUS-FNA) for diagnosis of solid pancreatic masses. Dig Endosc. 2011;23(Suppl 1): 29–33.
53. Matsubayashi H, Matsui T, Yabuuchi Y, et al. Endoscopic ultrasonography guided-fine needle aspiration for the diagnosis of solid pancreaticobiliary lesions: clinical aspects to improve the diagnosis. World J Gastroenterol. 2016;22:628–40.
54. Puli SR, Bechtold ML, Buxbaum JL, et al. How good is endoscopic ultrasound-guided fine-needle aspiration in diagnosing the correct etiology for a solid pancreatic mass? A meta-analysis and systematic review. Pancreas. 2013;42:20–6.
55. Chen J, Yang R, Lu Y, et al. Diagnostic accuracy of endoscopic ultrasound-guided fine-needle aspiration for solid pancreatic lesion: a systematic review. J Cancer Res Clin Oncol. 2012;138:1433–41.
56. Uehara H, Ikezawa K, Kawada N, et al. Diagnostic accuracy of endoscopic ultrasound-guided fine needle aspiration for suspected pancreatic malignancy in relation to the size of lesions. J Gastroenterol Hepatol. 2011;26:1256–61.

Evaluation of Resectability for Pancreatic Cancer Using Endoscopic Ultrasound

Masayuki Kitano, Mamoru Takenaka, Kosuke Minaga, Takeshi Miyata, and Ken Kamata

2.1 Introduction

Pancreatic cancer has one of the worst prognoses of all solid carcinomas. The 5-year overall survival is about 2%, with more than half of patients failing to survive for more than 1 year. Surgical resection presents the only chance of a cure for pancreatic cancer. If surgery achieves clear margins and negative lymph nodes, the 5-year survival rate approaches 25%. In the formulation of a treatment plan, pancreatic cancer is usually staged using the TNM system of the American Joint Committee on Cancer (AJCC), which divides it into three categories: "resectable," "borderline resectable," or "unresectable" [1]. However, laparotomy often shows pancreatic cancer to be of a more advanced stage than was originally thought [2, 3]. The staging procedure must be sufficiently accurate to ensure that patients with resectable disease are not classified as unresectable during surgery.

Previously, the modality for staging and assessing the resectability of pancreatic cancer was computed tomography (CT) because of its low cost and high availability [4]. Endoscopic ultrasonography (EUS) was developed in the 1980s to overcome the limitations of transabdominal US imaging of the pancreas, the limitations being caused by intervening gas, bone, and fat. The ability to position the transducer in direct proximity to the pancreas by means of the stomach and duodenum, combined with the use of high-frequency transducers, produces detailed high-resolution images of the pancreas that far surpass those of CT or magnetic resonance imaging (MRI). In a recent study, the sensitivity of EUS was indicated as being higher than that of

M. Kitano, M.D., Ph.D. (✉)
Second Department of Internal Medicine, School of Medicine, Wakayama Medical University, 811-1 Kimiidera, Wakayama 641-0012, Japan
e-mail: kitano@wakayama-med.ac.jp

M. Takenaka • K. Minaga • T. Miyata • K. Kamata
Department of Gastroenterology and Hepatology, Faculty of Medicine, Kindai University, 377-2 Ohno-higashi, Osaka-sayama, Japan

© Springer Science+Business Media Singapore 2017
H. Yamaue (ed.), *Innovation of Diagnosis and Treatment for Pancreatic Cancer*,
DOI 10.1007/978-981-10-2486-3_2

CT. EUS is believed to be highly accurate for the T- and N-staging of pancreatic cancer [5, 6], and may help to identify those patients who would benefit from surgical resection. EUS has become a standard component of the preoperative evaluation of patients with pancreatic cancer in many medical centers. This chapter focuses on the use of EUS for the evaluation of the resectability of pancreatic cancer.

2.2   EUS Diagnosis of Vascular Invasion in Pancreatic Cancer

The assessment of vascular invasion is key for T-staging in pancreatic cancer. EUS staging of pancreatic and other tumors follows the TNM system of the American Joint Committee on Cancer (AJCC) [1]. According to the AJCC-TNM staging classification for pancreatic cancer [1], the evaluation of tumor invasion of the portal venous system, celiac artery (CA), superior mesenteric artery (SMA), and superior mesenteric vein (SMV) is the key to accurate T-staging. The AJCC-TNM system classifies pancreatic cancer invading the portal venous (PV) system as T3, and tumors invading the CA or SMA as T4 [1]. Therefore, the diagnosis of vascular invasion is very important for evaluation of T-staging, as well as the resectability of pancreatic cancer.

The accuracy of EUS in evaluations of vascular invasion differs across published reports, probably due to operator-dependent differences in examination of the hepatopancreatobiliary zone [2–5], or the use of different assessment criteria for vascular invasion. EUS vascular involvement findings have been defined differently in various studies [2, 4, 6–8].

Several criteria have been used to describe EUS findings in the assessment of vascular invasion by pancreatic cancer; these include "rough-edged vessel with compression," "abnormal contour," "loss of interface between the tumor and the vessel wall," "close contact," "complete vascular obstruction," "venous collaterals," "tumor within the vessel," and "irregular vascular wall" [2, 4, 6–8]. To date, four different EUS criteria have been used to define vascular invasion in previous studies; these are "peripancreatic venous collaterals," "tumor within vessel lumen," "abnormal vessel contour," and "loss of the vessel-parenchymal interface" [9] (Figs. 2.1 and 2.2). Of these four different EUS criteria, "loss of interface between the tumor and the vessel wall," "tumor within the vessel," and "venous collaterals" are the most specific criteria [2]. The specificity for assessing vascular involvement using these three criteria is 100%. The findings, "peripancreatic venous collaterals" and "tumor within vessel lumen," are usually straightforward and easy to document, with a high specificity [10]. However, they are less prevalent and less sensitive when compared with "abnormal vessel contour" and "loss of the vessel-parenchymal interface." Furthermore, the diagnostic accuracy may differ between different vessels, with the superior mesenteric vein having been considered the most difficult to visualize on EUS [11]. It is noteworthy that the criteria for arterial invasion have not been standardized [10]. Whereas arterial involvement is obvious in cases of vessel wall irregularity or stenosis, in some reports, the loss of a hyperechoic interface may not be considered an absolute contraindication for surgical resection [10].

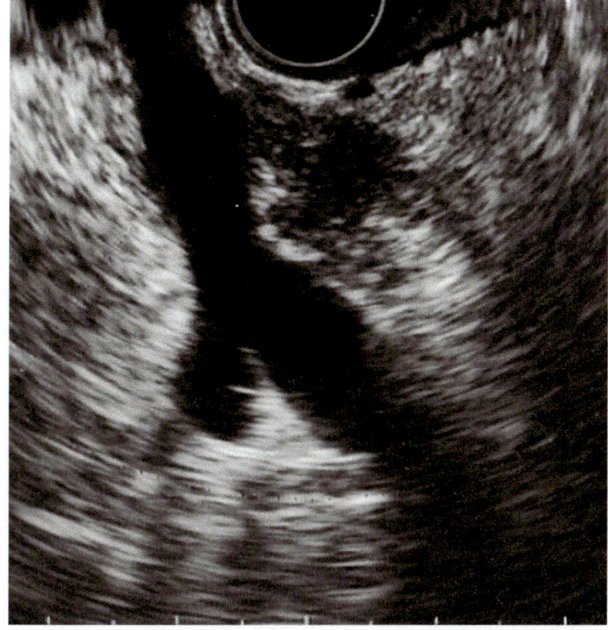

Fig. 2.1 A typical example of portal vein invasion on EUS. The finding "loss of the vessel-parenchymal interface" is observable

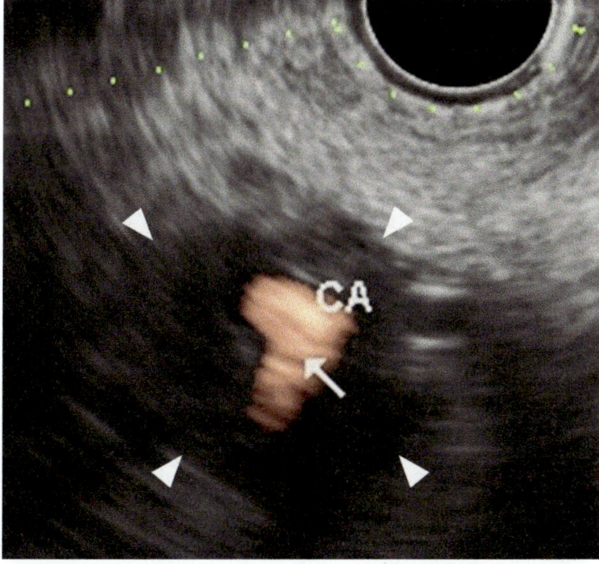

Fig. 2.2 A typical example of celiac artery invasion on color Doppler EUS. The finding "abnormal vessel contour" is observable

When the accuracy of EUS for diagnosis of vascular invasion by pancreatic cancer is compared with that of CT, the values should be separately compared for each vessel (PV, SMA, CA) because observation with EUS depends on the location of the vessels [4, 6, 8, 11, 12]. Tumor size may also affect the accuracy of EUS staging.

Attenuation of the ultrasound beam in large tumors lowers the accuracy. For this reason, tumors below 3 cm in size are more accurately staged with EUS [13]. Unlike radial EUS, linear EUS can show arterial vessels longitudinally with a linear image, and both the superior mesenteric and celiac arteries are more easily followed from the stomach with linear EUS. However, a recent meta-analysis of 29 studies on vascular invasion revealed no significant differences in the accuracy of radial and linear examinations [11].

In a recent meta-analysis assessing the performance characteristics of EUS in the staging of pancreatic cancer, which included 49 studies, the accuracy of EUS in the detection of vascular invasion ranged from 62 to 100%, with a pooled sensitivity of 85% and specificity of 91% [9]. EUS appeared to be more sensitive for detecting vascular invasion than CT although both CT and EUS revealed comparable specificities [9]. EUS has also been demonstrated to offer better results than angiography [14, 15]. EUS had a higher sensitivity for the detection of vascular involvement than selective venous angiography (86% vs 21%, respectively; $p = 0.0018$). The specificity and accuracy of EUS for detecting vascular involvement were 71% and 81%, respectively, while for selective venous angiography they were 71 and 38% [15].

In examinations according to vessel type, the sensitivity of EUS for tumor invasion of the portal vein (PV) has been reported as superior to that of CT [8, 12, 16, 17] and angiography [4, 8, 12, 16]. By contrast, EUS has shown low sensitivity in the SMV, SMA, and CA [3, 12, 17, 18]. Reported values for the sensitivity of EUS for tumor invasion of the PV range from 60 to 100%, with most studies demonstrating sensitivities over 80% [4, 6, 8, 12, 16, 19]. Yasuda et al. regarded a "rough-edged vessel with compression" as a marker of tumor invasion, and, using this criterion to evaluate tumor invasion of the PV, they found a sensitivity, a specificity, and an accuracy of 79%, 87%, and 81%, respectively [6]. Rösch et al. used "abnormal contour, loss of hyperechoic interface, and close contact" as a definition of tumor invasion, and using these criteria they found a sensitivity and specificity for the evaluation of tumor invasion of the PV of 43% and 91%, respectively.

Although the National Comprehensive Cancer Network guidelines for pancreatic cancer handle the invasion of the PV and arteries [20] separately, there are few reports that specifically examine the invasion of the CA; there may be several reasons for this. Firstly, it is difficult to obtain confirmation from surgical findings because in most cases where imaging modalities showed the invasion of the CA, the patient did not undergo surgical resection. Secondly, it is difficult to obtain histologic correlations with intraoperative findings in regard to vascular invasion. One report found the sensitivity of EUS for tumor invasion of the CA to be 57% although the sensitivity for tumor invasion of the SMA was only 17% [12]. A limitation of the radial scanning method employed with incomplete visualization of the SMA, and the sensitivity of EUS was found to be lower than that of CT. EUS evaluation of the SMA may be technically difficult due to either the inability to visualize the entire course of the vessel, or obscuration of the vessel by a large tumor in the uncinate or inferior portion of the pancreatic head [8].

Contrast-enhanced harmonic EUS (CH-EUS) has been developed for the diagnosis of pancreatic cancer; however, there are few reports on its use for the evaluation of vascular invasion by pancreatobiliary diseases. Imazu et al. evaluated

CH-EUS for T-staging in 26 patients with pancreatobiliary carcinomas and reported that the overall accuracy for T-staging of CH-EUS (92%) was significantly higher than that of conventional harmonic EUS (69%; $p < 0.05$) [21]. Further studies are warranted to confirm the utility of CH-EUS for T-staging of pancreatic cancer.

2.3 EUS Diagnosis of Node Metastasis in Pancreatic Cancer

As lymph node stage relates not only to the choice of treatment, but also to the prognosis, it is essential that the techniques used for N-staging are reliable [22, 23]. Pancreatic cancer patients with para-aortic lymph node (PALN) metastases have a poor prognosis [24]. A previous article reported that, in a multivariate analysis, the presence of PALN metastases was an independent factor with a significant association with mortality, and that 84% of those patients with positive PALN metastases died within 1 year [25]. If PALN metastases are detected, alternative treatment strategies should be considered. However, the diagnosis of malignant intra-abdominal lymph nodes is often challenging for endoscopists and radiologists [26]. A previous article evaluated the efficacy of ultrasonography (US), computed tomography (CT), endoscopic ultrasonography (EUS), and magnetic resonance imaging (MRI) in the assessment of lymph node metastases in pancreatic carcinoma, and EUS had an independent predictive value for tumor metastases in regional lymph nodes [27].

In EUS examinations, lymph nodes have been evaluated in terms of their size (i.e., the short and long axis lengths), shape (round or oval), edge characteristics (sharp or fuzzy), and echogenicity (hypo or hyper). A recent study reported that a short axis of 13 mm or longer and a long axis of 20 mm or longer had the best sensitivity and specificity for predicting malignancy [28]. Additionally, a round shape, a sharp edge, and hypoechogenicity were also found to be reliable parameters for predicting malignancy. Most studies have found no difference between CT and EUS in the prediction of resectability in relation to node involvement [6, 14, 29–31]. Only one study found EUS to be superior to CT for N-staging (EUS 93.1% vs CT 87.5%). Sawhney et al. [32] reported that the absence of a central intra-nodal vessel on color Doppler EUS is a strong and independent predictor of a metastatic lymph node (Fig. 2.3) although another article reported that the absence of such a vessel (Fig. 2.4) on color Doppler EUS did not predict malignancy better than the standard EUS variables [28].

Several studies have reported that although EUS (which has good spatial resolution) is useful for the differential diagnosis of malignant and benign lymph nodes, its diagnostic accuracy remains unsatisfactory [32–34]. By contrast, a cytopathological diagnosis via endoscopic ultrasonography-guided fine needle aspiration (EUS-FNA) is highly accurate. A recent study compared EUS-FNA and [18F]-Fluorodeoxyglucose positron emission tomography/computed tomography (PET/CT) for the diagnosis of PALN metastases [35], and found EUS-FNA to be superior to PET/CT for preoperative PALN staging in patients with pancreatobiliary cancers. Because of the clinical benefits of EUS-FNA for reducing unnecessary surgery, it should be considered a part of the standard preoperative examination for patients with pancreatobiliary cancers.

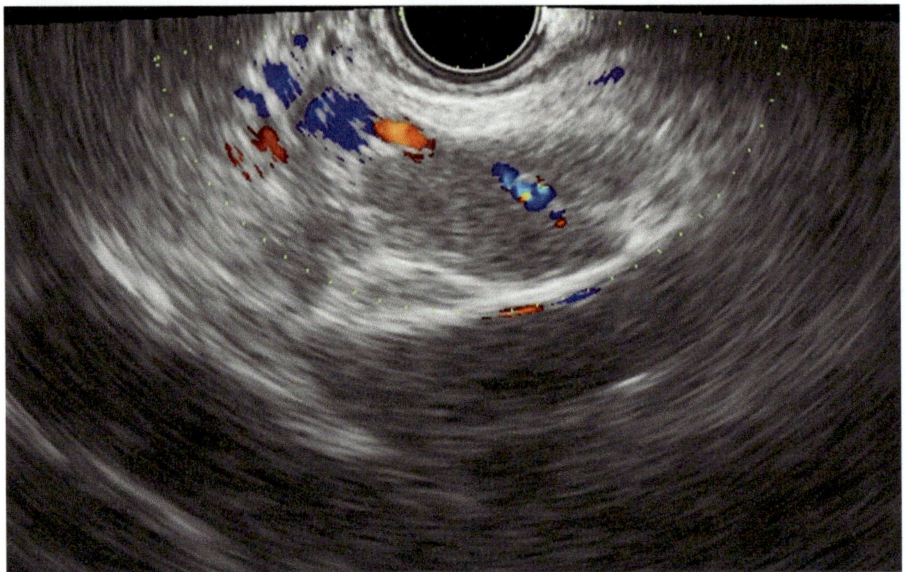

Fig. 2.3 A typical example of "central intra-nodal vessel" presence on color Doppler EUS

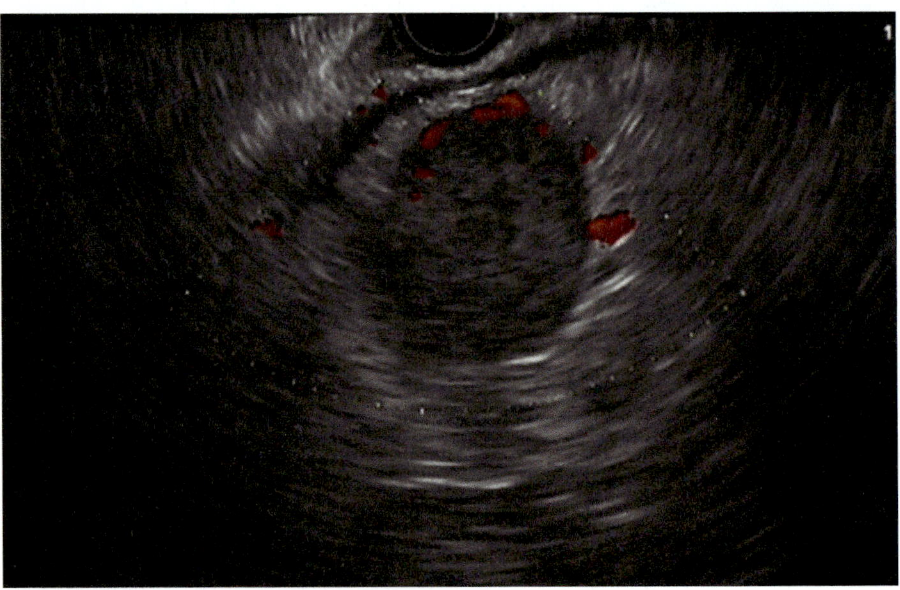

Fig. 2.4 A typical example of "central intra-nodal vessel" absence on color Doppler EUS

As EUS-FNA is highly accurate for the identification of malignant lymph nodes, most cases in which EUS-FNA reveals the presence of atypical cells in the lymph nodes do show malignancy of the lymph nodes [36]. However, false-positive and false-negative EUS-FNA results remain possible. Jason et al. [37] reported EUS-FNA false-positive and false-negative rates for intra-abdominal lymph node diagnosis as 0.7% and 5.8%, respectively. Additionally, EUS-FNA has another limitation, in that it cannot be performed in all cases, because of intervening vessels and/or the difficult location of the lymph node; this could, for example, lead to an excessively large scope angle or distance from the probe.

Thus, an accurate alternative evaluation method is needed for cases in which a lymph node cannot be accessed by EUS-FNA, or where EUS-FNA does not obtain adequate material for analysis. One such alternative method is EUS elastography. EUS elastography has been presented as a novel technique to assess tissue elasticity and has been used to differentiate between malignant and benign lymph nodes. Several different variables have been used as a measure of tissue elasticity in EUS elastography, including color patterns [38–43], strain ratio [44, 45], hue histogram analysis [46, 47], and computer analysis with artificial neural networks [48, 49]. Xu et al. [50] performed a meta-analysis that included seven articles and a large number of lymph nodes (368 patients with 431 lymph nodes). The sensitivity and specificity of EUS elastography were 88% and 85%, respectively, for the differential diagnosis of benign and malignant lymph nodes. The area under the summary receiver operating characteristic curve was 0.9456. However, the sensitivity and specificity of this method have varied greatly between studies [50].

Another alternative method is contrast-enhanced color Doppler EUS with a US contrast agent. Kanamori et al. [51] reported that, with the first generation of US contrast agent (Levovist; Nihon Schering Co., Ltd., Tokyo, Japan), defective enhancement on contrast-enhanced color Doppler EUS predicted lymph node malignancy significantly more accurate than standard EUS variables although the method suffered from Doppler-related artifacts. Recently, the combination of second-generation US contrast agents, including Sonazoid, SonoVue, and Definity, and low mechanical index imaging techniques, has led to CH-EUS being used for perfusion imaging, which facilitates the depiction of tumor vascularity [52–55]. The second-generation of US contrast agents resonate with a low acoustic power, and thus allow CH-EUS to be performed. A previous report demonstrated this method to have an excellent ability to differentiate malignant from benign lesions, without Doppler-related artifacts, even when lesions were small [56]. In a recent study [28], heterogeneous enhancement was observed in 39 of 47 (83%) malignant lymph nodes, and CH-EUS had a significantly higher diagnostic accuracy for malignant lymph nodes than most of the standard EUS variables (Figs. 2.5 and 2.6). The study also showed that CH-EUS was comparable to EUS-FNA for N-staging (88% vs 90%, $p = 0.50$). Additionally, in all the cases where EUS-FNA failed due to inadequate sampling or inaccessibility of the lymph nodes, CH-EUS resulted in correct N-staging. Thus, CH-EUS may be a useful modality for differentiating malignant

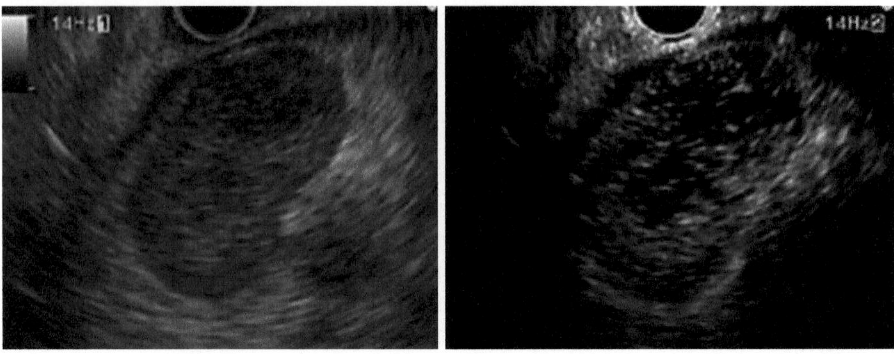

Fig. 2.5 A typical example of a lesion with heterogeneous enhancement (metastatic lymph node; the long axis is 25 mm and short axis 15 mm). Standard EUS (*left*) shows a round shape and sharp edge. CH-EUS (*right*) shows that this area exhibits heterogeneous enhancement

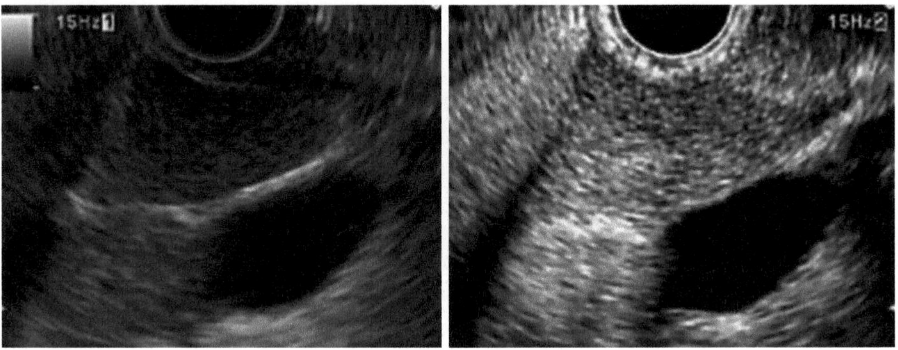

Fig. 2.6 A typical example of a lesion with homogeneous enhancement (benign lymph node; the long axis is 28 mm and short axis 18 mm). Standard EUS (*left*) shows an oval shape and sharp edge. CH-EUS (*right*) shows that this area exhibits homogeneous enhancement

from benign lymph nodes in patients with pancreatobiliary carcinomas, and may complement standard EUS, color Doppler EUS, and EUS-FNA, all of which have some limitations. It may also be helpful for determining which lymph nodes should be subjected to EUS-FNA. In view of its high accuracy, CH-EUS may help to avoid unnecessary surgery in the future. Hence, CH-EUS will play an important role in determining the optimal treatment for pancreatobiliary carcinomas.

2.4 EUS Diagnosis of Liver Metastases in Pancreatic Cancer

Most pancreatic cancers will develop liver metastases during the course of the disease [57]. Early detection of liver metastases in patients with known pancreatic cancer is important for therapeutic decision-making and is crucial to the prognosis for survival. In those patients who develop a recurrence following an apparently curative pancreatic resection, the high frequency of liver recurrence rates indicates that these metastases were present at the time of surgery, but remained "occult," i.e., undetected by preoperative imaging examinations. It is well recognized that patient outcome is highly dependent upon the ability to define the true extent of the metastatic disease; therefore, it is crucial to have a preoperative imaging modality with a high sensitivity for the detection of liver metastases. Traditionally, transabdominal US, and contrast-enhanced CT and/or MRI, have been used for staging in patients with pancreatic cancer, particularly for surveillance of liver metastases [58–60]. Unfortunately, these modalities are limited in their ability to detect liver lesions of less than 10 mm in diameter [61].

EUS was not traditionally thought to be clinically applicable to liver imaging until the first report appeared in 1999 [62]. Under EUS, the liver could be detected from the proximal stomach and/or distal esophagus to view the left lobe, and from the gastric antrum and/or duodenal bulb to view the portal hilum and proximal right lobe, including the major portion of the intrahepatic biliary tract. According to Bhatia et al., most liver segments can be visualized with EUS. The intrahepatic vascular landmarks include the major hepatic veins, PV radicals, and hepatic arterial branches, while the inferior vena cava, venosum, and teres ligaments form other important intrahepatic landmarks. The liver hilum and gallbladder serve as useful surface landmarks [63]. The caudate lobe lies in close proximity to the stomach and duodenum; therefore, EUS is superior to transabdominal US for imaging these regions. Conversely, EUS is limited in its ability to access the portion of the right lobe adjacent to the dome of the diaphragm, along with its lateral and inferior portions [64].

Nguyen et al. prospectively evaluated EUS images of the liver in 574 consecutive patients with a history or suspicion of gastrointestinal or pulmonary malignant tumors. Fifteen liver lesions (in 14 patients) were identified (5 were in the right lobe, 9 were in the left lobe) and underwent EUS-FNA; 14 of these were confirmed as malignant. Moreover, CT depicted liver lesions in only 3 of these 14 patients before EUS, with 12 of the 15 lesions being less than 20 mm [62]. Likewise, a retrospective study conducted by Prasad et al. revealed that EUS detected metastatic lesions missed by conventional cross-sectional imaging studies in 5 of 222 cases (2.3%), with EUS having sufficient resolution to detect lesions as small as 5 mm in diameter, although the technique was more operator dependent than other imaging modalities [65]. Awad et al. evaluated 14 consecutive patients with a history of a known liver mass. The patients underwent both contrast-enhanced CT and EUS. EUS not only allowed identification of the lesions in all 14 patients, but also led to the identification of four new lesions smaller than 5 mm, which had not been visualized by the preceding CT scan [61]. These studies suggest that EUS is a useful modality for detection of liver metastases, particularly small lesions.

Liver biopsy has traditionally been performed percutaneously under transabdominal US or CT guidance, and a transjugular fluoroscopy-guided approach is applied when a percutaneous approach is contraindicated because of coagulopathy or ascites [66]. Recently, liver biopsy under EUS guidance has emerged as an alternative to the percutaneous or transjugular approach, and its high diagnostic accuracy and safety have been described in many articles [61, 62, 65, 67–76]. EUS has an advantage over the other noninvasive imaging methods (CT or MRI), in that samples for pathological diagnosis can be obtained by subsequent EUS-FNA. In 2002, ten Berge et al. conducted a large retrospective international multicenter survey to evaluate the indications, complications, and findings of EUS-FNA of the liver [67]. The study revealed that the complication rate for EUS-FNA of the liver was only 4%, with a major complication rate of 1% in 167 cases. They also showed that EUS-FNA helped to diagnose malignancy in cases that could not be accessed by transabdominal US-guided FNA. The authors therefore concluded that EUS-FNA of the liver was a safe procedure, and that EUS-FNA should be considered when a hepatic lesion is difficult to access with transabdominal US or CT-guided FNA, or when these modalities are unable to result in a diagnosis [67]. Singh et al. prospectively compared the accuracy of EUS/EUS-FNA and CT scan for the detection of liver metastases, and revealed that there was a trend in favor of EUS/EUS-FNA, with a superior diagnostic accuracy in comparison with CT [71] (Fig. 2.7). A large multicenter prospective clinical trial that included 110 patients showed that the rate of definitive pathological diagnoses was 98%, and the overall complication rate was only 1%, which led the authors to conclude that EUS-FNA of the liver was a safe technique which provides a high diagnostic accuracy [75].

A recent article by Pineda et al. compared liver tissue yield between EUS-FNA, percutaneous liver biopsy, and the transjugular approach [76]. The study demonstrated that EUS-FNA using a 19-gauge needle produced specimens at least comparable with, and in some cases better than, percutaneous or transjugular biopsy. They suggested that, when EUS is performed for diagnosis, it is reasonable and feasible to perform EUS-FNA of the liver during the same endoscopic session in patients with known or suspicious pancreatic cancer. The ability to perform EUS-FNA during the same session will likely be one of the reasons for an increase in the use of EUS-FNA for investigation of liver lesions.

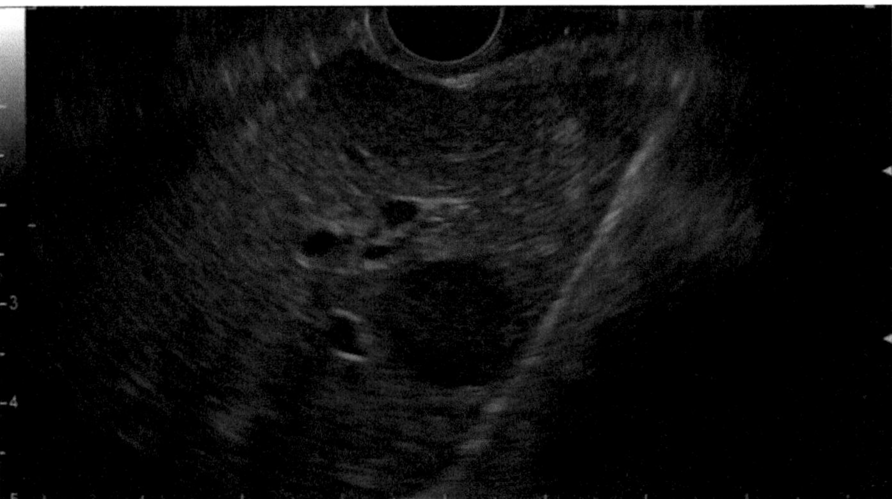

Fig. 2.7 A typical example of a liver metastasis on EUS. A low echoic nodule is observed in the left lobe of the liver

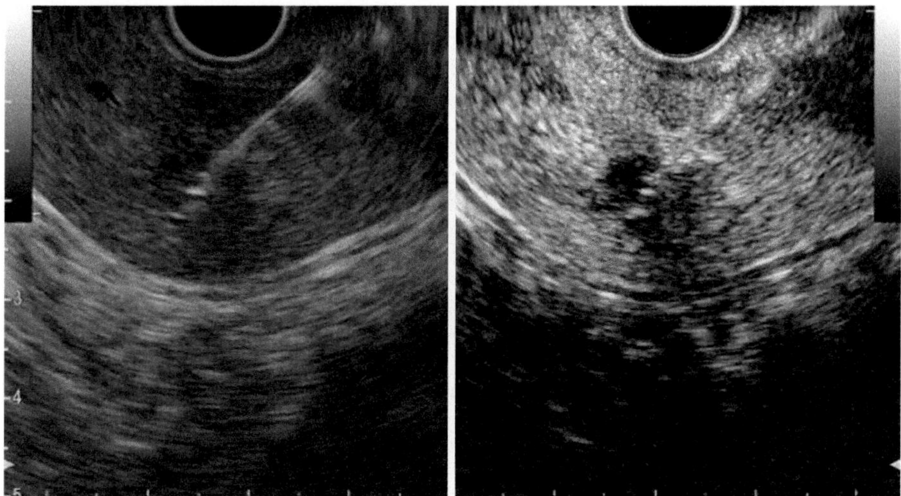

Fig. 2.8 A typical example of EUS-guided fine needle aspiration of a liver metastasis. Standard EUS (*left*) shows a subtle nodule in the left lobe of the liver. CH-EUS (*right*) shows that this nodule is more clearly identified, which facilitates EUS-guided fine needle aspiration

More recently, new EUS/EUS-FNA techniques, such as EUS elastography [77] and KRAS mutation analysis by next-generation sequencing from EUS-guided tissue sampling [78] for solid liver lesions, have been described; these appear to provide additional diagnostic yield. Another upcoming technique is contrast-enhanced EUS technology. This principle was already established for pancreatic tumors [52]. Under transabdominal US, contrast-enhanced US techniques play important roles in the diagnosis of liver lesions, and the accuracy of detection of metastatic liver lesions has been reported to be 91.2%, which was significantly higher than that for conventional US [79]. Therefore, contrast-enhanced EUS is expected to become a highly diagnostic modality for the detection of liver metastases (Fig. 2.8).

References

1. Edge S, Byrd DR, Compton CC, Fritz AG, Greene FL, Trotti A, editors. AJCC cancer staging manual. 7th ed. New York: Springer; 2010. p. 245–7.
2. Snady H, Bruckner H, Siegel J, et al. Endoscopic ultrasonographic criteria of vascular invation by potentially resectable pancreatic tumors. Gastrointest Endosc. 1994;40:326–33.
3. Buscail L, Pagès P, Berthélemy P, et al. Role of EUS in the management of pancreatic and ampullary carcinoma: a prospective study assessing resectability and prognosis. Gastrointest Endosc. 1999;50:34–40.
4. Brugge WR, Lee MJ, Kelsey PB, Schapiro RH, Warshaw AL. The use of EUS to diagnose malignant portal venous system invasion by pancreatic cancer. Gastrointest Endosc. 1996; 43:561–7.
5. Rivadeneira DE, Pochapin M, Grobmyer SR, et al. Comparison of linear array endoscopic ultrasound and helical computed tomography for the staging of periampullary malignancies. Ann Surg Oncol. 2003;10:890–7.

6. Yasuda K, Mukai H, Nakajima M, Kawai K. Staging of pancreatic carcinoma by endoscopic ultrasonography. Endoscopy. 1993;25:151–5.
7. Ahmad NA, Lewis JD, Ginsberg GG, Rosato EF, Morris JB, Kochman ML. EUS in preoperative staging of pancreatic cancer. Gastrointest Endosc. 2000;52:463–8.
8. Rösch T, Dittler HJ, Strobel K, Meining A, Schusdziarra V, Lorenz R, et al. Endoscopic ultrasound criteria for vascular invasion in the staging of cancer of the head of the pancreas: a blind reevaluation of videotapes. Gastrointest Endosc. 2000;52:469–77.
9. Nawaz H, Fan CY, Kloke J, et al. Performance characteristics of endoscopic ultrasound in the staging of pancreatic cancer: a meta-analysis. JOP. 2013;14:484–97.
10. Snady H. EUS criteria for vascular invasion: analyzing the meta-analysis. Gastrointest Endosc. 2007;65:798–807.
11. Puli SR, Singh S, Hagedorn CH, et al. Diagnostic accuracy of EUS for vascular invasion in pancreatic and periampullary cancers: a meta-analysis and systematic review. Gastrointest Endosc. 2007;65:788–97.
12. Rösch T, Dittler HJ, Lorenz R, et al. The endosonographic staging of pancreatic carcinoma. Dtsch Med Wochenschr. 1992;117:563–9.
13. Nakaizumi A, Uehara H, Iishi H, et al. Endoscopic ultrasonography in diagnosis and staging of pancreatic cancer. Dig Dis Sci. 1995;40:696–700.
14. Soriano A, Castells A, Ayuso C, et al. Preoperative staging and tumor resectability assessment of pancreatic cancer: prospective study comparing endoscopic ultrasonography, helical computed tomography, magnetic resonance imaging, and angiography. Am J Gastroenterol. 2004;99:492–501.
15. Ahmad NA, Kochman ML, Lewis JD, et al. Endosonography is superior to angiography in the preoperative assessment of vascular involvement among patients with pancreatic carcinoma. J Clin Gastroenterol. 2001;32:54–8.
16. Sugiyama M, Hagi H, Atomi Y, et al. Diagnosis of portal venous invasion by pancreatobiliary carcinoma: value of endoscopic ultrasonography. Abdom Imaging. 1997;22:434–8.
17. Midwinter MJ, Beveridge CJ, Wilsdon JB, et al. Correlation between spiral computed tomography, endoscopic ultrasonography and findings at operation in pancreatic and ampullary tumours. Br J Surg. 1999;86:189–93.
18. Mertz HR, Sechopoulos P, Delbeke D, et al. EUS, PET, and CT scanning for evaluation of pancreatic adenocarcinoma. Gastrointest Endosc. 2000;52:367–71.
19. Rösch T, Braig C, Gain T, et al. Staging of pancreatic and ampullary carcinoma by endoscopic ultrasonography. Comparison with conventional sonography, computed tomography, and angiography. Gastroenterology. 1992;102:188–99.
20. NCCN guidelines for Treatment of Cancer by Site. Pancreatic Adenocarcinomas. 2017. National Comprehensive Cancer Network. https://www.nccn.org/.
21. Imazu H, Uchiyama Y, Matsunaga K, et al. Contrast-enhanced harmonic EUS with novel ultrasonographic contrast (Sonazoid) in the preoperative T-staging for pancreaticobiliary malignancies. Scand J Gastroenterol. 2010;45:732–8.
22. Schomas DA, Quevedo JF, Donahue JM, Nichols 3rd FC, Romero Y, et al. The prognostic importance of pathologically involved celiac node metastases in node-positive patients with carcinoma of the distal esophagus or gastroesophageal junction: a surgical series from the Mayo Clinic. Dis Esophagus. 2010;23:232–9.
23. Natsugoe S, Yoshinaka H, Shimada M, Sakamoto F, Morinaga T, Nakano S, Kusano C, Baba M, Takao S, Aikou T, et al. Number of lymph node metastases determined by presurgical ultrasound and endoscopic ultrasound is related to prognosis in patients with esophageal carcinoma. Ann Surg. 2001;234:613–8.
24. Masui T, Kubota T, Aoki K, Nakanishi Y, Miyamoto T, Nagata J, et al. Long-term survival after resection of pancreatic ductal adenocarcinoma with para-aortic lymph node metastasis: case report. World J Surg Oncol. 2013;11:195.
25. Doi R, Kami K, Ito D, Fujimoto K, Kawaguchi Y, Wada M, et al. Prognostic implication of para-aortic lymph node metastasis in resectable pancreatic cancer. World J Surg. 2007; 31:147–54.

26. Sharma A, Fidias P, Hayman LA, Loomis SL, Taber KH, Aquino SL, et al. Patterns of lymphadenopathy in thoracic malignancies. Radiographics. 2004;24:419–39.
27. Tian YT, Wang CF, Wang GQ, Ahao XM, Ouyang H, Hao YZ, Chen Y, Zhang HM, Ahao P, et al. Prospective evaluation of the clinical significance of ultrasonography, helical computed tomography, magnetic resonance imaging and endoscopic ultrasonography in the assessment of vascular invasion and lymph node metastasis of pancreatic carcinoma. Zhonghua Zhong Liu Za Zhi. 2008;30:682–5.
28. Miyata T, Kitano M, Omoto S, Kadosaka K, Kamata K, Imai H, Sakamoto H, Nishida N, Harwani Y, Murakami T, Takeyama Y, Chiba Y, Kudo M, et al. Contrast-enhanced harmonic endoscopic ultrasonography for assessment of lymph node metastases in pancreatobiliary carcinoma. World J Gastroenterol. 2016;12:3381–91.
29. DeWitt J, Devereaux B, Chriswell M, McGreevy K, Howard T, Imperiale TF, et al. Comparison of endoscopic ultrasonography and multidetector computed tomography for detecting and staging pancreatic cancer. Ann Intern Med. 2004;141:753–63.
30. Arabul M, Karakus F, Alper E, Kandemir A, Celik M, Karakus V, et al. Comparison of multidetector CT and endoscopic ultrasonography in malignant pancreatic mass lesions. Hepato-Gastroenterology. 2012;59:1599–603.
31. Ramsay D, Marshall M, Song S, Zimmerman M, Edmunds S, Yusoff I, et al. Identification and staging of pancreatic tumours using computed tomography, endoscopic ultrasound and mangafodipir trisodium-enhanced magnetic resonance imaging. Australas Radiol. 2004;48:154–61.
32. Sawhney MS, Debold SM, Kratzke RA, Lederle FA, Nelson DB, Kelly RF, et al. Central intranodal blood vessel: a new EUS sign described in mediastinal lymph nodes. Gastrointest Endosc. 2007;65:602–8.
33. Eloubeidi MA, Wallace MB, Reed CE, Hadzijahic N, Lewin DN, Van Velse A, Leveen MB, Etemad B, Matsuda K, Patel RS, Hawes RH, Hoffman BJ, et al. The utility of EUS and EUSguided fine needle aspiration in detecting celiac lymph node metastasis in patients with esophageal cancer: a single-center experience. Gastrointest Endosc. 2001;54:714–9.
34. Bhutani MS, Hawes RH, Hoffman BJ. A comparison of the accuracy of echo features during endoscopic ultrasound (EUS) and EUS-guided fine-needle aspiration for diagnosis of malignant lymph node invasion. Gastrointest Endosc. 1997;45:474–9.
35. Kurita A, Kodama Y, Nakamoto Y, Isoda H, Minamiguchi S, Yoshimura K, et al. Impact of EUS-FNA for preoperative para-aortic lymph node staging in patients with pancreatobiliary cancer. Gastrointest Endosc. 2016;84:467–75.
36. Srinivasan R, Bhutani MS, Thosani N, et al. Clinical impact of EUS-FNA of mediastinal lymph nodes in patients with known or suspected lung cancer or mediastinal lymph nodes of unknown etiology. J Gastrointestin Liver Dis. 2012;21:145–52.
37. Jason K, Archana A, David E, et al. The role of endoscopic ultrasound-guided fine needle aspiration (EUS-FNA) for the diagnosis of intra-abdominal lymphadenopathy of unknown origin. J Interv Gastroenterol. 2012;2:172–6.
38. Giovannini M, Hookey LC, Bories E, Pesenti C, Monges G, Delpero JR, et al. Endoscopic ultrasound elastography: the first step towards virtual biopsy? Preliminary results in 49 patients. Endoscopy. 2006;38:344–8.
39. Jansen J, Schlorer E, Greiner L, et al. EUS elastgraphy of the pancreas: feasibility and pattern description of the normal pancreas, chronic pancreatitis, and focal pancreatic lesions. Gastrointest Endosc. 2007;65:971–8.
40. Giovannini M, Thomas B, Erwan B, Christian P, Fabrice C, Benjamin E, Geneviève M, Paolo A, Pierre D, Robert Y, Walter S, Hanz S, Carl S, Christoph D, Pierre E, Jean-Luc VL, Jacques D, Peter V, Andrian S, et al. Endoscopic ultrasound elastography for evaluation of lymph nodes and pancreatic masses: a multicenter study. World J Gastroenterol. 2009;15:1587–93.
41. Iglesias Garcia J, Larino Noia J, Abdulkader I, Forteza J, Dominguez Munoz JE, et al. EUS elastography for the characterization of solid pancreatic masses. Gastrointest Eodosc. 2009;70:1101–8.

42. Itokawa F, Itoi T, Sofuni A, Kurihara T, Tsuchiya T, Ishii K, Tsuji S, Ikeuchi N, Umeda J, Tanaka R, Yokoyama N, Moriyasu F, Kasuya K, Nagao T, Kamisawa T, Tsuchida A, et al. EUS slastography combined with the strain ratio of tissue elasticity for diagnosis of solid pancreatic masses. J Gastroenterol. 2011;46:843–53.

43. Hocke M, Ignee A, Dietrich CF, et al. Advanced endosonographic diagnostic tools for discrimination of focal chronic pancreatitis and pancreatic carcinoma- elastography, contrast enhanced high mechanical index (CEHMI) and low mechanical index (CELMI) endosonography in direct comparison. Z Gastroenterol. 2012;50:199–203.

44. Larsen MH, Fristrup CW, Mortensen MB, et al. Intra- and interobserver agreement of endoscopic sonoelastography in the evaluation of lymph nodes. Ultraschall Med. 2011;32:45–50.

45. Iglesias-Gacia J, Larino-Noia J, Abdulkader I, Forteza J, Dominguez-Munoz JE, et al. Quantitative endoscopic ultrasound elastography: an accurate method for the differentiation of solid pancreatic masses. Gastroenterology. 2010;139:1172–80.

46. Dawwas MF, Taha H, Leeds JS, Nayar MK, Oppong KW, et al. Diagnostic accuracy of quantitative EUS elastography for discriminating malignant from benign solid pancreatic masses: a prospective, single-center study. Gastrointest Endosc. 2012;76:953–61.

47. Saftoiu A, Iordache SA, Gheonea DI, Popescu C, Maloş A, Gorunescu F, Ciurea T, Iordache A, Popescu GL, Manea CT, et al. Combined contrast-enhanced power Doppler and real-time sonoelastography performed during EUS, used in the differential diagnosis of focal pancreatic masses (with videos). Gastrointest Endosc. 2010;72:739–47.

48. Saftoiu A, Vilman P, Gorunescu F, Janssen J, Hocke M, Larsen M, Iglesias-Garcia J, Arcidiacono P, Will U, Giovannini M, Dietrich C, Havre R, Gheorghe C, McKay C, Gheonea DI, Ciurea T, et al. Accuracy of endoscopic ultrasound elastography used for differential diagnosis of focul pancreatic masses: a multicenter study. Endoscopy. 2011;43:596–603.

49. Saftoiu A, Vilman P, Gorunescu F, Gheonea DI, Gorunescu M, Ciurea T, Popescu GL, Iordache A, Hassan H, Iordache S, et al. Neural network analysis of dynamic sequences of EUS elastography used for the differential diagnosis of chronic pancreatitis and pancreatic cancer. Gastrointest Endosc. 2008;68:1086–94.

50. Xu W, Shi J, Zeng X, Li X, Xie WF, Guo J, Lin Y, et al. EUS elastography for the differentiation of benign and malignant lymph nodes: a meta-analysis. Gastrointest Endosc. 2011;74:1001–9.

51. Kanamori A, Hirooka Y, Ito A, Hashimoto S, Kawashima H, Hara K, Uchida H, Goto J, Ohmiya N, Niwa Y, Goto H, et al. Usefulness of contrast-enhanced endoscopic ultrasonography in the differentiation between malignant and benign lymphadenopathy. Am J Gastroenterol. 2006;101:45–51.

52. Kitano M, Sakamoto H, Matsui U, Ito Y, Maekawa K, von Schrenck T, Kudo M, et al. A novel perfusion imaging technique of the pancreas: contrast-enhanced harmonic EUS (with video). Gastrointest Endosc. 2008;67:141–50.

53. Ding H, Kudo M, Onda H, Suetomi Y, Minami Y, Maekawa K, et al. Hepatocellular carcinoma: depiction of tumor parenchymal flow with intermittent harmonic power Doppler US during the early arterial phase in dual-display mode. Radiology. 2001;220:349–56.

54. Park BK, Kim B, Kim SH, Ko K, Lee HM, Choi HY, et al. Assessment of cystic renal masses based on Bosniak classification: comparison of CT and contrast-enhanced US. Eur J Radiol. 2007;61:310–4.

55. Kitano M, Kamata K, Imai H, Miyata T, Yasukawa S, Yanagisawa A, Kudo M, et al. Endoscopic ultrasonography and contrast-enhanced ultrasonography. Pancreatology. 2011;11(Suppl 2):28–33.

56. Kitano M, Kudo M, Yamao K, Takagi T, Sakamoto H, Komaki T, Kamata K, Imai H, Chiba Y, Okada M, Murakami T, Takeyama Y, et al. Characterization of small solid tumors in the pancreas: the value of contrast-enhanced harmonic endoscopic ultrasonography. Am J Gastroenterol. 2012;107:303–10.

57. Egawa S, Toma H, Ohigashi H, Okusaka T, Nakao A, Hatori T, et al. Japan pancreatic cancer registry; 30th year anniversary: Japan Pancreas Society. Pancreas. 2012;41:985–92.

58. Hein E, Albrecht A, Melzer D, Steinhöfel K, Rogalla P, Hamm B, et al. Computer-assisted diagnosis of focal liver lesions on CT images evaluation of the perceptron algorithm. Acad Radiol. 2005;12:1205–10.
59. Namasivayam S, Martin DR, Saini S. Imaging of liver metastases: MRI. Cancer Imaging. 2007;7:2–9.
60. Albrecht T, Blomley MJ, Burns PN, Wilson S, Harvey CJ, Leen E, et al. Improved detection of hepatic metastases with pulse-inversion US during the liver-specific phase of SHU 508A: multicenter study. Radiology. 2003;227:361–70.
61. Awad SS, Fagan S, Abudayyeh S, Karim N, Berger DH, Ayub K. Preoperative evaluation of hepatic lesions for the staging of hepatocellular and metastatic liver carcinoma using endoscopic ultrasonography. Am J Surg. 2002;184:601–64.
62. Nguyen P, Feng JC, Chang KJ. Endoscopic ultrasound (EUS) and EUS-guided fine-needle aspiration (FNA) of liver lesions. Gastrointest Endosc. 1999;50:357–61.
63. Bhatia V, Hijioka S, Hara K, Mizuno N, Imaoka H, Yamao K. Endoscopic ultrasound description of liver segmentation and anatomy. Dig Endosc. 2014;26:482–90.
64. Srinivasan I, Tang SJ, Vilmann AS, Menachery J, Vilmann P. Hepatic applications of endoscopic ultrasound: current status and future directions. World J Gastroenterol. 2015;21:12544–57.
65. Prasad P, Schmulewitz N, Patel A, Varadarajulu S, Wildi SM, Roberts S, Tutuian R, King P, Hawes RH, Hoffman BJ, Wallace MB. Detection of occult liver metastases during EUS for staging of malignancies. Gastrointest Endosc. 2004;59:49–53.
66. Kalambokis G, Manousou P, Vibhakorn S, Marelli L, Cholongitas E, Senzolo M, et al. Transjugular liver biopsy—indications, adequacy, quality of specimens, and complications—a systematic review. J Hepatol. 2007;47:284–94.
67. ten Berge J, Hoffman BJ, Hawes RH, Van Enckevort C, Giovannini M, Erickson RA, et al. EUS-guided fine needle aspiration of the liver: indications, yield, and safety based on an international survey of 167 cases. Gastrointest Endosc. 2002;55:859–62.
68. Hollerbach S, Willert J, Topalidis T, Reiser M, Schmiegel W. Endoscopic ultrasound-guided fine-needle aspiration biopsy of liver lesions: histological and cytological assessment. Endoscopy. 2003;35:743–9.
69. DeWitt J, LeBlanc J, McHenry L, Ciaccia D, Imperiale T, Chappo J, et al. Endoscopic ultrasound-guided fine needle aspiration cytology of solid liver lesions: a large single-center experience. Am J Gastroenterol. 2003;98:1976–81.
70. Crowe DR, Eloubeidi MA, Chhieng DC, Jhala NC, Jhala D, Eltoum IA. Fine-needle aspiration biopsy of hepatic lesions: computerized tomographic-guided versus endoscopic ultrasound-guided FNA. Cancer. 2006;108:180–5.
71. Singh P, Mukhopadhyay P, Bhatt B, Patel T, Kiss A, Gupta R, et al. Endoscopic ultrasound versus CT scan for detection of the metastases to the liver: results of a prospective comparative study. J Clin Gastroenterol. 2009;43:367–73.
72. Stavropoulos SN, Im GY, Jlayer Z, Harris MD, Pitea TC, Turi GK, et al. High yield of same-session EUS-guided liver biopsy by 19-gauge FNA needle in patients undergoing EUS to exclude biliary obstruction. Gastrointest Endosc. 2012;75:310–8.
73. Sey MS, Al-Haddad M, Imperiale TF, McGreevy K, Lin J, DeWitt JM. EUS-guided liver biopsy for parenchymal disease: a comparison of diagnostic yield between two core biopsy needles. Gastrointest Endosc. 2016;83:347–52.
74. Fally M, Nessar R, Behrendt N, Clementsen PF. Endoscopic ultrasound-guided liver biopsy in the hands of a chest physician. Respiration. 2016;92:53–5.
75. Diehl DL, Johal AS, Khara HS, Stavropoulos SN, Al-Haddad M, Ramesh J, et al. Endoscopic ultrasound-guided liver biopsy: a multicenter experience. Endosc Int Open. 2015;3:E210–5.
76. Pineda JJ, Diehl DL, Miao CL, Johal AS, Khara HS, Bhanushali A, et al. EUS-guided liver biopsy provides diagnostic samples comparable with those via the percutaneous or transjugular route. Gastrointest Endosc. 2016;83:360–5.

77. Rustemovic N, Hrstic I, Opacic M, Ostojic R, Jakic-Razumovic J, Kvarantan M, et al. EUS elastography in the diagnosis of focal liver lesions. Gastrointest Endosc. 2007;66:823–4.
78. Choi HJ, Moon JH, Kim HK, Lee YN, Lee TH, Cha SW, et al. KRAS mutation analysis by next-generation sequencing in endoscopic ultrasound-guided sampling for solid liver masses. J Gastroenterol Hepatol. 2016;32:154–62.
79. Dietrich CF, Kratzer W, Strobe D, Danse E, Fessl R, Bunk A, et al. Assessment of metastatic liver disease in patients with primary extrahepatic tumors by contrast-enhanced sonography versus CT and MRI. World J Gastroenterol. 2006;12:1699–705.

Evaluation of Resectability of Pancreatic Cancer by MDCT

3

Toshifumi Gabata

3.1 Introduction

Ninety-five percent of pancreatic cancers and pancreatic ductal cancers are adenocarcinomas, which are characterized by rich stromal parenchyma and an infiltrative growth pattern. Even on plain CT large advanced pancreatic cancers obviously invading peripancreatic adipose tissue and peripancreatic blood vessels (celiac artery~splenic artery and common hepatic artery, superior mesenteric artery, splenic vein~portal vein) can be identified in many cases. In contrast, relatively small tumors that do not exceed the pancreatic rim and are resectable are not detectable by plain CT. If pancreatic cancer occludes the main pancreatic duct, caudal pancreatic duct dilatation and atrophy of the pancreatic parenchyma, in other words tumor-associated chronic pancreatitis, are induced. Accordingly, when interpreting plain CT even more important than detection of the tumor itself is meticulous confirmation of the presence/absence of pancreatic duct dilatation and an atrophic, irregular pancreatic parenchyma. Furthermore, in some cases acute pancreatitis may be induced by pancreatic duct occlusion associated with growth of the pancreatic cancer. Especially various findings suggestive of acute pancreatitis such as increased adipose tissue density and exudate accumulation around the pancreas body and tail, and left perirenal fascial thickening can be observed on plain CT too. However, for the early detection of pancreatic cancer and determination of the extent of its spread plain CT, as well as only contrast-enhanced CT, is far from adequate. In this context, contrast-enhanced dynamic CT (dynamic CT) using MDCT is essential.

Recently, use of 16–256 multidetector row CT (MDCT) has become widespread, and indeed seems to have become the standard against which other modalities are measured. However, full advantage cannot be taken of the capabilities of MDCT for

T. Gabata
Department of Radiology, Kanazawa University Hospital,
Kanazawa, Ishikawa Prefecture, Japan
e-mail: tgabata@icloud.com

© Springer Science+Business Media Singapore 2017

29

H. Yamaue (ed.), *Innovation of Diagnosis and Treatment for Pancreatic Cancer*,
DOI 10.1007/978-981-10-2486-3_3

the diagnosis of pancreatic cancer if only past imaging methods used for contrast-enhanced CT are applied. To enhance the detectability of pancreatic cancer and the diagnosis of the extent of its spread, a sufficient volume of a high concentration iodinated contrast medium must be rapidly injected intravenously, a thin slice thickness selected, and multiphasic dynamic CT performed. Since unlike hepatocellular carcinoma it is not possible to establish a high-risk group for pancreatic cancer, if pancreatic cancer is overlooked on the initial CT, on subsequent examinations progression to unresectable advanced pancreatic cancer is almost inevitably found, and so imaging should be conducted using the highest possible quality CT, and every effort made not to overlook any of the early findings.

3.2   Method of Contrast-Enhanced Dynamic MDCT for Pancreas

At our Institution (Kanazawa University Hospital), imaging is performed with 64-row MDCT. In cases in which pancreatic cancer is suspected a contrast medium at a high concentration (350 mg/ml, 100–135 ml) is used, and the injection time of the contrast agent is fixed at 30 s (fixed injection time method) [1]. The volume of contrast medium used for contrast-enhanced dynamic CT is 1.8 ml/kg (108 ml if 60 kg; 126 ml if 70 kg), and the injection speed of the contrast agent is set at injection volume/30 s (3.6 ml/s if 60 kg; 4.2 ml/s if 70 kg) (Table 3.1). The reasons why we use a high iodinated concentration contrast medium at our institution include: (1) Use of a high iodine concentration contrast medium is advantageous to clearly depict the peripancreatic vasculature. (2) Since pancreatic cancer is ischemic, in the early phase by enhancing to the extent possible the staining of the pancreatic parenchyma with a high concentration of iodine, the depiction of the pancreatic cancer as

Table 3.1 Pancreas dynamic CT protocol using contrast, Iomeron 350 (135 ml) or Omnipaque 350 (100 ml)

	Range	Scan delay time (s)	Slice thickness (mm)	Additional slice (mm)	Reconstruction images
Precontrast	Liver ~ Kidney		2.5		
Early arterial phase	Liver ~ Kidney	25	2.5	1.25	3D (VR) MIP
Late arterial (pancreatic) phase	Liver ~ Kidney	40	2.5	1.25	MIP (3 mm · 1 mm space)
Portal phase	Liver ~ Kidney	70	2.5	1.25	MIP (3 mm · 1 mm space)
Equilibrium phase	Liver ~ Pelvis	180	2.5	1.25	MIP (3 mm · 1 mm space)

Contrast agent injection time: fixed at 30 s: fixed injection time method
350 mg/ml: 1.8 ml/kg: if 60 kg 108 ml; if 70 kg 126 ml
Injection speed: injection volume/30 s: if 60 kg 3.6 ml/s; if 70 kg 4.2 ml/s

a low density region is facilitated (i.e., depicted as negative). Also, in some small pancreatic cancers on dynamic early phase (arterial phase) no difference in density relative to the pancreas is apparent. In some of such cases, in the dynamic late phase (equilibrium phase) the tumor may show delayed enhancement and higher absorbance than the surrounding pancreas, making it possible to identify the tumor (Fig. 3.1) [2, 3]. Accordingly, by using a high concentration contrast medium the delayed enhancement of characteristic of pancreatic cancer becomes more prominent, which is expected to enhance its diagnosability.

Dynamic CT imaging requires imaging of at least four phases: early arterial phase (after 25 s), late arterial phase (pancreatic parenchyma phase) (after 40 s), venous phase (after 70 s), and equilibrium phase (after 180 s) [1]. From the arterial-dominant phase data 3D images (volume rendering: VR) can be prepared and facilitate evaluation of the arterial anatomy and arterial invasion (Fig. 3.2). Also, from the pancreatic parenchyma phase data, reconstruction images such as coronal, sagittal or oblique ones parallel to the pancreatic head and body/tail can be prepared and used to determine tumor spread and vessel invasion since it is also important to evaluate these factors from a viewpoint different from that of transverse images (Figs. 3.3 and 3.4) [4, 5]. Since on pancreas arterial phase dynamic CT images or slab MIP images superimposed with pancreatic parenchyma phase or portal vein phase four 2.5 mm thick slices (10 mm thick) or seven slices (17.5 mm thick) the peripancreatic arteries and veins are depicted continuously along their length in a single cross section, the preoperative vessel anatomy and presence/absence of anatomical variants can be instantly grasped (Fig. 3.5). slab MIP images in the portal

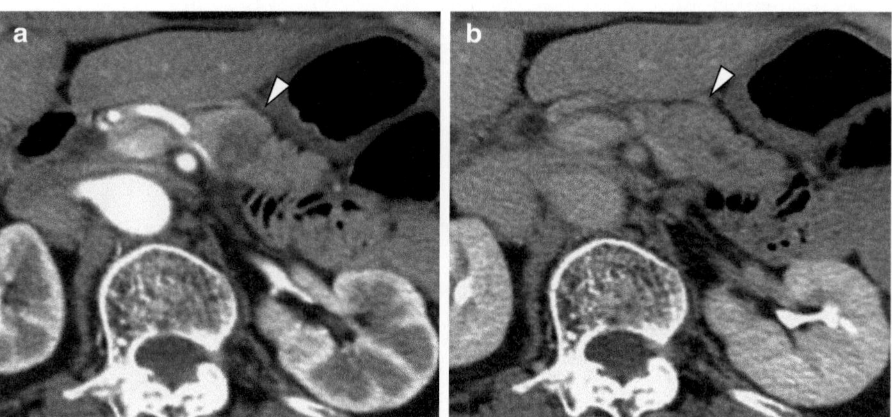

Fig. 3.1 Pancreatic body cancer showing isodensity on dynamic CT equilibrium phase. In dynamic CT arterial phase (**a**), an ischemic tumor in the pancreatic body (*arrowhead*) is pointed out. However, in the equilibrium phase (**b**) the tumor shows delayed staining and isodensity with the peripancreatic parenchyma. Only in the postcontrast equilibrium phase there is a danger of overlooking the tumor

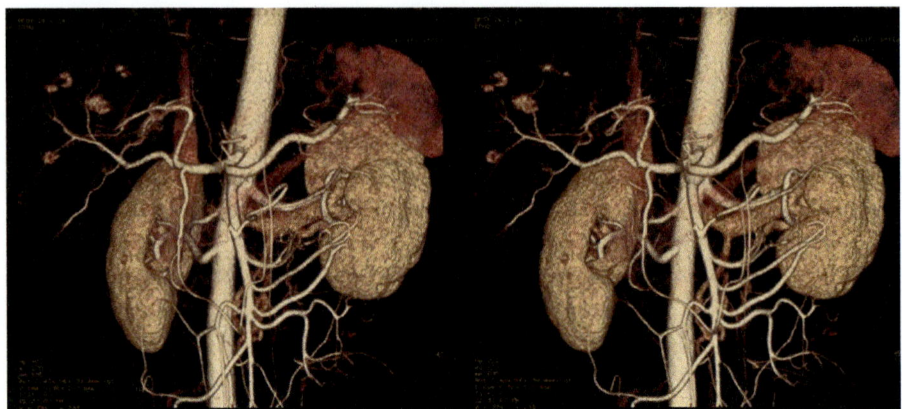

Fig. 3.2 By subjecting dynamic CT arterial phase 3D (VR) image and 3D VR (Volume Rendering) images to stereoscopic vision (cross-over method), the influence of vessel overlap can be made to disappear, thereby facilitating precise identification of the vasculature up to its distal portions. Stereoscopic vision is thus recommended for preoperative evaluation of the arterial anatomy

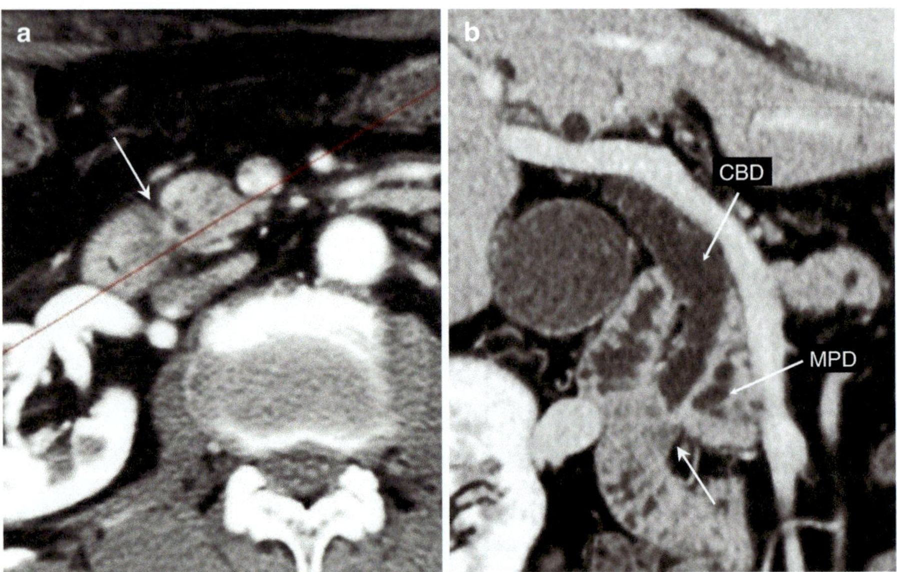

Fig. 3.3 Groove pancreatic cancer. In dynamic CT arterial phase (**a**), an ischemic tumor (*arrow*) is found in the groove region. On oblique coronal section images (**b**) reconstructed with a *red reference line*, occlusion by the groove tumor (*arrow*) of the common bile duct (CBD) and main pancreatic duct (MPD) can be evaluated on a single cross section

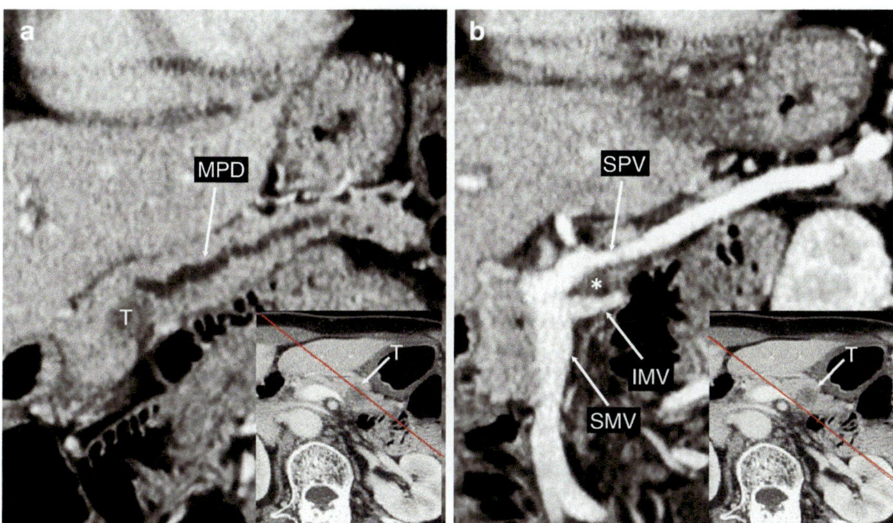

Fig. 3.4 Splenic vein and inferior mesenteric vein invasion by pancreatic body cancer. These are oblique sagittal section reconstruction images (**a**, **b**) taken parallel to the pancreatic body in the portal venous phase of dynamic CT. An ischemic tumor (T) occluding the main pancreatic duct (MPD) extends posteroinferiorly (*asterisk*), with findings suggestive of invasion of the inferior mesenteric vein (IMV) at the junction of the splenic vein (SPV) and superior mesenteric vein (SMV) noted

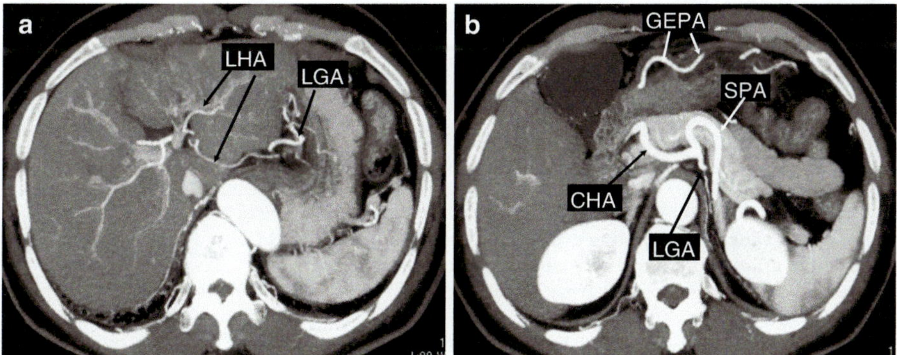

Fig. 3.5 Dynamic CT late arterial phase of normal pancreas, slab MIP image (12.5 mm thick). On slab MIP image (12.5 mm thick) (**a**, **b**) prepared by overlapping seven 2.5 mm thick slices, it can be easily noticed that the left hepatic artery (LHA) branches from the left gastric artery (LGA). Also, since the splenic artery (SPA) branching from the celiac artery (CA) and common hepatic artery (CHA) are depicted along their length in a single cross section the vessel anatomy can be well appreciated. The left gastric artery (LGA) that branches posterior to the celiac artery root and the gastro-epiploic artery (GEPA) that runs along the greater curvature side of the stomach can also be identified

venous phase are useful for the evaluation of the normal peripancreatic venous anatomy. They can identify the right colic vein that flows into the gastrocolic trunk (GCT), middle colic vein, jejunal vein that flows into the gastro-epiploic and superior mesenteric veins, and inferior mesenteric vein that flows into the splenic or superior mesenteric vein, as well as evaluate the presence/absence of tumor invasion and of venous dilatation indicating collaterals associated with venous stenosis or occlusion (Figs. 3.6 and 3.7).

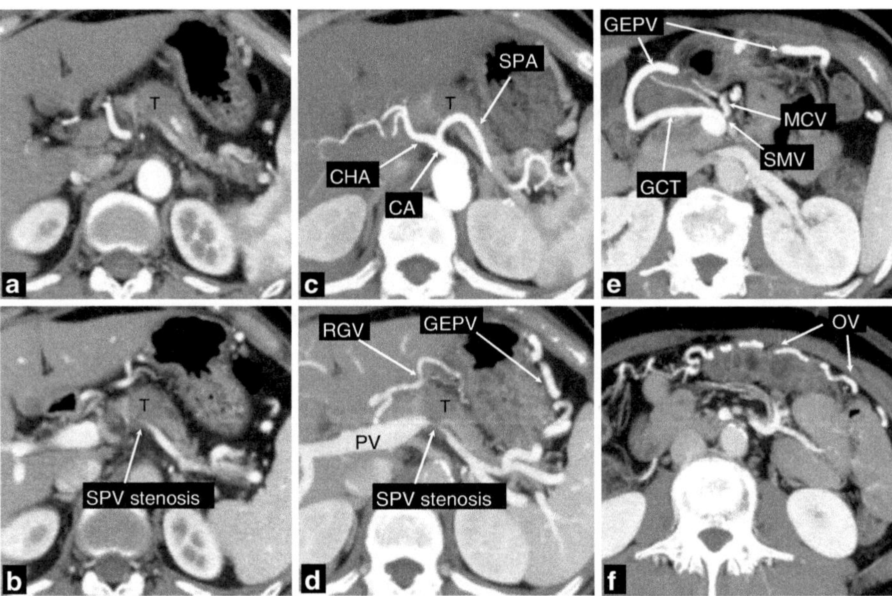

Fig. 3.6 Pancreatic body cancer with retroperitoneum invasion, splenic artery and splenic vein invasion, and collateral formation evaluated by slab MIP imaging (17.5 mm slice thickness). On dynamic CT arterial phase with 2.5 mm slice thickness (**a**), an ischemic tumor (T) is found in the pancreatic body. Invasion of the serous membrane and retroperitoneum is suspected. On the portal vein phase (**b**), stenosis of the splenic vein (SPV) is seen to have been induced by tumor invasion. In the arterial phase of 17.5 mm thick slab MIP (**c**), invasion by the tumor (T) of the splenic artery (SPA) branching from the celiac artery (CA) is clearly discernible, while invasion of the common hepatic artery (CHA) is not found. On slab MIP (17.5 mm thick) portal vein phase (**d–f**), the development due to splenic vein (SPV) stenosis of perigastric venous collaterals [short gastric vein ~ right gastric vein (RGV)~portal vein (PV) and gastroepiploic vein (GEPV)~GCT (gastrocolic trunk)~superior mesenteric vein (SMV), middle colic vein (MCV), omental vein (OV)] can be clearly grasped

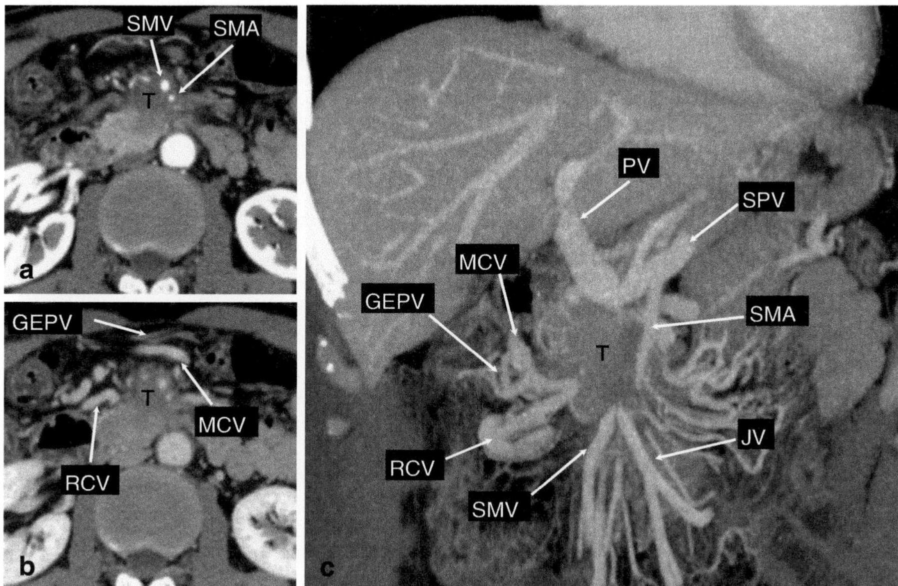

Fig. 3.7 Pancreas uncinate process cancer with superior mesenteric arteriovenous and mesentery root invasion. On dynamic CT arterial phase (**a**), an ischemic tumor (*arrow*) is found in the pancreatic head. The tumor extends anteriorly involving the superior mesenteric artery (SMA) and superior mesenteric vein (SMV). (**b**) Since GCT is occluded by invasion of the tumor, venous stasis is induced and the gastro-epipolic vein (GEPV), middle colic vein (MCV), and right colic vein (RCV) are dilated. In venous phase convolution on MIP images (coronal) (**c**), venous dilatation (RCV, GEPV, MCV) due to GCT occlusion is clearly seen. Occlusion is also noted of the jejunal vein (JV) at the juncture with the superior mesenteric vein (SMV). That the pancreatic head cancer has extensively invaded the mesocolon and mesentery can be clearly concluded from the venous occlusion

3.3   Diagnosis of Extent of Spread of Pancreatic Cancer

CT is central to the diagnosis of the extent of the local spread of pancreatic cancer, and as shown in Table 3.2 evaluation of eight factors is required.

Evaluation of intrapancreatic bile duct invasion (CH) depends directly on whether or not normal pancreatic tissue is interposed between the tumor and bile duct wall, and in practice is judged in most cases by the indirect finding of the presence/absence of bile duct dilatation. In some cases, pancreatic cancer invades along the bile duct wall and is depicted as thickening associated with contrast enhancement of the common bile duct wall (Fig. 3.8).

Table 3.2 Diagnosis of extent of spread of pancreatic cancer

Bile duct invasion	CH	
Duodenal invasion	DU	
Serosal invasion	S	Pancreatic serosa, omentum, mesentery, and mesocolon
Retroperitoneal invasion	RP	Retropancreatic connective tissue
Portal venous invasion	PV	Portal vein, superior mesenteric vein, splenic vein
Arterial system	A	Celiac artery, splenic artery, common hepatic artery, superior mesenteric artery
Perineural invasion	PL	Pancreatic head (I, II), celiac artery, superior mesenteric artery, splenic artery, common hepatic artery
Other organ invasion	OO	Inferior vena cava, kidney, adrenal gland, stomach, colon, spleen

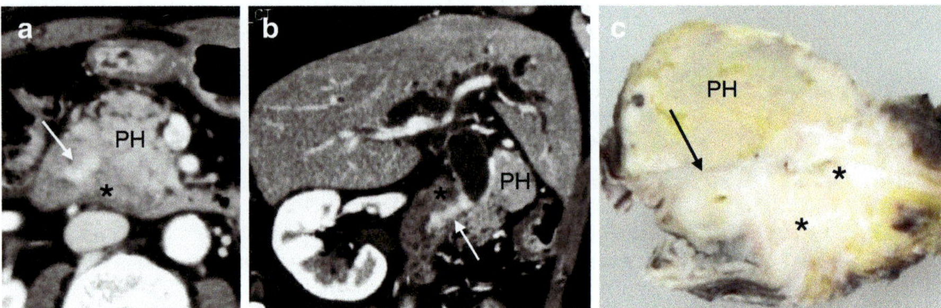

Fig. 3.8 Pancreatic head cancer with intrapancreatic bile duct invasion. On transverse (**a**) and oblique coronal images (**b**) of dynamic CT arterial phase, an ischemic mass (*asterisk*) is found in the pancreatic head. The intrapancreatic bile duct shows mural thickening and staining (*arrow*). In the resected specimen (**c**), pancreatic head cancer (*asterisk*) is seen to invade the intrapancreatic bile duct, and marked thickening (*arrow*) of the bile duct wall is found. *PH* pancreatic head

Evaluation of duodenal invasion (DU) depends directly on whether or not adipose tissue and normal pancreatic tissue are interposed between the tumor and duodenum. For this evaluation, MPR coronal section images are frequently useful (Fig. 3.9). Between the duodenal descending portion~horizontal portion junction and pancreatic head the superior and inferior pancreaticoduodenal venous system is present, and occlusion of these veins also suggests duodenal invasion. Also, pancreatic cancer that extends to the groove area may closely resemble groove pancreatitis in some cases, with this kind of tumor often invading the duodenum as well, and proof of malignancy often only obtained after repeated duodenal mucosal biopsies (Fig. 3.10) [6].

On evaluation of invasion into the pancreatic serosal (S) and retropancreatic tissues (RP), the diagnosis of "invasion absent" is limited to only those cases in which normal pancreatic parenchyma is present between the tumor and peripancreatic adipose tissue. Since the pancreas does not possess a thick fibrous capsule, any tumor that reaches the pancreas rim can easily invade outside the pancreas. Accordingly, when in the peripancreatic adipose tissue a structure showing a funicular shadow

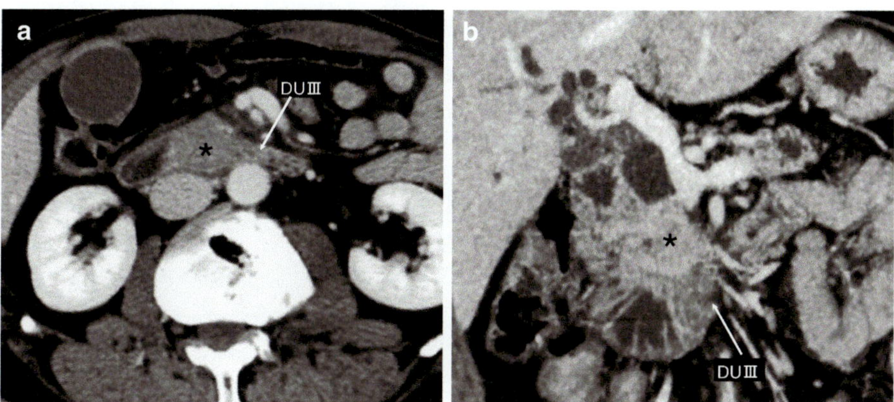

Fig. 3.9 Pancreas uncinate process cancer with duodenal invasion (horizontal limb). On transverse (**a**) and coronal images (**b**) of dynamic CT portal venous phase, an ischemic mass (*asterisk*) is found in the pancreas uncinate process. On coronal section images (**b**), the tumor invades the upper wall of the duodenal horizontal limb (DUIII), and the duodenal lumen is stenotic

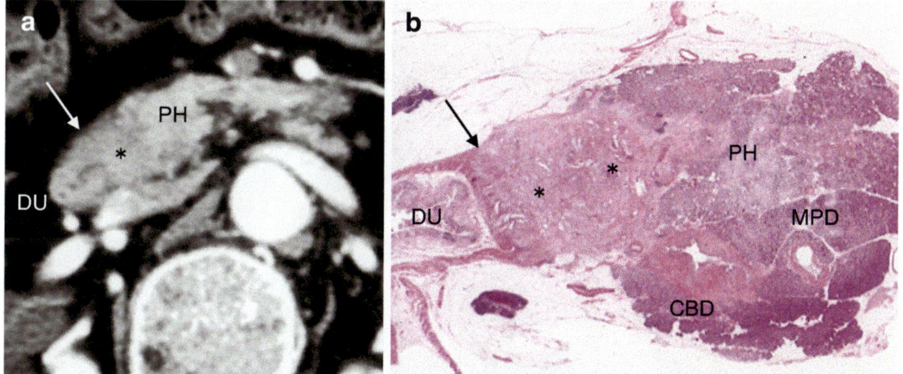

Fig. 3.10 Duodenal invasion by groove pancreatic cancer. On dynamic CT arterial phase (**a**), an ischemic mass (*asterisk*) is noted in the groove region between the pancreatic head (PH) and duodenum. The border with the internal wall of the duodenum (DU) is indistinct, and invasion is suspected (*arrow*). On endoscopy, an ulcer is found in the duodenal descending limb, and on biopsy adenocarcinoma is documented. In the resected specimen (**b**), the groove pancreatic cancer (*asterisk*) extends past the muscle layer of the duodenal internal wall and invades up to the mucosa (*arrow*)

and increased density is seen, even in the absence of any change in the density of the surrounding adipose tissue when normal pancreatic parenchyma is not interposed between the tumor and surrounding adipose tissue of course "invasion present" may reasonably be considered (Figs. 3.11 and 3.12). Since the presence/absence of invasion into the tissues located posterior to the pancreas is an extremely important determinant of operability and prognosis, this point requires an especially meticulous evaluation.

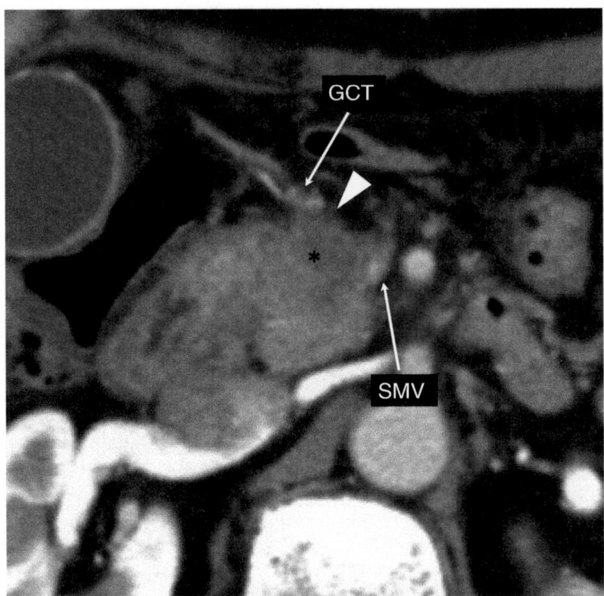

Fig. 3.11 Pancreatic head cancer with serous membrane invasion (S). On dynamic CT arterial phase, an ischemic tumor (*asterisk*) in the pancreatic head is seen to reach the serous membrane surface, and serous membrane invasion positive (S+) status is diagnosed. Invasion of the gastrocolic trunk (GCT) and superior mesenteric vein (SMV) is also noted

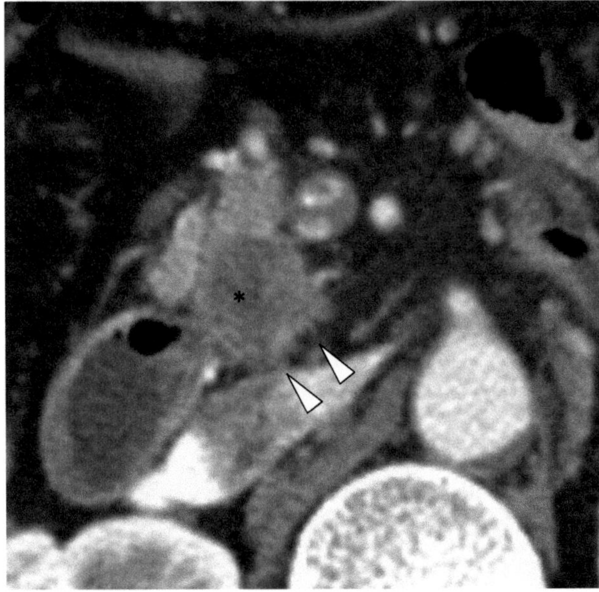

Fig. 3.12 Pancreatic head cancer with retroperitoneal invasion (Rp). On dynamic CT arterial phase protruding serrated (dentate) changes are found posterior to an ischemic tumor (*asterisk*), and make possible a diagnosis of retroperitoneal invasion (Rp+)

Invasion of the portal venous system (PV) is determined by evaluating the main trunk of the portal vein, superior mesenteric vein, and splenic vein. In cases in which there is marked stenosis or occlusion of the vascular lumen by the tumor, invasion is found [7] in ≥90% of cases when the tumor and vessel are in contact for ≥1/2 of the vessel circumference (Fig. 3.13). Evaluation of invasion of the portal

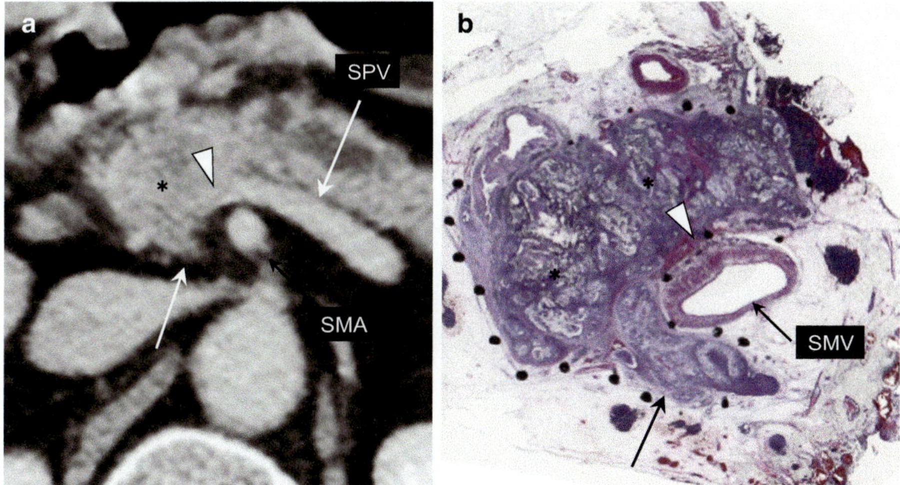

Fig. 3.13 Pancreatic head cancer with invasion of the superior mesenteric vein and neural plexuses around the superior mesenteric artery. On dynamic CT portal venous phase (**a**), an ischemic tumor (*asterisk*) was found in the pancreatic head. Compression stenosis (*arrowhead*) was seen at the junction of the superior mesenteric vein and splenic vein, and invasion was diagnosed. On the posterior surface of the pancreatic head, a club-like protrusion (*arrow*) was noted, and invasion of the nerve plexuses around the superior mesenteric artery was suspected. There was no problem in the adipose tissue around the superior mesenteric artery (SMA), and no invasion of the main trunk of the superior mesenteric artery was found. In the resected specimen (**b**), superior mesenteric vein (SMV) invasion (*arrowhead*) and nerve plexus invasion (*arrow*) were evident. *SPV* splenic vein

venous system is important for selection of the optimal surgical procedure, such as combined resection of affected vessel(s), and as a prognostic factor of hepatic metastasis recurrence, with the postoperative results unfavorable in cases with circumferential stenosis in the portal venous system.

Invasion of the arterial system (A) is determined by evaluation of the common hepatic, superior mesenteric, splenic, and celiac arteries. "Invasion present" is judged when stenosis or occlusion of the arterial lumen is seen or an artery is encased by tumor (Figs. 3.14, 3.15, and 3.16). In the case of the portal venous system, "contact between the tumor and vessel for $\geq 1/2$ of the vessel circumference" is a valid criterion to judge "invasion present," whereas in the arterial system because of the possibility of coexisting non-tumorous fibrosis false-positives are not uncommon [8]. For this reason, there is another method that judges invasion to be present when contact between the tumor and vessel exceeds 1/2 of the vessel circumference and thickening and/or irregularity of the arterial wall is observed [9]. However, the absence of histological vascular wall invasion and the nonpersistence of tumor cells after surgical resection are not equivalent, and some institutions aim for combined resection whenever possible when this finding is present. As a general rule, invasion of the celiac or superior mesenteric artery constitutes a contraindication to surgery. Also, regardless of the presence/absence of invasion, a preoperative grasp of the vessel anatomy is important for both the selection and safety of the surgical

Fig. 3.14 Invasion by pancreatic body cancer of the splenic artery via the celiac artery. In the arterial phase of dynamic CT, a pancreatic body tumor (*asterisk*) invades posterior to the pancreas. Clear encasement of the celiac artery (CA)~proximal splenic artery (SPA) is found, allowing a diagnosis of arterial invasion to be made

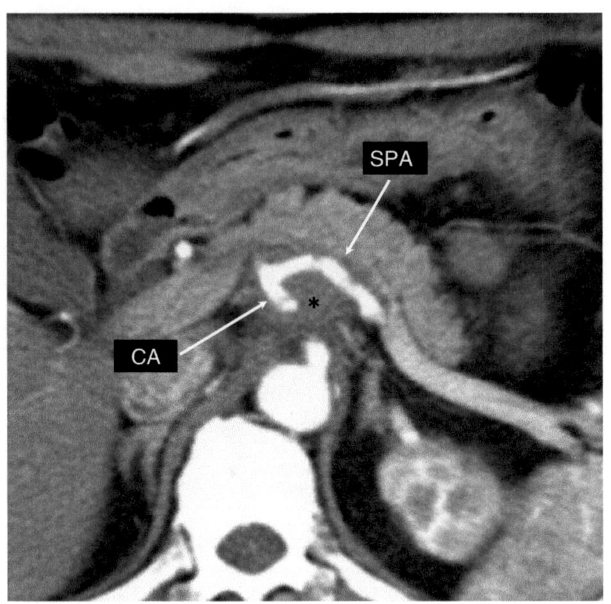

Fig. 3.15 Pancreatic body cancer with splenic artery invasion. On dynamic CT arterial phase slab MIP (17.5 mm thick) images, irregular encasement of the splenic artery (SPA) due to invasion by pancreatic body cancer (*asterisk*) is found

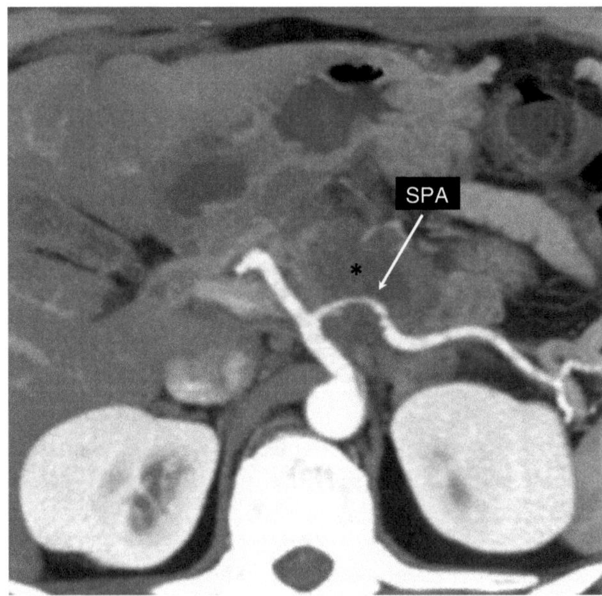

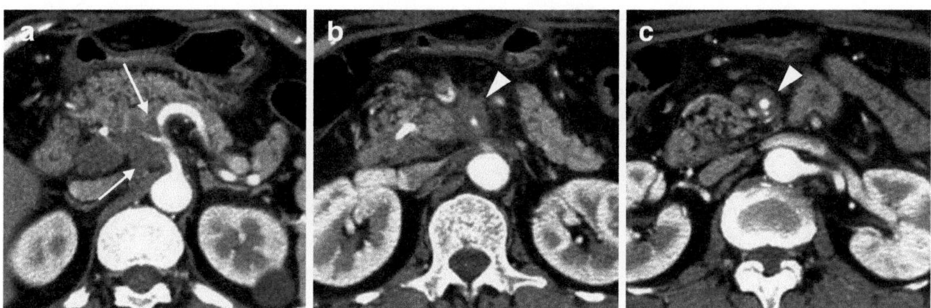

Fig. 3.16 Pancreas uncinate process cancer with periceliac and perisuperior mesenteric arterial neural plexus invasion. On dynamic CT arterial phase (**a–c**), there is marked invasion of the extra-pancreatic neural plexuses by pancreas uncinate process cancer, and formation of a mass that encases the celiac artery~common hepatic artery (*arrow*) and superior mesenteric artery (*arrowhead*)

procedure. With recent MDCT, almost all of the knowledge of vascular anatomy needed for surgery can be acquired by preparing MIP, slab MIP, and/or VR images.

Extrapancreatic neural plexus invasion (PL) is a major determinant of prognosis, and its accurate diagnosis is of vital importance in determining the extent of the dissection needed. Findings suggestive of neural plexus invasion include a serrated (dentate), funicular, or mass shadow facing the superior mesenteric or celiac artery from the pancreatic uncinate process; a funicular shadow or mass formation around the inferior pancreaticoduodenal artery and vein; and tumor-induced stenosis of the jejunal vein trunk [10] (Fig. 3.13). When a mass shadow continuous from a tumor encases the superior mesenteric artery in a donut-like manner, it is appropriate to diagnose neural plexus invasion (Fig. 3.16). Since the introduction of MDCT, considerable knowledge about the imaging findings of neural plexus invasion has been accumulated, but because of the interference of factors such as concomitant pancreatitis and non-tumorous fibrosis, an accurate diagnosis is still quite difficult to make.

The CT diagnosis of lymph node metastases from pancreatic cancer is basically the same as that of those from cancers of other organs, aiming for a short diameter of ≥ 1 cm. However, needless to say, with CT alone false-positives and false-negatives are common, and so the possibility of metastases must be kept in mind even when lesions measure less than 1 cm, especially those showing a globular shape, intense staining, and/or ring-like staining (Fig. 3.17). The extent of lymph node metastases is strongly correlated with prognosis, and the presence of para-aortic lymph node metastases is a contraindication to surgery [11, 12].

The diagnosis of hepatic metastases as well is fundamentally the same as that of hepatic metastases from cancer of other organs, but pancreatic cancer is characterized by a particularly high frequency of multiple small metastases, and the finding of AP shunt-like wedge-shaped staining on contrast-enhanced dynamic study (Figs. 3.18 and 3.19).

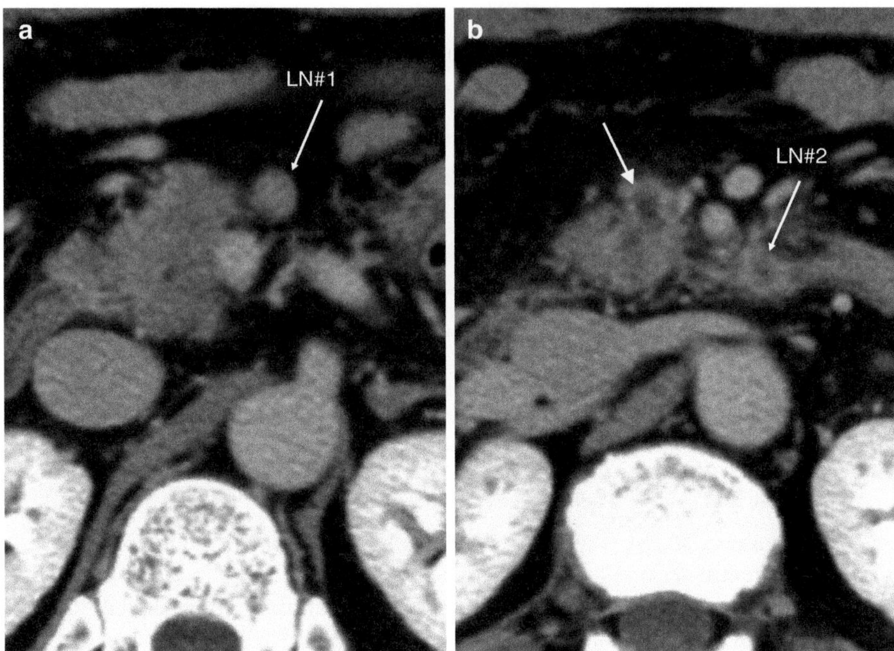

Fig. 3.17 Pancreatic head cancer with lymph node metastases. On dynamic CT equilibrium phase (**a, b**), an irregular tumor (**b:** *arrow*) is found in the pancreatic head, associated with two enlarged lymph nodes. The larger #1 lymph node is uniformly enhanced while an area of low absorption suggestive of necrosis is found in the interior of #2 lymph node. Histologically, metastasis was found only in #2 lymph node

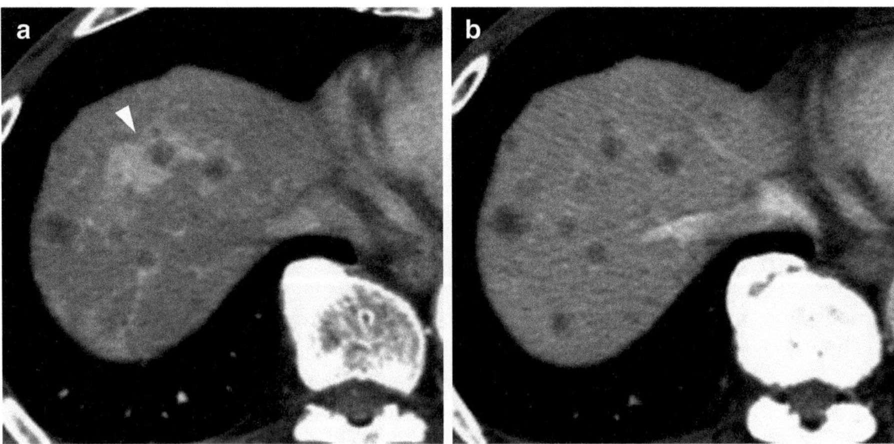

Fig. 3.18 Pancreas uncinate process cancer with multiple hepatic metastases and AP shunt-like staining. In the arterial phase of dynamic CT (**a**), multiple hepatic metastases showing ring-like staining are found in the hepatic right lobe. Around one of the hepatic metastases, an AP shunt-like stain is found. In the equilibrium phase (**b**), the hepatic metastatic foci showed low absorption, while the AP shunt staining has disappeared

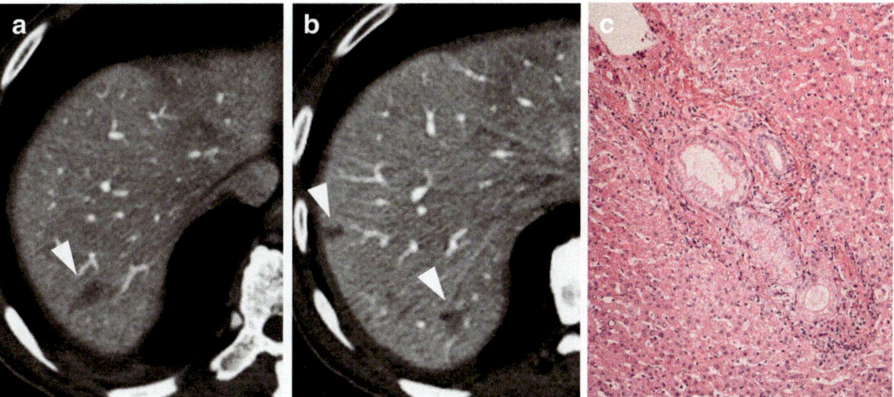

Fig. 3.19 Pancreatic head cancer with microscopic hepatic metastases and AP shunt-like change. In the dynamic CT arterial phase, the liver is somewhat uneven, but no obvious hepatic metastases could be pointed out. On CTAP (CT during arterial portography) (**a**, **b**), multiple wedge-shaped hepatic portal vein perfusion defects are present in the right lobe, and multiple AP shunts are suspected. Intraoperatively multiple microscopic hepatic metastases are noted on the liver surface. Histologically, (**c**) multiple tumor thrombi are identified in the microscopic portal vein branches in the distal hepatic Glisson's capsule and are thought to be the cause of the AP shunts

3.4   Final Remarks

Here, focusing mainly on personally experienced cases I outlined the dynamic CT evaluation of blood vessel invasion by pancreatic cancer. To achieve the most accurate evaluation of tumor extent and blood vessel invasion, further refinements will need to be made in dynamic CT and CT imaging methods. Observation relying on thin slices (1.25–2.5 mm thickness), high concentration, high-dose ionized contrast medium, optimal imaging timing (plain, early arterial phase, pancreatic parenchyma phase, portal vein phase, equilibrium phase), and multiplanar reconstruction images (MIP images) such as oblique coronal, and oblique sagittal images in addition to transverse ones is recommended. Since pancreatic cancer exhibits a strong tendency to invade periarterial neural plexuses, radiologists must also familiarize themselves with the CT findings of neural plexus invasion.

References

1. Yanaga Y, Awai K, Nakayama Y, et al. Pancreas: patient body weight tailored contrast material injection protocol versus fixed dose protocol at dynamic CT. Radiology. 2007;245(2): 475–82.
2. Fukukura Y, Hamada H, Kamiyama T, et al. Pancreatic adenocarcinoma: analysis of the effect of various concentrations of contrast material. Radiat Med. 2008;26(6):355–61.
3. Ishigami K, Yoshimitsu K, Irie H, et al. Diagnostic value of the delayed phase image for iso-attenuating pancreatic carcinomas in the pancreatic parenchymal phase on multidetector computed tomography. Eur J Radiol. 2009;69:139–46.

4. Takeshita K, Furui S, Takada K. Multidetector row helical CT of the pancreas: value of three-dimensional images, two-dimensional reformations, and contrast-enhanced multiphasic imaging. J Hepato-Biliary-Pancreat Surg. 2002;9:576–82.

5. Nino-Murcia M, Tamm EP, Charnsangavej C, et al. Multidetector-row helical CT and advanced postprocessing techniques for the evaluation of pancreatic neoplasms. Abdom Imaging. 2003;28:366–77.

6. Gabata T, Kadoya M, Terayama N, et al. Groove pancreatic carcinomas: radiological and pathological findings. Eur Radiol. 2003;13:1679–84.

7. Lu DS, Reber HA, Krasny RM, et al. Local staging of pancreatic cancer: criteria for unresectability of major vessels as revealed by pancreatic-phase, thin-section helical CT. AJR Am J Roentgenol. 1997;168:1439–43.

8. Nakayama Y, Yamashita Y, Kadota M, et al. Vascular encasement by pancreatic cancer: correlation of CT findings with surgical and pathologic results. J Comput Assist Tomogr. 2001;25:337–42.

9. Li H, Zeng MS, Zhou KR, et al. Pancreatic adenocarcinoma: the different CT criteria for peripancreatic major arterial and venous invasion. J Comput Assist Tomogr. 2005;29:170–5.

10. Mochizuki K, Gabata T, Kosaka K, et al. MDCT findings of extrapancreatic nerve plexus invasion by pancreas head carcinoma: correlation with en bloc pathological specimens and diagnostic accuracy. Eur Radiol. 2010;20:1757–67.

11. Sakai M, Nakao A, Kaneko T, et al. Para-aortic lymph node metastasis in carcinoma of the head of the pancreas. Surgery. 2005;137:606–11.

12. Capussotti L, Massucco P, Ribero D, et al. Extended lymphadenectomy and vein resection for pancreatic head cancer: outcomes and implications for therapy. Arch Surg. 2003;138:1316–22.

Evaluation of Effect of Neoadjuvant Therapy Using Positron Emission Tomography

4

Ik Jae Lee and Jinsil Seong

4.1 Introduction

Pancreatic cancer is one of the most common gastrointestinal tumors and the fourth leading cause of cancer-related mortality in the United States [1]. Early diagnosis of pancreatic cancer, which allow curative resection, is crucial to a great clinical outcome. However, only 10–30% of pancreatic cancers are resectable at the initial diagnosis [2]. The majority of patients presents borderline resectable or locally advanced pancreatic cancers, which might fall into poor outcome unless resection performed. Neoadjuvant therapy with induction chemotherapy or concurrent chemoradiotherapy (CRT) could provide a change converting tumors to resectable status as several prospective studies have demonstrated the benefits of neoadjuvant therapy [3].

18F-fluorodeoxyglucose (FDG) positron emission tomography (PET) is a very useful and noninvasive tool for imaging tumor glucose metabolic activity in the management and prediction of survival of numerous malignant disorders [4]. There has been a growing evidence showing importance of metabolic imaging for predicting clinical outcome after the introduction of PET-computed tomography (CT) and application in oncology [5]. However, despite the increasing use of PET, the significance of changes of PET in patients with locally advanced pancreatic cancer after neoadjuvant therapy is not well defined.

In this chapter, we review the role of PET in patients with pancreatic cancer in terms of differential diagnosis, staging malignant lesions, detection of recurrence, and assessment of tumor response to neoadjuvant therapy.

I.J. Lee, M.D., Ph.D.
Department of Radiation Oncology, Gangnam Severance Hospital, Yonsei
University College of Medicine, 211 Eonju-ro, Gangnam-gu, Seoul, 06273, Korea

J. Seong, M.D., Ph.D. (✉)
Department of Radiation Oncology, Yonsei Cancer Center, Yonsei University College of
Medicine, 50-1 Yonsei-ro, Seodaemun-gu, Seoul 03722, Korea
e-mail: jsseong@yuhs.ac

© Springer Science+Business Media Singapore 2017

45

H. Yamaue (ed.), *Innovation of Diagnosis and Treatment for Pancreatic Cancer*,
DOI 10.1007/978-981-10-2486-3_4

4.2 PET-CT: Diagnostic Efficacy in the Detection and Differential Diagnosis of Pancreatic Cancer

4.2.1 Diagnostic Efficacy

PET has been reported to be a high-sensitivity and relatively low-specificity (87–95% and 80.1–100%, respectively) technique [6–8], and Asagi et al. also reported that the diagnostic accuracy rate of PET-CT was more than 80% for most factors in local invasion and 94% for distant metastasis, but only 42% for lymph node metastasis in the initial workup for staging in patients with resectable pancreatic cancer [9]. However, the inadequate capability of FDG imaging to provide anatomic accuracy remains a significant limitation. Therefore, CT and magnetic resonance imaging (MRI) are the most essential modalities in the diagnosis and staging of pancreatic disease, as they are the most accurate methods of evaluating vascular and adjacent structures. To improve the sensitivity and diagnostic accuracy, Sun et al. further analyzed PET-CT combined with tumor marker such as CA19-9 level. They demonstrated better diagnostic value when mean maximum standard uptake values (SUV_{max}) and CA19-9 are combined [10].

PET is more accurate than conventional imaging tools such as CT and MRI for differentiating benign from malignant cystic lesions of the pancreas and intraductal papillary mucinous neoplasm (IPMNs). In a prospective study of patients with suspected cystic pancreatic tumors, the sensitivity, specificity, positive and negative predictive values, and accuracy of PET for differentiating malignant disease were 94%, 94%, 89%, 97%, and 94%, respectively, compared with 65%, 88%, 73%, 83%, and 80%, respectively, for CT scanning [11].

In a series of 64 patients with suspected IPMN, the sensitivity of PET was 80% (4/5) for carcinoma in situ and 95% (20/21) for invasive carcinoma, both superior to CT or MRI, which were strongly suggestive of invasive carcinoma in only 62% of patients who had invasive carcinoma [12]. FDG uptake was absent in all adenomas ($n = 13$) and 87% (7/8) of borderline IPMNs. A positive PET influenced the management of ten patients with malignant IPMNs. Yoshiok et al. suggested that the optimal cutoff value for differentiating benign IMPN from malignant IPMN was 2.5 [13].

However, the differential diagnosis between pancreatic carcinoma and chronic pancreatitis remains a challenge. While PET imaging cannot differentiate exactly between tumor and inflammation, dynamic and delayed CT imaging appear to be able to differentiate malignant from benign disease and to detect diabetes mellitus and other tumors. Therefore, integrated PET-CT fusion images can improve the localization of FDG uptake and are valuable in the accurate diagnosis of pancreatic cancer prior to neoadjuvant treatment.

PET may also be very useful for evaluating indistinct abnormalities in the resected tumor bed seen on CT, which is difficult to differentiate from surgery- or radiotherapy-induced fibrosis after neoadjuvant therapy; for detecting and determining the extent of distant liver and other metastases of pancreatic cancer; and for restaging patients with increased tumor marker levels and negative follow-up images with conventional tools.

18F-FDG may be affected by various conditions that alter normal tissue metabolism, such as hyper/hypoglycemia, local inflammation or infection, diabetes mellitus, and administration of insulin or oral hypoglycemic agents. Chung et al. reported that the SUV_{max} of diabetes mellitus patients were significantly lower than those of non-diabetes mellitus patients ($p = 0.001$). The sensitivity of SUV_{max} (cutoff value 4.0) was significantly lower in the diabetes mellitus patients than in the non-diabetes mellitus patients (49.3% vs. 75.5%, $p < 0.001$) and lower in the normoglycemic diabetes mellitus group ($n = 24$) than in the non-diabetes mellitus group (54.2% vs. 75.5%, $p = 0.038$). Therefore, PET-CT results should be interpreted carefully when used for evaluating pancreatic cancer in diabetes mellitus patients.

Recurrence rates after definitive treatment of pancreatic cancer with a curative aim are as high as 42–68% within 2 years. The most common recurrence sites are liver, local, peritoneum, lung, and lymph nodes in descending order of occurrence [14]. Recurrent tumors are usually unresectable, and prognosis is very poor. However, recent therapeutic advances could potentially alter survival rates in selected patients. As such, early detection and treatment of the recurrent disease is critical in selected patients with good performance status. Follow-ups every 3–6 months with physical examination, tumor markers such as CA19-9, and conventional imaging tools (CT and MRI) are recommended for these patients.

Several studies have assessed the efficacy of PET-CT in detecting recurrent pancreatic cancer. PET identifies recurrence earlier than CT, with higher sensitivity (83.3–98%) and specificity (90%) than CT and MRI [15–17]. Kitajima et al. reported an added value of abdominal contrast-enhanced (CE) CT to PET-CT in their retrospective study of 45 patients who underwent surgical resection of pancreatic cancer [15]. They reported improved sensitivity, specificity, and accuracy (91.7%, 95.2%, and 93.3%, respectively) compared with non-enhanced PET-CT (83.3%, 90.5%, and 86.7%, respectively). Hamidian Jahromi et al. suggested that a combination of CA19-9 with CT or PET-CT was 100% accurate in detecting cancer recurrence [18]. The conventional imaging tools present an irradiation problem that is reflected in a larger gross tumor volume (GTV) on image compared with PET-CT [19]. Asagi et al. [9] reported that regarding the detection of postoperative recurrence, PET-CECT correctly detected local recurrence in all 11 cases of recurrence, whereas abdominal CECT detected only 7 of the 11 cases, suggesting that PET-CECT is superior in this context.

4.2.2 Usefulness of PET for Selecting Initial Treatment

Pancreatic cancer is one of the most threatening disease in oncology with higher mortality due to the much higher percentage (40–45%) of patients show metastatic disease at initial diagnosis and aggressive metastatic potential [20]. The MD Anderson Cancer Center performed neoadjuvant CRT for locally advanced pancreatic cancer, and 25% of patients had evidence of metastatic disease on preoperative restaging after CRT [21]. In this study, 9 (82%) of 11 patients who did not undergo resection have died of disease at a median time after restaging of 4 months. Chang et al. found that integrating PET-CT with conventional imaging tools

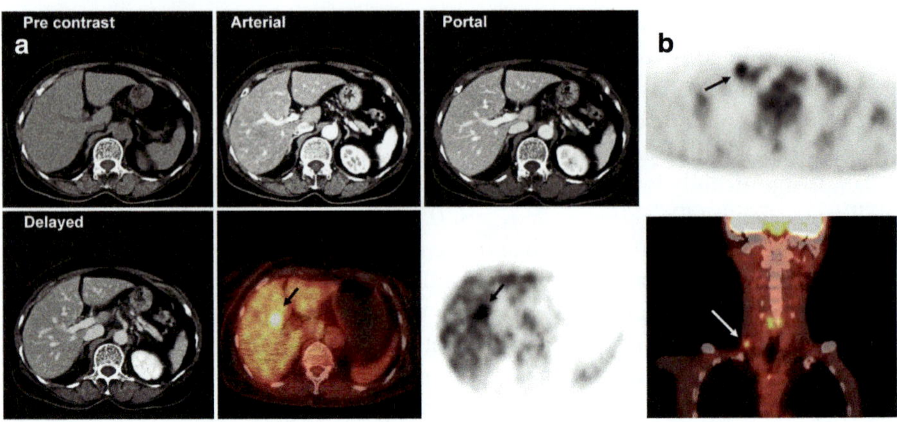

Fig. 4.1 (**a**) Computed tomography (CT) and positron emission tomography (PET) images of a 74-year-old woman diagnosed with locally advanced pancreatic cancer on conventional imaging. No definite mass is seen in the liver on CT images. PET scan reveals a focus of fluorodeoxyglucose (FDG) uptake to S4 of the liver, suggestive of metastasis (*arrow*). (**b**) PET images of a 73-year-old man. PET scan shows a focus of increased FDG uptake in the right supraclavicular fossa (*arrow*). A pathological examination of each specimen revealed metastatic adenocarcinoma from the pancreas

facilitated the detection of 33% of unsuspected distant metastasis (DM) in locally advanced pancreatic cancer (LAPC) patients before CRT [22]. This means that those patients with occult metastatic form could be spared from the unnecessary and potentially harmful treatment. Therefore, the patient selection process is the most critical step in the application of radiotherapy (RT) in LAPC patients. Thus, proper patient selection for CRT is required in order to exclude patients in whom it can be anticipated that uncontrollable widespread DM will develop (Fig. 4.1). The development of early widespread DMs in locally advanced pancreatic cancer is conventionally thought to be due to treatment failure, which allows for the escape of coexisting tumor cells with more aggressive behavior. However, it might also be largely due to detection errors in discovering occult DM concealed by conventional imaging tools (MRI, CT).

Delbeke et al. reported that PET is more accurate than CT for detecting primary pancreatic cancers and for identifying hepatic and distant metastases [23]. They described PET-detected occult DMs in 14% of all patients and changed the clinical decision in 43% (28 of 65) of patients. These metastatic patients demonstrated a significantly worse overall survival (OS) than patients without metastatic disease (median OS, 9.1 vs. 14.6 months, $p < 0.001$). In recent studies, the addition of PET-CT changed the planned surgical treatment in 10–16% of cases as a result of detecting occult metastatic disease [24, 25]. The proportion of change in management was significantly higher in patients who were considered to have borderline resectable compared with resectable disease (17% vs. 7%, $p = 0.019$). Topkan et al. restaged with PET-CT before CRT in 71 patients with unresectable LAPC, and 19 patients (26.8%) were found to have DMs that were not identified initially on conventional imaging [26]. The treatment intent for these patients was changed from curative to palliative. Chang et al. [22] reported that integrating PET with conventional imaging tools facilitated the detection of 33% of unsuspected DMs in LAPC patients and allowed them to receive systemic chemotherapy (Fig. 4.1).

4.3   Determining Prognosis According to PET-CT Parameters and Assessment of Metabolic Response by Neoadjuvant Treatment

Before beginning neoadjuvant therapy such as chemotherapy and radiation therapy, accurate tumor staging is required. Conventional staging of patients scheduled to receive neoadjuvant therapy is based on CT or MRI. PET improves staging because of its high sensitivity and specificity in identifying tumor extent and metastasis. Recent data has suggested that PET-CT might be able to predict treatment response to CRT in patients with pancreatic cancer. Bang et al. reported that PET-detected treatment response, whereas CT could not detect any treatment response due to fibrotic changes after CRT [27]. In addition, the authors suggested that CT was not an accurate method for evaluating tumor response because CT cannot assess the viability of tumor cells directly. Treatment of aim, radiotherapy dose, and volume seem to be affected in many patients, according to emerging data incorporating PET into the RT-planning process. Conventional RT planning based only on CT or MRI findings is likely to miss regions of macroscopic tumors in some patients, resulting in a treatment volume that is too small, and leads to the irradiation of unnecessarily large treatment volumes in other patients. In addition, anatomic imaging is inadequate in patients with uncertain tumor boundaries. Delineating target volume in this setting is fraught with a large degree of interobserver variability. PET appears to be very useful as a molecular imaging method in these situations. Conversely, PET cannot be used alone for treatment planning, due to the very limited anatomic information available on PET scans. Thus, combining PET-CT in the RT-planning process, performing scanning in the RT position, may be very beneficial. Previously, PET and CT images were made on two independent scanners and required software co-registration of images. While most studies using combined PET and CT images have been of RT for lung cancer, the efficacy of this method for other tumors, such as head and neck, gynecologic, and anorectal cancers, has recently been demonstrated. PET-CT imaging can now be performed on combined in-line PET-CT scanners providing hardware co-registered data. This method facilitates the integration of PET imaging data into the treatment-planning process. The available data has suggested that the addition of PET improves target delineation, thereby leading to a reduction in interobserver variability and missed tumors within the RT field, whereas organ-at-risk (OAR) volumes are smallest on MRI. To compare differences in target volume delineation and RT dose distribution between PET-CT and CECT, Li et al. evaluated the sparing of OARs in the treatment plan of locally advanced pancreatic cancer [19]. Mean non-CE GTV_{CT}, GTV_{PET}, and GTV_{PET-CT} were 76.9 ± 47.8, 47.0 ± 40.2, and 44.5 ± 34.7 cm^3 (mean $\pm$ standard deviation), respectively. Non-CE GTV_{PET-CT} was significantly smaller than non-CE GTV_{CT} ($p < 0.001$), and CE GTV_{PET-CT} was significantly smaller than CE GTV_{CT} ($p = 0.033$). In OARs, there were significant differences between non-CE CT and non-CE PET-CT in the intestine D_{max} ($p = 0.023$) and right kidney D_{mean} ($p = 0.029$). Like other studies, this study suggested that co-registration of ^{18}F-FDG PET with CECT might improve the accuracy of GTV delineation in LAPC and might reduce the adverse effects of irradiation. Parlak et al. [28] grouped cases into GTV less (GTVL) versus greater (GTVG) than cutoff value determined by receiver operating characteristic analysis, and they compared OS, locoregional relapse-free survival (LRRFS), and progression-free survival (PFS). In their study, patients in the GTVL group had significantly better OS, LRRFS, and PFS than the GTVG group. Parlak et al. used three-dimensional tumor volume to define the tumor, based on studies suggesting that one-dimensional tumor measurements might not be as representative of real tumor volume measurement, especially in variable tumor shapes. Titola et al. [29] proposed that one-dimensional volume estimation of irregularly shaped tumor-like phantoms should be replaced by computer-based tumor volume measurement. The favorable OS, LRPFS, and PFS observed in the GTVL patients compared with the GTVG patients suggests a potential for PET-CT-defined GTV size in predicting outcomes of LAPC patients treated with definitive CRT, which needs to be validated by further studies with prospective cohorts. The current studies have demonstrated the use of PET as a predictive imaging tool in managing pancreatic cancer patients with CRT. Some of the prognostic factors they evaluated included performance status, GTV, SUV, and pre-CRT CA19-9 levels. Bjerregaard et al. suggested that good performance status with small tumors was also indicative of a favorable prognosis [30].

4.3.1   The Clinical Implications of SUV Values

Evidence of the association between SUV_{max} and survival can be found in other various ways, and Table 4.1 shows that the cutoff values of SUV_{max} for predicting survival are variable (3.4–7.0). It is suggested that SUV_{max} indicates the activity and grade of cancer. Ahn et al. evaluated histopathological differentiation grades and

Table 4.1 Prognostic value of PET parameters of pancreatic cancer according to time of scanning

Scanning time	SUV_{max}	MTV	TLG	GTV	% change
Before treatment	3.4–7.0 [34, 35, 40, 46–49]	3.0–57.45 [31–34]	10–70.9 [32–34]	100 [28]	
At recurrence	3.0–3.3 [35, 36]				
After neoadjuvant CRT					50–63.7% change in SUV_{max} [22, 37, 38]

Abbreviations: *SUVmax* maximum standardized uptake value, *MTV* metabolic tumor volume, *TLG* total lesion glycolysis, *GTV* gross tumor volume, *CRT* chemoradiotherapy

SUVs in pancreatic cancer and found that there was a significant correlation between SUV and pathological grade ($p < 0.01$) [39]. There was also a significant correlation between SUV and survival ($p < 0.01$), with better prognosis in the lower SUV group. Topkan et al. [37] stratified patients into two groups according to median difference between pre- and post-treatment SUV_{max} as a value of response for comparison, and they suggested that the difference in SUV_{max} values was the predictive value for OS, PFS, and LRPFS. Schellenberg et al. [31] grouped patients into high-SUV_{max} versus low-SUV_{max} subgroups by placing them above or below the median SUV_{max}. Their results showed that median survival was 9.8 vs. 15.3 months for the high- and low-SUV_{max} subgroups ($p < 0.01$). On multivariate analysis, clinical SUV_{max} was an independent predictor for OS ($p = 0.03$) and PFS ($p = 0.03$). Thus, there is consensus that poorer survival is associated with high-SUV_{max} values [40]. On the other hand, Asagi et al. [9] suggested that categorizing benign and malignant pancreatic tumors based on the SUV_{max} is difficult, as SUV_{max} sometimes overlapped in these situation. In addition, they reported that the values for different stages were not significantly different, except that the SUV_{max} of invasive pancreatic ductal cancer tended to be higher than those of other pancreatic tumor diseases, excluding benign pancreatic endocrine tumors. Overall, there is still no consensus or standard on defining the threshold for PET-based tumor volume delineation. In predicting pancreatic cancer recurrence, a SUV_{max} of 3.0 was the cutoff value for predicting tumor recurrence. To determine the effect of blood glucose level correction on SUV, Lee et al. stated that blood glucose level-corrected SUV (SUV_{gluc}) was calculated as $SUV_{max} \times$ blood glucose level/100, and they suggested that a SUV_{gluc} of 4.8 was the cutoff value for predicting tumor recurrence [35].

4.3.2   SUV Value After Neoadjuvant Therapy

There have been several studies regarding the analysis of SUV after neoadjuvant therapy [22, 27, 38]. Treatment response after chemotherapy or RT in pancreatic cancer is usually assessed within 4–12 weeks after treatment (Fig. 4.2). The correlation between metabolic regression (% change in SUV_{max}) and pathological response was demonstrated by evaluating a pathological specimen after surgery; a high regression index (≥ 0.46) was shown, with 71% in the pathological response group versus 26% in the pathological nonresponse group ($p = 0.01$) [41]. In addition, initial metabolic response was shown to be proportional to size change during subsequent follow-up [42]. In LAPC patients, median SUV_{max} significantly decreased after 6 weeks of CRT (pre-CRT median $SUV_{max} = 8$, range 0–15.6; post-CRT median $SUV_{max} = 3.6$, range 0–7.9; $p = 0.009$) [43]. In Fig. 4.3, Chang et al. showed mean SUV_{max} values for primary tumors, and the baseline SUV (3.5) and decline in SUV (60%) were significant factors in predicting 1-year OS (sensitivity, 82.9% and 92.3%; specificity, 42.1% and 22.6%, respectively). The decline in SUV from before to after CRT was a median of 37% (range, -100–93%) [22]. However, there were no significant differences ($p = 0.853$) in mean SUV_{max} among the response groups, and there were no significant differences in response after the initial 1–2 cycles of chemotherapy according to SUV_{max} ($p = 0.807$) [44].

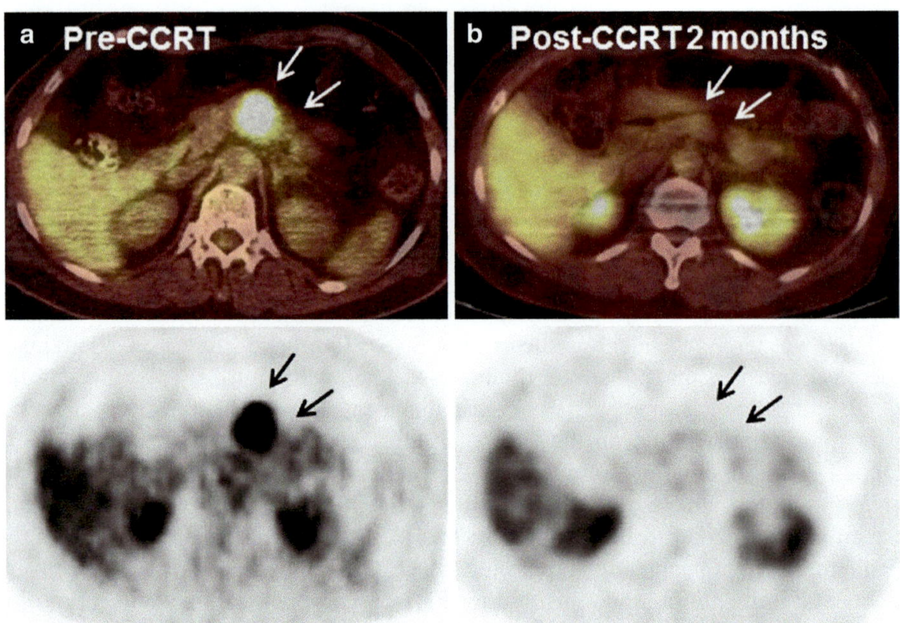

Fig. 4.2 (**a**) Initial PET image of 64-year-old woman diagnosed with locally advanced pancreatic body cancer (cT3N0M0, with splenic artery, splenic vein, and dorsal pancreatic artery invasion). PET scan shows an about 2.7 cm size mass with intense FDG uptake (mean maximum standard uptake values, SUV_{max} = 17.34) in the pancreas body, suggestive of malignancy (*arrow*). (**b**) PET image of the same patient 2 months after gemcitabine-based concurrent chemoradiotherapy (CCRT). Post-CCRT PET scan reveals further decrease in size of primary pancreatic cancer with significantly decreased FDG uptake (SUV_{max} = 1.01), suggestive of favorable treatment response (*arrow*). This patient was judged as having resectable tumor 2 months after initial treatments, and distal pancreatectomy was successfully done. Resected specimen consisted of only fibrosis and ductal dilatation with no residual carcinoma

4.3.3   Volumetric and Other Parameters (GTV, MTV, TLG)

Volumetric parameters such as GTV, metabolic tumor volume (MTV), and total lesion glycolysis (TLG) were also studied for prediction of survival [32]. Metabolic tumor volume is defined as the volume of tumor that shows increased FDG uptake over a set threshold, and TLG is representative of metabolic activity throughout the entire cancer lesion. Schellenberg et al. reported that MTV was prognostic of overall survival in LAPC patients undergoing CRT [31]. Choi et al. [33] used a fixed SUV threshold of 2.5 and demonstrated that MTV and TLG had prognostic significances. The authors considered this threshold to be an optimal point for differentiating benign lesions from malignant lesions and for minimizing the inclusion of unwanted physiological FDG uptake in normal tissues. There was a linear

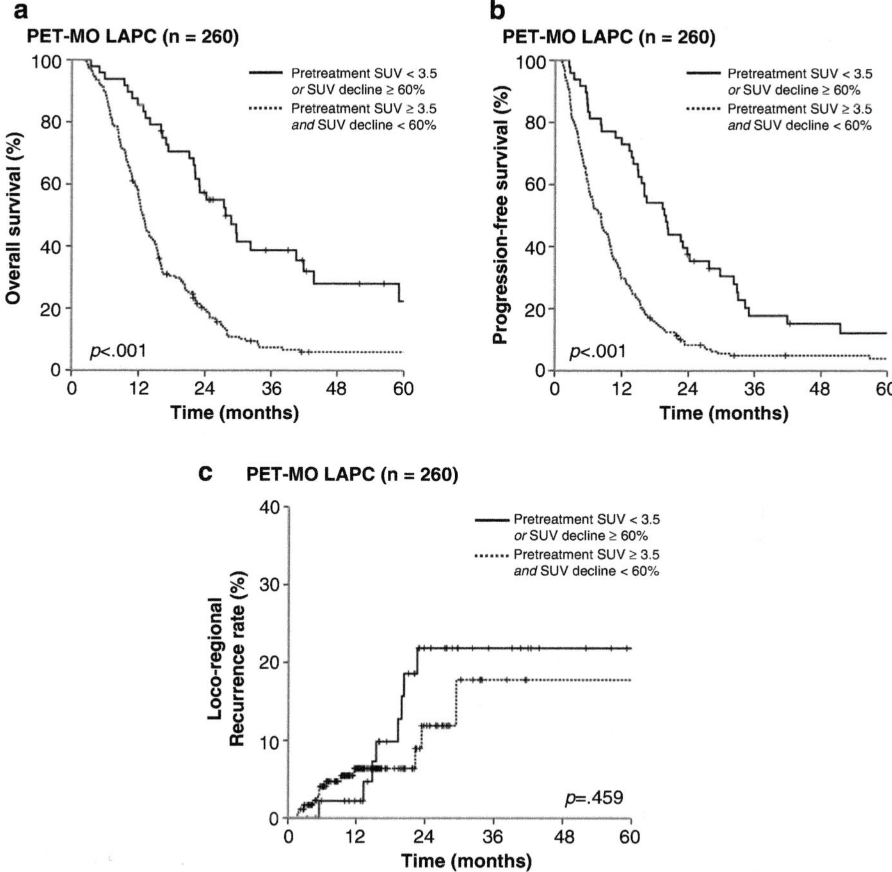

Fig. 4.3 (**a**) Overall survival for 388 patients with no metastasis as shown by CT (CT-M0) locally advanced pancreatic cancer according to the presence of unsuspected metastasis by PET. (**b**) Actuarial probability of locoregional recurrence rate of 260 patients with no metastasis as shown by positron emission tomography (PET-M0) patients treated with upfront chemoradiation therapy. (**c**) Overall and progression-free survival of 260 PET-M0 patients treated with upfront chemoradiation therapy (reprinted with permission from Elsevier. Adapted from: Chang et al., Clinical usefulness of (18)F-fluorodeoxyglucose-positron emission tomography in patients with locally advanced pancreatic cancer planned to undergo concurrent chemoradiation therapy. *Int J Radiat Oncol Biol Phys* 2014, 90:126–133)

correlation between MTV and TLG and tumor markers such as CA19-9 and CA125 [45]. Chirindel et al. reported that SUV_{max}, peak SUV, and TLG of pancreatic cancer are associated with PFS, and that TLG is associated with OS in patients with pancreatic cancer [46]. Before stereotactic body radiotherapy, high MTV and TLG values were associated with poorer OS and higher recurrence rates, suggesting that hypoxia within tumors might contribute to this phenotype [32, 34]. However, there is a wide spectrum of MTV and TLG thresholds in these studies.

4.4 Current Research Gaps and Possible Future Work

PET-CT evaluation at initial staging and follow-up after definitive treatment such as neoadjuvant therapy is very useful. When combined with abdominal CT and CA19-9, a PET-CT evaluation prior to curative resection might be more accurate in predicting survival and detecting occult DMs before neoadjuvant therapy and tumor recurrences, including distant recurrence involving areas not covered by abdominal CT. These findings suggest that PET-CT should be the preferred method for patients at initial staging and follow-up status. The correlation between PET imaging and tumor response after neoadjuvant treatment has been published in several tumor types [47–49]. However, there is little information about the role of PET-CT after neoadjuvant therapy in pancreatic cancer. The limited number of studies, small number of patients who underwent follow-up PET imaging, and the various time intervals from completion of neoadjuvant therapy could limit the significance of clinical outcomes. Thus, future clinical research attempts should determine an optimal time point of PET-CT after neoadjuvant therapy based on larger number of patients, and the value of follow-up PET parameters could be measured to increase the clinical applicability as decision-making tools for further treatment. Therefore, personalized treatment approach is expected to promote better clinical outcomes by wide utilization of PET-CT, reduce the number of unnecessary treatment and related complications after neoadjuvant therapy.

As discussed above, a number of studies have investigated how to utilize PET-CT for the prognosis and neoadjuvant therapy of pancreatic cancer [5, 22, 33, 35, 40]. Meanwhile, some of the challenges are being faced. One of them is that there is no consensus or standardization on defining the threshold for metabolic tumor volume delineation and the value of SUV_{max}. Moreover, the analysis of GTV size and delineation of target volume using PET-CT for radiotherapy planning is also challenging to improve clinical outcomes. Lastly, the lack of a comparator group of patients who have not undergone follow-up PET after neoadjuvant therapy results in limited information with which to evaluate the benefits of incorporating PET in RT planning. Nevertheless, the future of PET-CT is bright. Li et al. [19] stated that although it is challenging to implement, individually adapted treatment planning for radiation therapy of LAPC based on PET-CT is practical and highly promising.

In the near future, the development of PET imaging techniques and other PET-based parameters besides SUV, and new radioisotopes should be investigated in order to increase the diagnostic and predictive accuracy of PET after neoadjuvant therapy.

References

1. Siegel RL, Miller KD, Jemal A. Cancer statistics, 2016. CA Cancer J Clin. 2016;66:7–30.
2. Faria SC, Tamm EP, Loyer EM, Szklaruk J, Choi H, Charnsangavej C. Diagnosis and staging of pancreatic tumors. Semin Roentgenol. 2004;39:397–411.
3. Moertel CG, Frytak S, Hahn RG, O'Connell MJ, Reitemeier RJ, Rubin J, Schutt AJ, Weiland LH, Childs DS, Holbrook MA, Lavin PT, Livstone E, Spiro H, Knowlton A, Kalser M, Barkin J,

Lessner H, Mann-Kaplan R, Ramming K, Douglas Jr HO, Thomas P, Nave H, Bateman J, Lokich J, Brooks J, Chaffey J, Corson JM, Zamcheck N, Novak JW. Therapy of locally unresectable pancreatic carcinoma: a randomized comparison of high dose (6000 rads) radiation alone, moderate dose radiation (4000 rads + 5-fluorouracil), and high dose radiation + 5-fluorouracil: the Gastrointestinal Tumor Study Group. Cancer. 1981;48:1705–10.

4. Nunna P, Sheikhbahaei S, Ahn S, Young B, Subramaniam RM. The role of positron emission tomography/computed tomography in management and prediction of survival in pancreatic cancer. J Comput Assist Tomogr. 2016;40:142–51.

5. Wang XY, Yang F, Jin C, Fu DL. Utility of PET/CT in diagnosis, staging, assessment of resectability and metabolic response of pancreatic cancer. World J Gastroenterol. 2014;20: 15580–9.

6. Tang S, Huang G, Liu J, Liu T, Treven L, Song S, Zhang C, Pan L, Zhang T. Usefulness of 18F-FDG PET, combined FDG-PET/CT and EUS in diagnosing primary pancreatic carcinoma: a meta-analysis. Eur J Radiol. 2011;78:142–50.

7. Wu LM, Hu JN, Hua J, Liu MJ, Chen J, Xu JR. Diagnostic value of diffusion-weighted magnetic resonance imaging compared with fluorodeoxyglucose positron emission tomography/ computed tomography for pancreatic malignancy: a meta-analysis using a hierarchical regression model. J Gastroenterol Hepatol. 2012;27:1027–35.

8. Pakzad F, Groves AM, Ell PJ. The role of positron emission tomography in the management of pancreatic cancer. Semin Nucl Med. 2006;36:248–56.

9. Asagi A, Ohta K, Nasu J, Tanada M, Nadano S, Nishimura R, Teramoto N, Yamamoto K, Inoue T, Iguchi H. Utility of contrast-enhanced FDG-PET/CT in the clinical management of pancreatic cancer: impact on diagnosis, staging, evaluation of treatment response, and detection of recurrence. Pancreas. 2013;42:11–9.

10. Sun Y, Duan Q, Wang S, Zeng Y, Wu R. Diagnosis of pancreatic cancer using (1)(8)F-FDG PET/CT and CA19-9 with SUVmax association to clinical characteristics. J BUON. 2015;20:452–9.

11. Sperti C, Pasquali C, Decet G, Chierichetti F, Liessi G, Pedrazzoli S. F-18-fluorodeoxyglucose positron emission tomography in differentiating malignant from benign pancreatic cysts: a prospective study. J Gastrointest Surg. 2005;9:22–8. Discussion 28–9

12. Sperti C, Bissoli S, Pasquali C, Frison L, Liessi G, Chierichetti F, Pedrazzoli S. 18-fluorodeoxyglucose positron emission tomography enhances computed tomography diagnosis of malignant intraductal papillary mucinous neoplasms of the pancreas. Ann Surg. 2007;246:932–7. Discussion 937–9

13. Yoshioka M, Uchinami H, Watanabe G, Sato T, Shibata S, Kume M, Ishiyama K, Takahashi S, Hashimoto M, Yamamoto Y. F-18 fluorodeoxyglucose positron emission tomography for differential diagnosis of pancreatic tumors. Springerplus. 2015;4:154.

14. Staley CA, Lee JE, Cleary KR, Abbruzzese JL, Fenoglio CJ, Rich TA, Evans DB. Preoperative chemoradiation, pancreaticoduodenectomy, and intraoperative radiation therapy for adenocarcinoma of the pancreatic head. Am J Surg. 1996;171:118–24. Discussion 124–5

15. Kitajima K, Murakami K, Yamasaki E, Kaji Y, Shimoda M, Kubota K, Suganuma N, Sugimura K. Performance of integrated FDG-PET/contrast-enhanced CT in the diagnosis of recurrent pancreatic cancer: comparison with integrated FDG-PET/non-contrast-enhanced CT and enhanced CT. Mol Imaging Biol. 2010;12:452–9.

16. Sperti C, Pasquali C, Bissoli S, Chierichetti F, Liessi G, Pedrazzoli S. Tumor relapse after pancreatic cancer resection is detected earlier by 18-FDG PET than by CT. J Gastrointest Surg. 2010;14:131–40.

17. Ruf J, Lopez Hanninen E, Oettle H, Plotkin M, Pelzer U, Stroszczynski C, Felix R, Amthauer H. Detection of recurrent pancreatic cancer: comparison of FDG-PET with CT/MRI. Pancreatology. 2005;5:266–72.

18. Hamidian Jahromi A, Sangster G, Zibari G, Martin B, Chu Q, Takalkar A, Shi R, Shokouh-Amiri H. Accuracy of multi-detector computed tomography, fluorodeoxyglucose positron emission tomography-CT, and CA 19-9 levels in detecting recurrent pancreatic adenocarcinoma. JOP. 2013;14:466–8.

19. Li XX, Liu NB, Zhu L, Yuan XK, Yang CW, Ren P, Gong LL, Zhao LJ, Xu WG, Wang P. Consequences of additional use of contrast-enhanced (18)F-FDG PET/CT in target volume delineation and dose distribution for pancreatic cancer. Br J Radiol. 2015;88:20140590.
20. Willett CG, Czito BG, Bendell JC, Ryan DP. Locally advanced pancreatic cancer. J Clin Oncol. 2005;23:4538–44.
21. Evans DB, Rich TA, Byrd DR, Cleary KR, Connelly JH, Levin B, Charnsangavej C, Fenoglio CJ, Ames FC. Preoperative chemoradiation and pancreaticoduodenectomy for adenocarcinoma of the pancreas. Arch Surg. 1992;127:1335–9.
22. Chang JS, Choi SH, Lee Y, Kim KH, Park JY, Song SY, Cho A, Yun M, Lee JD, Seong J. Clinical usefulness of (1)(8)F-fluorodeoxyglucose-positron emission tomography in patients with locally advanced pancreatic cancer planned to undergo concurrent chemoradiation therapy. Int J Radiat Oncol Biol Phys. 2014;90:126–33.
23. Delbeke D, Rose DM, Chapman WC, Pinson CW, Wright JK, Beauchamp RD, Shyr Y, Leach SD. Optimal interpretation of FDG PET in the diagnosis, staging and management of pancreatic carcinoma. J Nucl Med. 1999;40:1784–91.
24. Burge ME, O'Rourke N, Cavallucci D, Bryant R, Francesconi A, Houston K, Wyld D, Eastgate M, Finch R, Hopkins G, Thomas P, Macfarlane D. A prospective study of the impact of fluorodeoxyglucose positron emission tomography with concurrent non-contrast CT scanning on the management of operable pancreatic and peri-ampullary cancers. HPB (Oxford). 2015;17: 624–31.
25. Kim R, Prithviraj G, Kothari N, Springett G, Malafa M, Hodul P, Kim J, Yue B, Morse B, Mahipal A. PET/CT fusion scan prevents futile laparotomy in early stage pancreatic cancer. Clin Nucl Med. 2015;40:e501–5.
26. Topkan E, Parlak C, Yapar AF. FDG-PET/CT-based restaging may alter initial management decisions and clinical outcomes in patients with locally advanced pancreatic carcinoma planned to undergo chemoradiotherapy. Cancer Imaging. 2013;13:423–8.
27. Bang S, Chung HW, Park SW, Chung JB, Yun M, Lee JD, Song SY. The clinical usefulness of 18-fluorodeoxyglucose positron emission tomography in the differential diagnosis, staging, and response evaluation after concurrent chemoradiotherapy for pancreatic cancer. J Clin Gastroenterol. 2006;40:923–9.
28. Parlak C, Topkan E, Onal C, Reyhan M, Selek U. Prognostic value of gross tumor volume delineated by FDG-PET-CT based radiotherapy treatment planning in patients with locally advanced pancreatic cancer treated with chemoradiotherapy. Radiat Oncol. 2012;7:37.
29. Tiitola M, Kivisaari L, Tervahartiala P, Palomaki M, Kivisaari RP, Mankinen P, Vehmas T. Estimation or quantification of tumour volume? CT study on irregular phantoms. Acta Radiol. 2001;42:101–5.
30. Bjerregaard JK, Mortensen MB, Jensen HA, Nielsen M, Pfeiffer P. Prognostic factors for survival and resection in patients with initial nonresectable locally advanced pancreatic cancer treated with chemoradiotherapy. Int J Radiat Oncol Biol Phys. 2012;83:909–15.
31. Schellenberg D, Quon A, Minn AY, Graves EE, Kunz P, Ford JM, Fisher GA, Goodman KA, Koong AC, Chang DT. [18]Fluorodeoxyglucose PET is prognostic of progression-free and overall survival in locally advanced pancreas cancer treated with stereotactic radiotherapy. Int J Radiat Oncol Biol Phys. 2010;77:1420–5.
32. Lee JW, Kang CM, Choi HJ, Lee WJ, Song SY, Lee JH, Lee JD. Prognostic value of metabolic tumor volume and Total lesion glycolysis on preoperative (1)(8)F-FDG PET/CT in patients with pancreatic cancer. J Nucl Med. 2014;55:898–904.
33. Choi HJ, Lee JW, Kang B, Song SY, Lee JD, Lee JH. Prognostic significance of volume-based FDG PET/CT parameters in patients with locally advanced pancreatic cancer treated with chemoradiation therapy. Yonsei Med J. 2014;55:1498–506.
34. Dholakia AS, Chaudhry M, Leal JP, Chang DT, Raman SP, Hacker-Prietz A, Su Z, Pai J, Oteiza KE, Griffith ME, Wahl RL, Tryggestad E, Pawlik T, Laheru DA, Wolfgang CL, Koong AC, Herman JM. Baseline metabolic tumor volume and total lesion glycolysis are associated with survival outcomes in patients with locally advanced pancreatic cancer receiving stereotactic body radiation therapy. Int J Radiat Oncol Biol Phys. 2014;89:539–46.

35. Lee SM, Kim TS, Lee JW, Kim SK, Park SJ, Han SS. Improved prognostic value of standardized uptake value corrected for blood glucose level in pancreatic cancer using F-18 FDG PET. Clin Nucl Med. 2011;36:331–6.
36. Jung W, Jang JY, Kang MJ, Chang YR, Shin YC, Chang J, Kim SW. The clinical usefulness of 18F-fluorodeoxyglucose positron emission tomography-computed tomography (PET-CT) in follow-up of curatively resected pancreatic cancer patients. HPB (Oxford). 2016;18:57–64.
37. Topkan E, Parlak C, Kotek A, Yapar AF, Pehlivan B. Predictive value of metabolic 18FDG-PET response on outcomes in patients with locally advanced pancreatic carcinoma treated with definitive concurrent chemoradiotherapy. BMC Gastroenterol. 2011;11:123.
38. Choi M, Heilbrun LK, Venkatramanamoorthy R, Lawhorn-Crews JM, Zalupski MM, Shields AF. Using 18F-fluorodeoxyglucose positron emission tomography to monitor clinical outcomes in patients treated with neoadjuvant chemo-radiotherapy for locally advanced pancreatic cancer. Am J Clin Oncol. 2010;33:257–61.
39. Ahn SJ, Park MS, Lee JD, Kang WJ. Correlation between 18F-fluorodeoxyglucose positron emission tomography and pathologic differentiation in pancreatic cancer. Ann Nucl Med. 2014;28:430–5.
40. Hwang JP, Lim I, Chang KJ, Kim BI, Choi CW, Lim SM. Prognostic value of SUVmax measured by fluorine-18 fluorodeoxyglucose positron emission tomography with computed tomography in patients with pancreatic cancer. Nucl Med Mol Imaging. 2012;46:207–14.
41. Kittaka H, Takahashi H, Ohigashi H, Gotoh K, Yamada T, Tomita Y, Hasegawa Y, Yano M, Ishikawa O. Role of (18)F-fluorodeoxyglucose positron emission tomography/computed tomography in predicting the pathologic response to preoperative chemoradiation therapy in patients with resectable T3 pancreatic cancer. World J Surg. 2013;37:169–78.
42. Yoshioka M, Sato T, Furuya T, Shibata S, Andoh H, Asanuma Y, Hatazawa J, Shimosegawa E, Koyama K, Yamamoto Y. Role of positron emission tomography with 2-deoxy-2-[18F]fluoro-D-glucose in evaluating the effects of arterial infusion chemotherapy and radiotherapy on pancreatic cancer. J Gastroenterol. 2004;39:50–5.
43. Wilson JM, Mukherjee S, Chu KY, Brunner TB, Partridge M, Hawkins M. Challenges in using (1)(8)F-fluorodeoxyglucose-PET-CT to define a biological radiotherapy boost volume in locally advanced pancreatic cancer. Radiat Oncol. 2014;9:146.
44. Moon SY, Joo KR, So YR, Lim JU, Cha JM, Shin HP, Yang YJ. Predictive value of maximum standardized uptake value (SUVmax) on 18F-FDG PET/CT in patients with locally advanced or metastatic pancreatic cancer. Clin Nucl Med. 2013;38:778–83.
45. Shi S, Ji S, Qin Y, Xu J, Zhang B, Xu W, Liu J, Long J, Liu C, Liu L, Ni Q, Yu X. Metabolic tumor burden is associated with major oncogenomic alterations and serum tumor markers in patients with resected pancreatic cancer. Cancer Lett. 2015;360:227–33.
46. Chirindel A, Alluri KC, Chaudhry MA, Wahl RL, Pawlik TM, Herman JM, Subramaniam RM. Prognostic value of FDG PET/CT-derived parameters in pancreatic adenocarcinoma at initial PET/CT staging. AJR Am J Roentgenol. 2015;204:1093–9.
47. Wieder HA, Brucher BL, Zimmermann F, Becker K, Lordick F, Beer A, Schwaiger M, Fink U, Siewert JR, Stein HJ, Weber WA. Time course of tumor metabolic activity during chemoradiotherapy of esophageal squamous cell carcinoma and response to treatment. J Clin Oncol. 2004;22:900–8.
48. Bokemeyer C, Kollmannsberger C, Oechsle K, Dohmen BM, Pfannenberg A, Claussen CD, Bares R, Kanz L. Early prediction of treatment response to high-dose salvage chemotherapy in patients with relapsed germ cell cancer using [(18)F]FDG PET. Br J Cancer. 2002;86:506–11.
49. Joye I, Deroose CM, Vandecaveye V, Haustermans K. The role of diffusion-weighted MRI and (18)F-FDG PET/CT in the prediction of pathologic complete response after radiochemotherapy for rectal cancer: a systematic review. Radiother Oncol. 2014;113:158–65.
50. Okamoto K, Koyama I, Miyazawa M, Toshimitsu Y, Aikawa M, Okada K, Imabayashi E, Matsuda H. Preoperative 18[F]-fluorodeoxyglucose positron emission tomography/computed tomography predicts early recurrence after pancreatic cancer resection. Int J Clin Oncol. 2011;16:39–44.

51. Maemura K, Takao S, Shinchi H, Noma H, Mataki Y, Kurahara H, Jinnouchi S, Aikou T. Role of positron emission tomography in decisions on treatment strategies for pancreatic cancer. J Hepato-Biliary-Pancreat Surg. 2006;13:435–41.
52. Yamamoto T, Sugiura T, Mizuno T, Okamura Y, Aramaki T, Endo M, Uesaka K. Preoperative FDG-PET predicts early recurrence and a poor prognosis after resection of pancreatic adenocarcinoma. Ann Surg Oncol. 2015;22:677–84.
53. Kitasato Y, Yasunaga M, Okuda K, Kinoshita H, Tanaka H, Okabe Y, Kawahara A, Kage M, Kaida H, Ishibashi M. Maximum standardized uptake value on 18F-fluoro-2-deoxy-glucose positron emission tomography/computed tomography and glucose transporter-1 expression correlates with survival in invasive ductal carcinoma of the pancreas. Pancreas. 2014;43:1060–5.

Liquid Biopsy for Early Detection of Pancreatic Cancer

5

Erina Takai and Shinichi Yachida

5.1   Implications of Early Diagnosis in Pancreatic Cancer

Pancreatic ductal adenocarcinoma (PDAC) is the most common type of pancreatic cancer. It is a devastating disease with a 5-year survival rate of only approximately 4–7%, and this figure has not been improved in recent decades. Although surgical resection is the only curative treatment for PDAC, only 15–20% of patients present with resectable disease and the majority of patients are diagnosed with locally advanced or metastatic cancer, which is not eligible for surgical resection. This situation is mainly a consequence of the aggressive nature of this disease and the lack of an efficient method for detection of early-stage pancreatic cancer. Furthermore, since some patients who receive potentially curative resection suffer from recurrent cancer, effective methods for early detection of relapse are also needed.

The molecular genetics landscape of PDAC has been studied by whole-genome or exome sequencing and somatic alterations associated with this disease have been identified. Four genes, *KRAS*, *CDKN2A*, *TP53*, and *SMAD4*, are commonly mutated or modified epigenetically in PDAC, and dozens of candidate driver genes are altered at low frequency (<5%). Clonal evolution of pancreatic cancer has also been investigated. Although PDAC is a highly aggressive disease, mathematical modeling of the rate of mutation acquisition suggests that there is 11.7-year period from acquisition of the initiating mutation to full transformation in a pancreatic cell, and another 6.8 years are needed to develop the first metastatic subclone [1]. This model implies that there is a substantial time window for early detection of PDAC.

Currently, the detection and diagnosis of pancreatic cancer largely rely on imaging modalities, including ultrasonography, computed tomography (CT), magnetic resonance imaging (MRI), and endoscopic ultrasonography (EUS). However,

E. Takai (✉) • S. Yachida
Division of Cancer Genomics, National Cancer Center Research Institute,
5-1-1 Tsukiji, Chuo-ku, Tokyo 104-0045, Japan
e-mail: ertakai@ncc.go.jp

© Springer Science+Business Media Singapore 2017
H. Yamaue (ed.), *Innovation of Diagnosis and Treatment for Pancreatic Cancer*,
DOI 10.1007/978-981-10-2486-3_5

early-stage pancreatic cancers are difficult to detect even if combinations of these modalities are employed. In addition, these modalities require expensive equipment and specialist technicians. Therefore, imaging technologies are not likely to be suitable for routine pancreatic cancer screening, at least at present. Diagnosis of early-stage pancreatic cancer by means of imaging technologies is discussed in detail elsewhere in this book.

On the other hand, some blood-based tumor biomarkers, such as carcinoembryonic antigen (CEA) and carbohydrate antigen (CA) 19-9, are used for detection of pancreatic cancer. But, although blood-based testing is simple and minimally invasive, these currently used tumor biomarkers are not sufficiently sensitive or specific for early detection of pancreatic cancer. Despite recent progress in understanding of the disease at the molecular level, no reliable blood-based biomarker for screening of pancreatic cancer is yet clinically available.

5.2   Liquid Biopsy in Cancer

5.2.1   Cell-Free DNA

Cell-free DNA (cfDNA) consists of small double-stranded DNA fragments found in blood. In 1948, Mandel and Metais firstly reported the presence of cfDNA in the circulation [2]. Tumor-derived cfDNA, now commonly known as circulating tumor DNA (ctDNA), was described in 1989 [3]. The clinical utility of cfDNA in plasma and serum has been an active area of research in a variety of clinical settings. Indeed, evaluation of fetal cfDNA in the circulation of pregnant women is becoming a routine diagnostic test for high-risk patients in clinics. In oncology, ctDNA is expected to provide a less-invasive approach for cancer diagnosis, monitoring of chemotherapy-resistant mutations, and overcoming the problem of tumor heterogeneity [1, 4, 5] (Fig. 5.1). The concept of detecting tumor-specific molecular alterations by analysis of bodily fluids, including peripheral blood, of cancer patients is termed "liquid biopsy." To date, cfDNA has been the main target of liquid biopsy for cancer detection, together with exosomes, microRNA (miRNA), and circulating tumor cells (CTCs).

5.2.2   Origin of cfDNA

It has been suggested that cancer patients have higher levels of cfDNA than healthy individuals [6]. Levels of cfDNA are also increased in a variety of other physiological and pathological conditions, including exercise, inflammation, smoking, sepsis, and trauma [7]. cfDNA is shed into the bloodstream via apoptosis, necrosis, direct release from viable cells, and lysis of circulating cells, but the major sources are now thought to be apoptotic and necrotic cells. In fact, the length of cfDNA fragments in the circulation often shows a characteristic laddering pattern with multiples of 170–180 base pairs, which is a well-known feature of apoptosis [6].

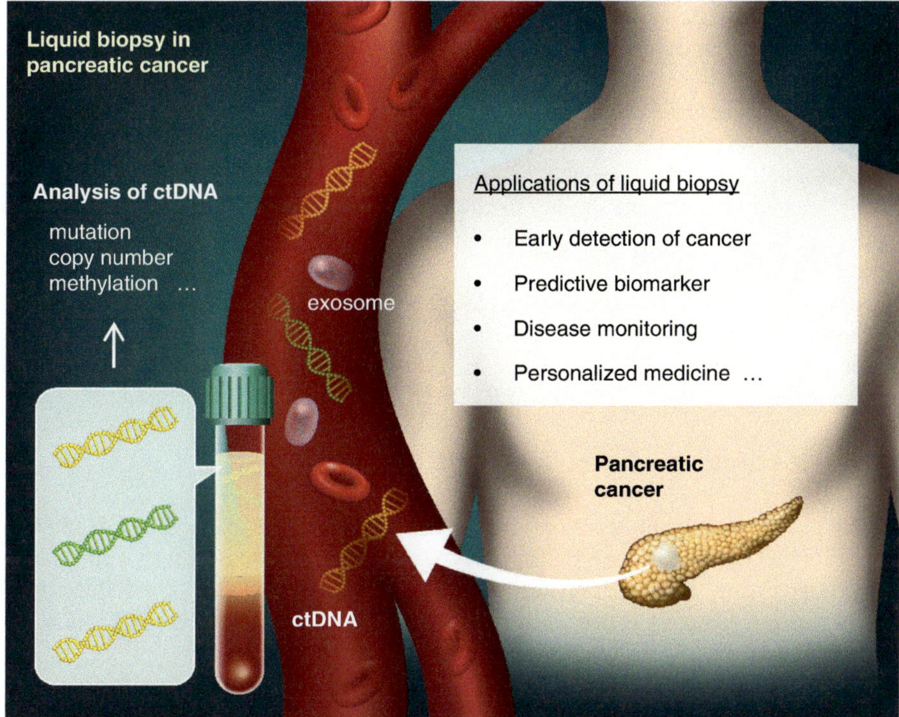

Fig. 5.1 Liquid biopsy in pancreatic cancer. Tumor-specific alterations can be detected in circulating tumor DNA (ctDNA) in blood. Detecting ctDNA in plasma or serum serves as a "liquid biopsy," which would be useful for a variety of clinical applications for pancreatic cancer

Apoptosis is programmed even for many normal cells on a daily basis. It has been suggested that a large fraction of cfDNA is derived from bone marrow and liver in healthy individuals [8]. But, in a tumor mass, hyperproliferation and rapid cellular turnover of cancer cells can lead to increased programmed cell death. Intratumoral microenvironments such as hypoxia may also lead to necrosis. Cellular debris of apoptotic or necrotic cells is normally phagocytozed by infiltrating macrophages and the cellular components are cleared. However, this clearance mechanism does not proceed effectively in a tumor mass, leading to the accumulation of cellular debris, including DNA, and its release into the circulation of patients.

5.2.3 cfDNA as a Biomarker for Cancer

Although cfDNA is generally increased in patients with cancer, its sensitivity and specificity for cancer detection are low, and the utility of total cfDNA level as a cancer biomarker is questionable. On the other hand, tumor DNA can be discriminated from normal cfDNA by detecting tumor-specific somatic mutations that exist only in the genomes of cancer cells or precancerous cells, but not in the genomes of matched normal cells. This assures the specificity of ctDNA as a cancer biomarker.

However, detection of ctDNA has been challenging, since the percentage of ctDNA is very low (<1.0% in many cases) in total cfDNA. Traditional sequencing methods such as Sanger sequencing or pyrosequencing can detect mutations of tumor-derived DNA fragment only in patients with a high tumor burden and a large amount of ctDNA. However, recent advances in sequencing technologies, including digital polymerase chain reaction and next-generation sequencing, have made it possible to detect ctDNA present at relatively low frequencies in blood, and there has recently been an explosive increase of studies to detect ctDNA in blood from patients with cancer and to investigate the clinical utility of ctDNA.

5.2.4 Methods for Detection of ctDNA

Digital polymerase chain reaction (dPCR) is now one of the major methods to sensitively detect genomic alterations in cfDNA. In 2003, a PCR-based digital approach, named BEAMing (Beads, Emulsion, Amplification, and Magnetics), was described [9]. Using emulsion PCR and flow cytometry, BEAMing can efficiently identify rare mutations with allele fractions as low as 0.01%.

Nowadays several dPCR systems, including droplet-based platforms, are commercially available. Generally, the sensitivity of a droplet dPCR system depends on the number of droplets. One of the most widely used droplet dPCR devices, QX200 Droplet Digital PCR System (Bio-Rad Laboratories) generates 20,000 nanoliter-sized droplets. The RainDrop Digital PCR System (RainDance Technologies) can perform "single-molecule" PCR in up to ten million picoliter-sized droplets, and therefore, possesses very high sensitivity. In addition, multiplex assays are possible in the RainDrop system by using combinations of two color probes at different concentrations (up to ten targets) [10].

Next-generation sequencing (NGS) is also widely used to analyze genomic alterations in cfDNA. Unlike dPCR, NGS techniques can analyze multiple, broad regions of interest. Even whole-genome sequencing or whole-exome sequencing of cfDNA from advanced cancer patients has been reported, and various alterations, including single nucleotide variants (SNV), copy number alterations (CNA) and structural alterations of DNA, were detected. However, only genomic alterations with high allele frequencies may be detectable with these platforms, since deep genome-wide analysis, especially whole-genome sequencing, is quite costly and not feasible in the routine clinical context. Therefore, these global genomic analyses can be applied for only cfDNA samples from advanced cancer patients with high tumor burden. On the other hand, targeted sequencing can be performed at relatively low cost. By focusing on clinically important genes, mutations can be detected with higher sensitivity compared to the genome-wide analyses.

Amplicon sequencing is one of the major techniques for analyzing mutations in specific genomic regions. Ion AmpliSeq Technology (Thermo Fisher Scientific) is a widely used targeted sequencing platform. Highly multiplex PCR followed by NGS, such as Ion PGM, allows deep sequencing of target regions from as little as 10 ng input DNA at low cost and with a short turnaround time. However, the Ion Ampliseq system has some issues such as relatively high error rate and false-negatives in detection of small insertions and deletions (indels).

Target enrichment techniques, target capture-based platforms, are widely used for analyzing gene alterations of cancer. In principle, fragmented genomic DNA is hybridized with DNA/RNA probes designed for capturing targeted regions, and the enriched DNA libraries are analyzed by NGS. The SureSelect Target Enrichment System (Agilent Technologies) is widely used for targeted sequencing in combination with the Illumina paired-end sequencing platform, which has quite a low error rate among high-throughput sequencing instruments. Although the manufacturer's protocol for the SureSelect Target Enrichment System requires at least 200 ng of input DNA, the amount of input DNA can be reduced by using particular library preparation kits, such as KAPA Hyper Prep Kit (KAPA Biosystems) [11].

In addition to these commercially available technologies, various highly sensitive sequencing methods have been developed for detecting ctDNA. In an amplicon-based system, Safe-SeqS (Safe-Sequencing System), individual DNA molecules are tagged with a unique identifier, then amplified and sequenced. According to the original paper, the error rate could be lowered to 9×10^{-6} by taking into account the unique identifiers [12]. Forshew et al. reported a method termed Tam-Seq (Tagged-Amplicon deep Sequencing) in 2012. They detected somatic mutations in cfDNA at 2% allele frequencies [13]. In the case of non-small cell lung cancer, another method for profiling ctDNA, CAPP-Seq (Cancer Personalized Profiling by deep Sequencing), has been described [14]. In addition to methods for detecting SNVs, PARE (Personalized Analysis of Rearranged Ends) identifies cancer-specific genome rearrangements, and it has been shown that these alterations can be used as personalized cancer biomarkers [15].

5.3 Liquid Biopsy in Pancreatic Cancer Diagnosis

The clinical utility of ctDNA has been investigated in various types of cancer. For cancer diagnosis, the most commonly mutated genes are probably best suited for analysis as blood-based biomarkers. However, even within a single tumor type, the mutation profile generally varies from patient to patient. Even if a single gene is commonly mutated in a particular cancer type, the altered loci can vary, especially in tumor suppressor genes such as *TP53*. For this reason, among others, it is not easy to utilize tumor-derived DNA in plasma for diagnosis of many cancer types without information about mutations in the tumor tissues.

On the other hand, point mutations of *KRAS* are commonly observed in PDAC and 90% of all *KRAS* mutations occur in codon 12 or 13 in PDAC. A number of studies have, therefore, investigated *KRAS* mutations in cfDNA from PDAC patients, although detection methods are diverse. To date, many studies have confirmed that mutant *KRAS* can be detected in plasma or serum from patients with PDAC.

In the 2000s, several research groups investigated the potential use of *KRAS* mutation in cfDNA as a biomarker of pancreatic cancer. Some of them found that mutant *KRAS* is more frequently detected in blood of PDAC patients than in that of chronic pancreatitis patients [16, 17]. It has also been suggested that sensitivity and specificity for detection of PDAC can be improved by combining detection of *KRAS* mutation in blood with detection of increased CA19-9 level [16, 17]. Furthermore, it has been reported that the presence of mutant *KRAS* in the circulation is associated with poor prognosis of patients with pancreatic cancer [11, 18–21]. Thus, *KRAS* mutant cfDNA could be useful as a predictive biomarker in patients with pancreatic cancer.

One of the major potential applications of ctDNA is disease monitoring. Tjensvoll et al. reported that changes in mutant *KRAS* levels in the circulation were correlated with radiological imaging data and CA19-9 levels during the course of chemotherapy [20]. They suggested that detection of *KRAS* mutation in plasma could be useful for monitoring treatment efficacy and tumor progression in pancreatic cancer patients.

It is noteworthy that various other cancer-related genes are mutated at relatively low frequencies in PDAC. Importantly, it has been indicated that 20% of patients with pancreatic cancer have somatic alterations in genes that are potential targets of therapies approved by the U.S. Food and Drug Administration (FDA) for oncologic indications or therapies in published prospective clinical studies [22]. This suggests that genomic profiling in pancreatic cancer could be useful to design precision treatment strategies. Due to improvements of sequencing technologies, global or highly multiplexed genomic analysis of ctDNA is becoming feasible using NGS. Analyzing ctDNA has also been proposed as an alternative method to tissue biopsy in the setting of precision medicine. Investigating mutations of actionable genes in cancer cells is essential for precision medicine. Although tumor tissue biopsies are generally used for molecular screening of cancer, it may be difficult in some patients to obtain sufficient amounts of tissues with a high tumor fraction. Indeed, obtaining adequate biopsy tissues for molecular diagnosis is often difficult in pancreatic cancer patients. Most importantly, tissue biopsies are invasive and are therefore not without clinical complications. Zill et al. analyzed 54 genes in tumor tissues and cfDNA samples using a commercially available gene panel and demonstrated that a large proportion of mutations detected in tumor biopsies can also be detected by sequencing of cfDNA in pancreatic and biliary cancer [23]. Although 35% of patients had an insufficient quantity or quality of tissue biopsy sample for sequencing analysis in their cohort, sequencing of cfDNA identified somatic mutations in many of these patients. We have also reported targeted deep sequencing analysis of cfDNA using a modified SureSelect-Illumina platform and an original gene panel for pancreatic cancer [11]. Our gene panel consisted of 60 genes, including 17 potentially actionable genes. As prescreening for sequencing analysis, dPCR assay was firstly performed to determine the mutational status of *KRAS* in plasma cfDNA of 259 patients with PDAC. We then carried out targeted deep sequencing in 48 patients including 43 cases that were considered to have ≥1% tumor DNA in total cfDNA based on dPCR *KRAS* assay and 5 cases with obvious distant organ metastasis, even though they were negative for *KRAS* mutation in plasma on dPCR assay. We found somatic mutations in potentially targetable genes in 14 of 48 patients (29.2%). In addition, we analyzed somatic copy number alterations using targeted sequencing data of cfDNA, and potentially targetable gene amplifications, such as *CCND1* and *ERBB2*, were also detected. Thus, previous studies indicate that liquid biopsy has great potential for diagnosis and treatment design in pancreatic cancer in diverse clinical settings.

5.4   Challenges Facing Early Detection of Pancreatic Cancer by Liquid Biopsy

As described above, clinical screening for early detection of PDAC currently has only limited effectiveness, and liquid biopsy appears to be a promising approach to meet this need. In general, however, detection of ctDNA is still challenging in early-stage cancer patients because of the high background levels of normal cfDNA. *KRAS* mutation, which is the most common somatic mutation in PDAC, has been proposed as a biomarker in cfDNA for early detection of PDAC, but in early-stage malignant disease (and also in some metastatic cancers), ctDNA may be an extremely rare population in total cfDNA (0.001% or less). Although many analyses of ctDNA have been reported in various cancer types, the vast majority of those studies were analyses of advanced cancer patients, with metastasis or high tumor burden, and the usefulness of detecting ctDNA in patients with early-stage cancer has been poorly investigated.

A multicenter study of liquid biopsies in 846 patients with 15 cancer types (including PDAC), using digital technologies and ~5 mL plasma, reported a detection rate of ctDNA of 80% in patients with advanced cancer, but only 47% in cases of localized cancer [24]. This finding implies that current technologies for ctDNA analysis are still insufficiently sensitive for reliable detection of early-stage cancers. Novel detection methods with much higher sensitivity are required. That study also demonstrated that the detection rates of ctDNA differ depending on the type of cancer [24]. The factors determining ctDNA levels are still not completely understood, but may include tumor burden and spatial proximity to vasculature, in addition to tumor type. Detailed analyses and accumulation of larger numbers of experimental data for patients with pancreatic cancer in various clinical situations are needed to develop ctDNA analysis that would be practical for early diagnosis of pancreatic cancer.

Although analyzing samples from patients with early-stage disease is particularly important for investigating the feasibility of utilizing ctDNA for early diagnosis, pancreatic cancer patients are rarely diagnosed at an early stage, and this remains an issue in the development of novel approaches for early detection of pancreatic cancer. In addition to acquisition of samples from early-stage disease, prospective follow-up and sequential blood sampling of individuals at high risk of pancreatic cancer (e.g., those with family history of pancreatic cancer or chronic pancreatitis) might be helpful for development of screening tests for early detection of pancreatic cancer. In addition to peripheral blood, other body fluids such as pancreatic juice may be a secondary source of tumor DNA for liquid biopsy. Collection of pancreatic juice is invasive, as it is collected endoscopically. But, although endoscopic techniques are more intricate than simple blood drawing, pancreatic juice is expected to contain a higher concentration of tumor DNA, compared to blood. Indeed, mutant *KRAS* has been detected in pancreatic juice from pancreatic cancer patients [25, 26].

Not only genetic alterations, but also epigenetic aberrations, such as DNA hypermethylation, occur during pancreatic carcinogenesis. Aberrant DNA methylations seem to occur in early-stage tumors, resulting in inactivation of tumor suppressor genes or gain-of-function of oncogenic signaling pathways. Genes that are aberrantly methylated in a high proportion of pancreatic cancer patients could be biomarkers for cancer screening. Methylation of several genes (including *NPTX2*, *SFRP1*, and *SPAK*) has been detected in pancreatic juice samples, and patients with pancreatic cancer were distinguished from patients with chronic pancreatitis or normal individuals by using these methylation markers [27]. Detecting tumor-specific epigenetic alterations in cfDNA could be an attractive option for diagnosis of pancreatic cancer by means of a liquid biopsy approach, since epigenetic markers, including aberrant DNA methylation, can be also found in ctDNA. Indeed, Joo et al. demonstrated the possibility of detecting promoter methylation of *BNC1* and *ADAMTS1* in cfDNA as potential serum biomarkers for early detection of pancreatic cancer [28].

In addition, it has been suggested that cancer-derived exosomes, which are defined by glypican-1 positivity, could also be a candidate target in serum for non-invasive diagnosis of early-stage pancreatic cancer [29].

In the future, it may be worth investigating the feasibility of utilizing combinatorial approaches with multiple blood-based biomarkers, including genomic mutations in ctDNA, epigenetic alterations in ctDNA, and cancer-specific exosomes, as a strategy to improve sensitivity and specificity in the diagnosis of early-stage pancreatic cancer.

5.5   Conclusions and Future Directions

Although pancreatic cancer is a highly lethal disease with limited treatment options, a novel diagnostic test able to accurately detect the disease at an early stage, when curative surgery may be feasible, would greatly improve the prognosis of patients. Less-invasive blood tests might also be useful for cancer screening. In this context, ctDNA present in circulation of cancer patients is expected to be a highly specific biomarker of cancer, compared to conventional tumor biomarkers in blood. Indeed, a number of studies have detected genomic alterations in blood from patients with pancreatic cancer, confirming the potential value of liquid biopsy approaches.

However, at present there is insufficient evidence of the utility of ctDNA analysis for early detection of pancreatic cancer, and several issues need to be addressed. One of the most urgent is improvement of sensitivity. In this regard, the prospects for technological developments and analytical improvements seem promising.

However, implementation of new ctDNA analyses for pancreatic cancer screening will also require demonstration of analytic and clinical validity in large prospective studies. Another issue is the diverse range of methods used so far for processing of blood samples and extraction of cfDNA. It will be important to standardize preanalytical processes of cfDNA analysis, such as blood sample acquisition, plasma separation, sample storage, and cfDNA quantification. This issue has only just begun to be discussed. In view of the potential benefit to patients of a liquid biopsy approach using ctDNA for early detection of pancreatic cancer, we believe work to address these issues will proceed rapidly.

References

1. Yachida S, Jones S, Bozic I, Antal T, Leary R, Fu B, et al. Distant metastasis occurs late during the genetic evolution of pancreatic cancer. Nature. 2010;467:1114–7.
2. Mandel P, Metais P. Les acides nucléiques du plasma sanguin chez l'homme. C R Seances Soc Biol Fil. 1948;142:241–3.
3. Stroun M, Anker P, Maurice P, Lyautey J, Lederrey C, Beljanski M. Neoplastic characteristics of the DNA found in the plasma of cancer patients. Oncology. 1989;46:318–22.
4. Diaz Jr LA, Bardelli A. Liquid biopsies: genotyping circulating tumor DNA. J Clin Oncol. 2014;32:579–86.
5. Campbell PJ, Yachida S, Mudie LJ, Stephens PJ, Pleasance ED, Stebbings LA, et al. The patterns and dynamics of genomic instability in metastatic pancreatic cancer. Nature. 2010;467:1109–13.
6. Jahr S, Hentze H, Englisch S, Hardt D, Fackelmayer FO, Hesch RD, et al. DNA fragments in the blood plasma of cancer patients: quantitations and evidence for their origin from apoptotic and necrotic cells. Cancer Res. 2001;61:1659–65.
7. Schwarzenbach H, Hoon DS, Pantel K. Cell-free nucleic acids as biomarkers in cancer patients. Nat Rev Cancer. 2011;11:426–37.
8. Sun K, Jiang P, Chan KC, Wong J, Cheng YK, Liang RH, et al. Plasma DNA tissue mapping by genome-wide methylation sequencing for noninvasive prenatal, cancer, and transplantation assessments. Proc Natl Acad Sci U S A. 2015;112:E5503–12.
9. Dressman D, Yan H, Traverso G, Kinzler KW, Vogelstein B. Transforming single DNA molecules into fluorescent magnetic particles for detection and enumeration of genetic variations. Proc Natl Acad Sci U S A. 2003;100:8817–22.
10. Baker M. Digital PCR hits its stride. Nat Methods. 2012;9:541–4.
11. Takai E, Totoki Y, Nakamura H, Morizane C, Nara S, Hama N, et al. Clinical utility of circulating tumor DNA for molecular assessment in pancreatic cancer. Sci Rep. 2015;5:18425.
12. Kinde I, Wu J, Papadopoulos N, Kinzler KW, Vogelstein B. Detection and quantification of rare mutations with massively parallel sequencing. Proc Natl Acad Sci U S A. 2011;108:9530–5.
13. Forshew T, Murtaza M, Parkinson C, Gale D, Tsui DW, Kaper F, et al. Noninvasive identification and monitoring of cancer mutations by targeted deep sequencing of plasma DNA. Sci Transl Med. 2012;4:136ra68.
14. Newman AM, Bratman SV, To J, Wynne JF, Eclov NC, Modlin LA, et al. An ultrasensitive method for quantitating circulating tumor DNA with broad patient coverage. Nat Med. 2014;20:548–54.
15. Leary RJ, Kinde I, Diehl F, Schmidt K, Clouser C, Duncan C, et al. Development of personalized tumor biomarkers using massively parallel sequencing. Sci Transl Med. 2010;2:20ra14.
16. Maire F, Micard S, Hammel P, Voitot H, Lévy P, Cugnenc PH, et al. Differential diagnosis between chronic pancreatitis and pancreatic cancer: value of the detection of KRAS2 mutations in circulating DNA. Br J Cancer. 2002;87:551–4.

17. Däbritz J, Preston R, Hänfler J, Oettle H. K-ras mutations in the plasma correspond to computed tomographic findings in patients with pancreatic cancer. Pancreas. 2012;41:323–5.
18. Chen H, Tu H, Meng ZQ, Chen Z, Wang P, Liu LM. K-ras mutational status predicts poor prognosis in unresectable pancreatic cancer. Eur J Surg Oncol. 2010;36:657–62.
19. Kinugasa H, Nouso K, Miyahara K, Morimoto Y, Dohi C, Tsutsumi K, et al. Detection of K-ras gene mutation by liquid biopsy in patients with pancreatic cancer. Cancer. 2015;121: 2271–80.
20. Sausen M, Phallen J, Adleff V, Jones S, Leary RJ, Barrett MT, et al. Clinical implications of genomic alterations in the tumour and circulation of pancreatic cancer patients. Nat Commun. 2015;6:7686.
21. Tjensvoll K, Lapin M, Buhl T, Oltedal S, Steen-Ottosen Berry K, et al. Clinical relevance of circulating KRAS mutated DNA in plasma from patients with advanced pancreatic cancer. Mol Oncol. 2015;10:635–43.
22. Jones S, Anagnostou V, Lytle K, Parpart-Li S, Nesselbush M, Riley DR, et al. Personalized genomic analyses for cancer mutation discovery and interpretation. Sci Transl Med. 2015;7: 283ra53.
23. Zill OA, Greene C, Sebisanovic D, Siew LM, Leng J, Vu M, et al. Cell-free DNA next-generation sequencing in pancreatobiliary carcinomas. Cancer Discov. 2015;5:1040–8.
24. Bettegowda C, Sausen M, Leary RJ, Kinde I, Wang Y, Agrawal N, et al. Detection of circulating tumor DNA in early- and late-stage human malignancies. Sci Transl Med. 2014;6:224ra24.
25. Shi C, Fukushima N, Abe T, Bian Y, Hua L, Wendelburg BJ, et al. Sensitive and quantitative detection of KRAS2 gene mutations in pancreatic duct juice differentiates patients with pancreatic cancer from chronic pancreatitis, potential for early detection. Cancer Biol Ther. 2008;7:353–60.
26. Eshleman JR, Norris AL, Sadakari Y, Debeljak M, Borges M, Harrington C, et al. KRAS and guanine nucleotide-binding protein mutations in pancreatic juice collected from the duodenum of patients at high risk for neoplasia undergoing endoscopic ultrasound. Clin Gastroenterol Hepatol. 2015;13:963–9.
27. Matsubayashi H, Canto M, Sato N, Klein A, Abe T, Yamashita K, et al. DNA methylation alterations in the pancreatic juice of patients with suspected pancreatic disease. Cancer Res. 2006;66:1208–17.
28. Yi JM, Guzzetta AA, Bailey VJ, Downing SR, Van Neste L, Chiappinelli KB, et al. Novel methylation biomarker panel for the early detection of pancreatic cancer. Clin Cancer Res. 2013;19:6544–55.
29. Melo SA, Luecke LB, Kahlert C, Fernandez AF, Gammon ST, Kaye J, et al. Glypican-1 identifies cancer exosomes and detects early pancreatic cancer. Nature. 2015;523:177–82.

Part II

Pancreaticoduodenectomy for Pancreatic Cancer: Indications and Procedure

Standard Resection and Extended Resection

6

Jin-Young Jang

6.1 Introduction

Pancreatic ductal adenocarcinoma (PDAC) is a malignant neoplasm with the poorest prognosis among periampullary cancers with a 5-year survival rate of approximately 20% even after curative resection. PDAC is a well-known systemic disease; however, currently there is no definitive systemic therapy for PDAC [1–3].

Considering the fact that the majority of pancreatic cancers occur in the head of the pancreas, pancreaticoduodenectomy is considered as a main treatment strategy for pancreatic cancer. Since the first en bloc resection of part of the pancreatic head, extrahepatic bile duct, and duodenum by Kausch in 1909, there has been tremendous developments in surgical techniques and perioperative care followed by marked decrease in operative mortality. Despite immense improvement in surgical safety, oncological long-term outcome after pancreaticoduodenectomy has been disappointing.

Under the existing scenario, numerous surgeons have tried to increase the survival of patients with PDAC through aggressive surgery. Following Fortner's regional pancreatectomy, several surgical methods have been applied in an effort to increase the extent of surgery with a purpose of increasing curability [4–6].

Actually speaking, some retrospective studies have demonstrated improved resectability following promising outcome through extended surgery; however, there are no reliable reports showing increase in long-term survival based on prospective studies [7, 8].

Although the definition of extended resection is not clearly defined, many surgeons have employed extended resection focusing on wider extent of

J.-Y. Jang, M.D., Ph.D.
Department of Surgery, Seoul National University College of Medicine,
101 Daehak-ro, Jongno-gu, Seoul 03080, Republic of Korea
e-mail: jangjy4@snu.ac.kr

© Springer Science+Business Media Singapore 2017
H. Yamaue (ed.), *Innovation of Diagnosis and Treatment for Pancreatic Cancer*,
DOI 10.1007/978-981-10-2486-3_6

lymphadenectomy with resection of peripancreatic nerve plexus. Some have also used extended resection regarding vessel resection around the pancreas. The issues of vessel resection will be addressed in other chapters. In this chapter, the role of extended resection based on recent evidences is described.

6.2   Comparison Between Standard and Extended Resection

6.2.1   Rationale for Dissection of Lymph Node and Nerve Plexus

Pancreatic cancer is a well-known extremely aggressive neoplasm. Even for small sized tumors, lymph nodes metastasis is frequently detected at the peripancreatic area as well as the para-aortic spaces. Lymph node status is one of the main prognostic factors in patients with pancreatic head cancer [9].

The Japanese Pancreatic Association reported that not only the presence but the site of metastatic lymph nodes is prognostic of early recurrence and long-term survival [10].

The high incidence of local recurrence after conventional pancreaticoduodenectomy was considered to result from incomplete clearance of these lymph nodes, with previous studies showing that standard pancreatoduodenectomy removes 80% of the lymph node sites which are most frequently involved [8, 11].

These findings suggest that more extensive lymph node dissection may enhance survival outcomes. Some surgeons and especially Japanese surgeons suggested that en bloc resection of lymph node including para-aortic spaces could improve survival in PDAC [6, 11].

Neural invasion is another important prognostic factor to be considered in pancreatic carcinoma. The postoperative survival rate of patients with extrapancreatic nerve plexus (PLX) invasion is significantly worse as compared with the patients without PLX invasion. About 60–80% of PDAC has combined perineural involvement of tumor. In a recent literature, the concept of a tumor-neural microenvironment in which the cancer cells and nerves constitute a microenvironment for mutual promotion or proliferation and inhibition of apoptosis has been proposed [12]. To improve survival, complete removal of nerve plexus around the pancreas was advocated by several surgeons [13].

Some reports have demonstrated that lymph nodes metastases are limited to areas along the SMA when a PDAC is almost entirely confined to the ventral pancreas. On the contrary, lymph nodes metastases are limited to areas along the common hepatic artery and the hepatoduodenal ligament when a PDAC is almost entirely confined to the dorsal pancreas. The researchers suggest that it is necessary to alter the extent of the nerve plexus and lymph node dissection according to the primary tumor location [13, 14].

Clearing the retroperitoneal nerve plexus, especially the SMA peripheral nerve plexus, during surgical treatment of pancreatic cancer has a neuroanatomical basis. Analysis of the recurrence patterns of pancreatic cancer after pancreaticoduodenectomy showed that retroperitoneal recurrence caused by perineural invasion is one of the important events except metastasis. Several surgeons tried to achieve complete clearance of the connective tissues surrounding the SMA. However, complete removal of nerve plexus can provoke intractable diarrhea followed by malnutrition and immunologic dysfunction. Considering the quality of life, only a right sided semicircular clearance of the SMA nerve plexus is recommended by other research groups [15].

6.2.2 Extent of Pancreaticoduodenectomy

Many pancreatic surgeons have tried to improve resectability and survival adopting aggressive extended resection on pancreatic cancer like extended lymphadenectomy and dissection of nerve plexus around major vessels based on the already established theoretical advantages [16–18].

Some retrospective studies showed better survival outcomes by adopting extended lymphadenectomy. Ishikawa et al. reported 3-year survival rates after radical resection as 38%, which was superior to that of standard resection (13%). However, many other retrospective studies have shown conflicting results. Considering selection bias in retrospective studies, it would be better to focus on well-designed RCT on the extent of resection in pancreatic head cancer.

Until now, five prospective randomized controlled trials (RCTs) have compared standard and extended resection with its main focus on lymphadenectomy, but each study had different extent of resection with respect to lymph node and nerve plexus (Table 6.1) [8, 19–23].

In two RCTs, dissection around the SMA was considered as nerve plexus dissection. Rates of diarrhea were reported to be 42–84% after circumferential dissection and 15% after semi-circumferential dissection of the SMA nerve plexus. However, the R0 resection rate and overall survival were not affected by the extent of SMA nerve plexus dissection. Therefore, it is proposed that circumferential dissection of the SMA is oncologically not necessary, as it only worsens QOL after pancreaticoduodenectomy.

Operative outcome according to the extent of surgery is summarized in Table 6.2. Mean operative time was significantly longer for extended pancreaticoduodenectomy in four studies. Blood transfusion rate was higher for extended than for standard pancreaticoduodenectomy in one trial. The R0 resection rates were similar in the standard (72.5–94.1%) and extended (78.0–93.0%) pancreaticoduodenectomy groups. In all five studies, the number of retrieved lymph nodes was significantly higher in the extended than in the standard pancreaticoduodenectomy group. However, lymph node metastasis rates in all five studies were similar in patients who underwent extended (43.2–68.0%) and standard (45.9–68.7%) pancreaticoduodenectomy [8, 19–23].

6.2.3 Results of Our Randomized Controlled Study

Previous to our RCT, four studies have already reported the optimal extent of pancreaticoduodenectomy. However, each study has been criticized due to the small number of patients, absence of objectively controlled operative techniques, no

Table 6.1 Extent of lymph node and nerve plexus dissection in five randomized controlled trials

	Pedrazzoli et al. [19]	Yeo et al. [20]	Farnell et al. [21]	Nimura et al. [22]	Jang et al. [23]
Standard operation	• Anterior/posterior pancreaticoduodenal • Pyloric • Biliary duct • Superior/inferior pancreatic head and body	• Anterior/posterior pancreaticoduodenal • Hepatoduodenal ligament • Right lateral aspect of the SMA and SMV	• Gastric lesser/greater curvature • Pyloric • Right of the hepatoduodenal ligament • Anterior/posterior pancreaticoduodenal • Right of the SMA • Anterior to the CHA	• Anterior/posterior pancreaticoduodenal	• Anterior/posterior pancreaticoduodenal • Bile duct and cystic duct
Extended operation	• Hepatic hilum • Along the aorta from the diaphragmatic hiatus to the IMA • Laterally to both renal hilus	• Gastric lesser/greater curvature • Superior/inferior pyloric • Celiac origin • Celiac to left renal vein • Left renal vein to IMA	• Between bilateral renal hilum • Hepatoduodenal ligament skeletonization up to the liver • Hepatic artery and celiac axis • Para-aortic from celiac axis to IPM • Circumferential dissection of the SMA	• Common hepatic artery • Celiac artery • Hepatoduodenal ligament skeletonization • SMA • Para-aortic from the origin of celiac axis to IMA	• Common hepatic artery • Celiac axis • Hepatoduodenal ligament skeletonization • SMA • Para-aortic between celiac axis and IMA
Nerve plexus dissection in extended operation				• Circumferentially around the CHA and SMA, semi-circumferentially on the right lateral aspect of the celiac axis	• Right side of the celiac axis and SMA semi-circumferentially

statistical calculation for required number of enrolled patients, mixed cases with non-pancreatic ductal adenocarcinoma, insufficient clearance of retroperitoneal tissue and lymph node, and no consideration of nerve plexus dissection or extensive dissection of nerve plexus provoking uncontrolled diarrhea [19–23]. To overcome the abovementioned pitfalls of previous RCTs, we designed and executed our own RCT on pancreatic ductal adenocarcinoma based on larger sample size with standardized method of operation and with focus on dissection of nerve plexus as well as lymph node.

In standard resection, lymph node around pancreas head (LN 13, 17) and gallbladder (LN 12c) were only removed without nerve dissection around hepatic artery or superior mesenteric artery (SMA). For extended resection, lymph node around common hepatic artery (LN 8), celiac axis (CA) (LN 9), peripancreatic area (LN 13, 17), hepatoduodenal ligament (LN 12), SMA (LN 14), and para-aortic area (LN16) between CA and inferior mesenteric artery were dissected. All

Table 6.2 Operative outcome of five RCTs according to type of surgery

		Pedrazzoli et al. [19]		Yeo et al. [20]		Farnell et al. [21]		Nimura et al. [22]		Jang et al. [23]	
		SPD	EPD	SPD	EPD	SPD	EPD	SPD	EPD	SPD	EPD
N		40	41	146	148	40	39	51	50	83	86
Operative time (min)	Mean ± SEM	371.9 ± 49.8	396.7 ± 49.9	354	384	378	450	426	547	355.5 ± 12.4	419.6 ± 13.0
Blood transfusion (U)	Mean ± SD	1.95 ± 0.2	2.07 ± 0.2	0.5 ± 0.1	0.5 ± 0.1	22%	44%	2.1	2.4	0.1 ± 0.05	0.25 ± 0.09
PD/PPPD/SSPPD	N	20/20/0	18/23/0	21/125/0	148/0/0	40/0/0	39/0/0	13/19/19	11/23/16	21/62/0	26/60/0
Portal vein resection	N (%)	–	–	4 (3%)	4 (3%)	–23%	–21%	24 (47%)	24 (48%)	17 (20.5%)	23 (26.7%)
No. of lymph node retrieved	Mean	13.3	19.8	17	28.5	15	34	13.3	40.1	17.3	33.7
LN (+) (%)	N (%)	24 (60.0%)	24 (58.5%)	67 (45.9%)	64 (43.2%)	–55%	–68%	32 (63%)	30 (60%)	57 (68.7%)	57 (66.3%)
R0 resection (%)	N (%)	29 (72.5%)	32 (78.0%)	128 (88%)	138 (93%)	–76%	–82%	48 (94.1%)	45 (90%)	71 (85.5%)	78 (90.7%)
Postoperative hospital stay (days)	Mean ± SD	22.7 ± 1.41	19.3 ± 1.11	11.3 ± 0.51	14.3 ± 0.81	13	16	43.8	42.4	19.7 ± 9.4	22.8 ± 17.1

SPD standard pancreaticoduodenectomy, *EPD* extended pancreaticoduodenectomy

the soft tissues around hepatoduodenal ligament were completely dissected and skeletonized. Nerve plexus or ganglion right side to CA and SMA were dissected semi-circumferentially (Fig. 6.1). Differences in extent of resection between two groups are summarized in Table 6.3 [23].

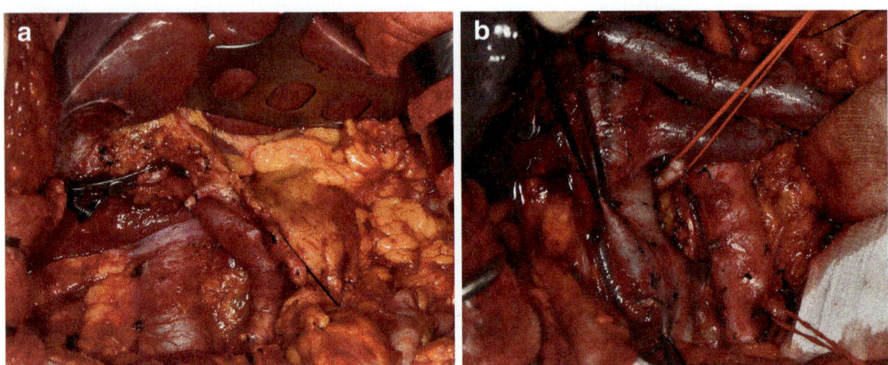

Fig. 6.1 Extent of resection in pancreaticoduodenectomy. (**a**) Standard and (**b**) Extended resection

Table 6.3 Summary of differences in surgical extents according to the type of surgery [23]

Tissues	Location	Standard pancreatectomy	Extended pancreatectomy
Lymph node	Superior pyloric (5)	×	○
	Inferior pyloric (6)	×	○
	Common hepatic artery (8)	×	○
	Celiac axis (9)	×	○
	Hepatoduodenal ligament (12)	△	○
	12a: proper hepatic artery	×	○
	12p: portal vein	×	○
	12b: bile duct	○	○
	12c: cystic duct	○	○
	12h: hilar area	×	○
	Posterior pancreaticoduodenal (13)	○	○
	Superior mesenteric artery (14)	×	○
	14a: origin of SMA	×	○
	14b: right side of SMA	×	○
	14c: anterior SMA at middle colic	×	○
	14d: left side of SMA	×	○
	Aortocaval nodes (16)	×	○
	16a2: celiac to left renal vein	×	○
	16b1: left renal vein to IMA	×	○
	Anterior pancreaticoduodenal (17)	○	○
Soft tissue	Gerota's fascia	×	○
	Vascular skeletonization	×	○
Nerve plexus	Celiac and SMA plexus	×	○

Morbidity of the extended resection group was 43%, which is slightly higher than that of standard resection group (32.5%); however, there was no statistical difference ($p = 0.160$).

There were no specific differences in complications related to surgical extent in our study. Postoperative diarrhea was found only in 13 patients (15.1%), which signifies that right side 180° dissection of nerve plexus imparted no major effect on changes in intestinal motility.

In the standard group, there was no postoperative mortality. However, there were two cases of mortality in the extended group due to pneumonia and sepsis in association with SMA pseudoaneurysm.

The overall median survival of enrolled patients ($n = 167$) except for postoperative death was 18.7 months. The 2-, 3-, and 5-year survival rate was 39.9%, 25.8%, and 18.8%, respectively. No survival difference could be found according to type of surgery (Fig. 6.2a). There was also no difference in disease specific survival rate between the two groups.

Although there was no statistical difference ($p = 0.358$), the 2-year survival rate and median survival of the standard group were 44.5% and 18.8 months, which are slightly higher than those of the extended group (35.7%/16.5 months). We could not see any survival differences even in the lymph node metastasis cases as well as in the negative cases (Fig. 6.2b). In cases of lymph node metastasis, median survival of the extended group was 18 months, which was similar to that (17.4 months) of standard group ($p = 0.523$).

Improved survival in the patients who received adjuvant chemoradiation was observed. Median survival of patients with adjuvant treatment ($n = 114$) was 20.8 months, which was higher than that (14.0 months) of no adjuvant treatment group ($n = 53$). Especially, the effect of adjuvant treatment was more prominent in the standard group ($p = 0.016$) (Fig. 6.2c).

Our study showed that extended pancreaticoduodenectomy including dissection of extensive lymph node and nerve plexus does not improve long-term outcome of pancreatic ductal adenocarcinoma. Considering early recovery with less morbidity, standard pancreatic resection followed by adjuvant treatment is a better option with respect to safety and effectiveness.

6.2.4 Meta-Analyses on Optimal Extent of Resection

Meta-analyses on five RCTs showed that delayed gastric emptying and pancreatic fistula rates tended to be higher in patients who underwent extended pancreaticoduodenectomy. However, meta-analyses of every morbidity using a random effects model revealed no significant differences. The rate of postoperative diarrhea (17.3% vs. 6.7%, $p = 0.08$) and overall postoperative morbidity (38.8% vs. 30.3%, $p = 0.160$) tended to be higher in patients who underwent extended pancreatoduodenectomy (Fig. 6.3). The odds ratio for mortality in the EPD group was 1.02 (95% CI: 0.38–2.69), but the difference was not statistically significant.

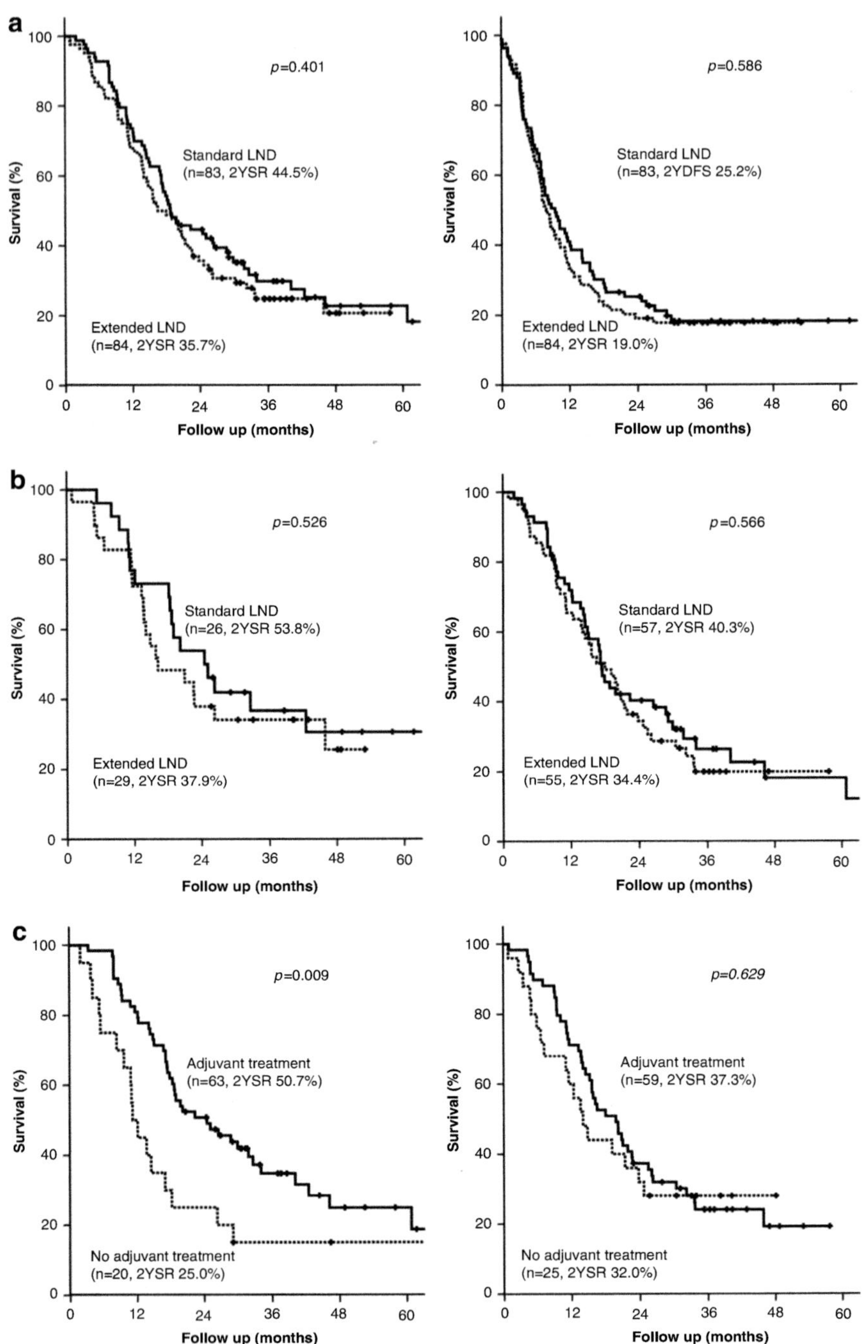

Fig. 6.2 (**a**) Overall and disease-free survival curves according to the type of surgery. (**b**) Survival curves according to the type of surgery without or with lymph node metastasis. (**c**) Survival curves according to the adjuvant treatment in standard and extended group

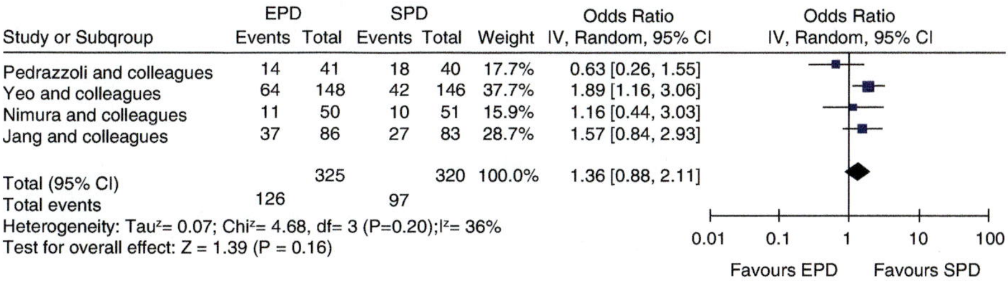

Study or Subgroup	EPD Events	EPD Total	SPD Events	SPD Total	Weight	Odds Ratio IV, Random, 95% CI
Pedrazzoli and colleagues	14	41	18	40	17.7%	0.63 [0.26, 1.55]
Yeo and colleagues	64	148	42	146	37.7%	1.89 [1.16, 3.06]
Nimura and colleagues	11	50	10	51	15.9%	1.16 [0.44, 3.03]
Jang and colleagues	37	86	27	83	28.7%	1.57 [0.84, 2.93]
Total (95% CI)		325		320	100.0%	1.36 [0.88, 2.11]
Total events	126		97			

Heterogeneity: Tau²= 0.07; Chi²= 4.68, df= 3 (P=0.20);I²= 36%
Test for overall effect: Z = 1.39 (P = 0.16)

Favours EPD   Favours SPD

Fig. 6.3 Operative morbidity after standard (SPD) and extended (EPD) pancreaticoduodenectomy

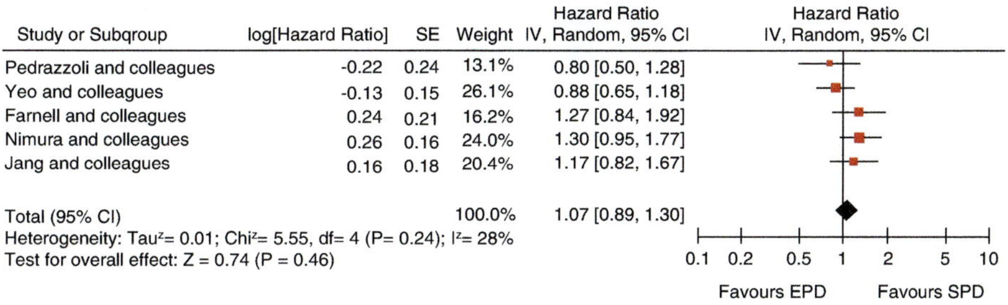

Study or Subgroup	log[Hazard Ratio]	SE	Weight	Hazard Ratio IV, Random, 95% CI
Pedrazzoli and colleagues	-0.22	0.24	13.1%	0.80 [0.50, 1.28]
Yeo and colleagues	-0.13	0.15	26.1%	0.88 [0.65, 1.18]
Farnell and colleagues	0.24	0.21	16.2%	1.27 [0.84, 1.92]
Nimura and colleagues	0.26	0.16	24.0%	1.30 [0.95, 1.77]
Jang and colleagues	0.16	0.18	20.4%	1.17 [0.82, 1.67]
Total (95% CI)			100.0%	1.07 [0.89, 1.30]

Heterogeneity: Tau²= 0.01; Chi²= 5.55, df= 4 (P= 0.24); I²= 28%
Test for overall effect: Z = 0.74 (P = 0.46)

Favours EPD   Favours SPD

Fig. 6.4 Overall survival after standard (SPD) and extended (EPD) pancreaticoduodenectomy

The rates of overall postoperative morbidity tended to be higher in patients who underwent extended pancreaticoduodenectomy, but pooled analyses showed no significant differences (38.8% vs. 30.3%, $p = 0.160$).

Regarding survival, meta-analyses showed that overall survival was not affected by the extent of surgery in pancreatic cancer. The pooled hazard ratio across all five trials was 1.07 (95% CI: 0.89–1.30, $p = 0.460$) (Fig. 6.4).

Overall survival was not affected by the extent of surgery (pooled hazard ratio 1.07, 95% CI: 0.89–1.30, $p = 0.460$).

In all five RCTs, R0 resection rates were similar, suggesting that extended pancreaticoduodenectomy does not guarantee more complete tumor removal followed by similar overall survival rate between standard and extended surgery. Moreover, it is proposed that adjuvant treatment rather than surgical extent may improve survival outcomes after curative resection [23, 24].

6.3 Vascular Resection

Since the first suggestion by Dr. Fortner, many surgeons believed that a more radical resection could improve survival by enhanced tumor clearance, especially tumor adhered to main vessels such as portal vein (PV)/superior mesenteric vein (SMV) or adjacent arteries. Few researchers were influenced with an assumption that aggressive surgery could overcome barrier of unresectability by en bloc resection of major vessels. A few retrospective data showed promising survival outcome [25, 26].

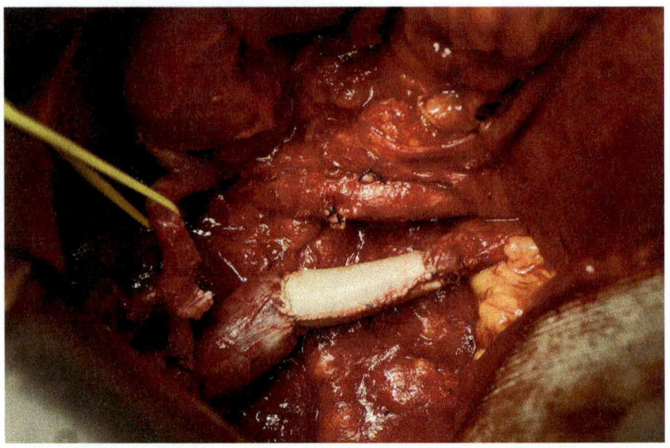

Fig. 6.5 Using bovine patch graft, long segment of PV/SMV was resected and anastomosed in patients with PDAC that invaded SMV and splenic vein confluence area

In an era of organ transplantation, vessel resection and anastomosis are not major concerns. Using autologous veins or several other materials, long segmental resection is technically possible (Fig. 6.5).

Based on some previous promising data, criteria for PV/SMV invasion as advanced T stage was eliminated from the 6th version of AJCC staging unlike other GI tract malignancy with a conviction that PV/SMV invasion is a matter of tumor location and not tumor aggressiveness. However, recent meta-analysis showed that patients undergoing PV–SMV resection had an increased risk of postoperative mortality [risk difference (RD) 0.01, 95% CI 0.00–0.03; $p = 0.02$] and of R1/R2 resection (RD 0.09, 0.06–0.13; $p < 0.001$) as compared to those undergoing standard surgery. Also, 1-, 3- and 5-year survival were worse in the PV–SMV resection group with hazard ratio as 1.23 (95% CI 1.07–1.43; $p = 0.005$), 1.48 (1.14–1.91; $p = 0.004$), and 3.18 (1.95–5.19; $p < 0.001$), respectively [27, 28] (Fig. 6.6).

In high volume centers equipped with vascular surgery, there is a possibility that perioperative mortality and morbidity in PV–SMV resection group could be similar with non-vessel resection group.

However, in cases of histological tumor infiltration into the tunica media or intima of PV–SMV, researchers reported that worse prognosis and long-term survival were hardly anticipated [29].

While performing pancreatectomy, indication of PV–SMV resection must be cautiously selected according to the hospitals' facilities and experience considering morbidity. In case of definite invasion of tumor into vessels, neoadjuvant treatment rather than upfront surgery would be a better option to avoid early recurrence and metastasis after surgery and reduce tumor infiltration into the vessels.

Unlike PV–SMV, resection of hepatic artery, SMA, and celiac trunk could not be recommended in spite of technical feasibility. No data supports improved survival after arterial resection which is inevitably followed by high morbidity.

a

	Overall morbidity				
Reference	Vein resection	Standard procedure	Weight (%)	Odds ratio	Odds ratio
Bachellier et al.[28]	8 of 21	30 of 66	4.7	0.74 (0.27, 2.02)	
Carrère et al.[29]	25 of 45	56 of 88	7.1	0.71 (0.34, 1.48)	
Castleberry et al.[30]	112 of 281	1099 of 3301	14.4	1.33 (1.03, 1.70)	
Chakravarty et al.[31]	6 of 12	30 of 75	3.5	1.50 (0.44, 5.09)	
Fuhrman et al.[32]	7 of 23	10 of 36	3.9	1.14 (0.36, 3.59)	
Fukuda et al.[33]	12 of 37	32 of 84	6.2	0.78 (0.34, 1.77)	
Gong et al.[46]	28 of 119	37 of 447	9.6	3.41 (1.99, 5.86)	
Hartel et al.[34]	18 of 68	45 of 203	8.3	1.26 (0.67, 2.38)	
Kelly et al.[47]	36 of 70	139 of 422	10.1	2.16 (1.29, 3.59)	
Kurosaki et al.[35]	12 of 35	10 of 42	4.8	1.67 (0.62, 4.52)	
Murakami et al.[48]	22 of 61	14 of 64	6.5	2.01 (0.91, 4.44)	
Ouaissi et al.[39]	35 of 59	45 of 82	7.8	1.20 (0.61, 2.36)	
Riediger et al.[41]	22 of 53	84 of 169	8.4	0.72 (0.38, 1.34)	
Shibata et al.[42]	9 of 28	12 of 46	4.6	1.34 (0.48, 3.76)	
Total	352 of 912	1643 of 5125	100.0	1.34 (1.03, 1.73)	

Heterogeneity: $\tau^2 = 0.10$; $\chi^2 = 25.87$, 13 d.f., $P = 0.02$; $I^2 = 50\%$
Test for overall effect: $Z = 2.21$, $P = 0.03$

0.01 0.1 1 10 100
Favours vein resection Favours standard procedure

b

Reference	Log[hazard ratio]	Standard error	Weight (%)	Hazard ratio	Hazard ratio
Murakami et al.[48]	2.186	1.095	5.2	8.90 (1.04, 76.15)	
Ouaissi et al.[39]	1.515	0.456	29.9	4.55 (1.86, 11.13)	
Riediger et al.[41]	0.051	0.577	18.7	1.05 (0.34, 3.26)	
Shimada et al.[43]	1.258	0.367	46.3	3.52 (1.72, 7.22)	
Total			100.0	3.18 (1.95, 5.19)	

Heterogeneity: $\chi^2 = 5.25$, 3 d.f., $P = 0.15$; $I^2 = 43\%$
Test for overall effect: $Z = 4.64$, $P < 0.001$

0.01 0.1 1 10 100
Favours vein resection Favours standard procedure

Fig. 6.6 Comparison of morbidity (**a**) and 5-year overall survival (**b**) after pancreatic resection with versus without PV–SMV resection. (Data collected from a meta-analysis by Giovinazzo et al., Br J Surg 2016 Feb; 103(3):179–91). (**a**) Comparison of overall morbidity rates after pancreatic resection with versus without portal–superior mesenteric vein resection. (**b**) Comparison of 5-year overall survival after pancreatic resection with versus without portal–superior mesenteric vein resection

Conclusion

Although achieving R0 resection is still the most important factor to guarantee curative surgery and long-term survival in pancreatic cancer, extended surgery alone cannot improve oncological curability. Recent meta-analyses showed that standard pancreaticoduodenectomy with R0 resection was a satisfactory operation with comparable survival outcomes and better morbidity, mortality and quality of life as compared to extended pancreaticoduodenectomy in patients with pancreatic cancer. According to the tumor location and severity, there might be room for extended surgery to obtain a marginally negative resection, but routine extended pancreatic surgery is not needed to increase survival rate. Surgical strategies could be customized considering the patients' condition and disease. Therefore, pancreaticoduodenectomy with dissection of peritumoral lymph nodes including LN 12, 13, 8, and 17 may be extended to further lymphadenectomy, depending on the tumor location and severity of disease. For peripancreatic nerve plexus, routine dissection is not needed but can be performed with a maximum of 180° to get R0 resection and to preserve QOL after operation, if the tumor is located in close proximity to the SMA. While performing pancreatectomy for pancreatic cancer, surgeons must bear in mind that surgery is only a component of the multimodality treatments provided for pancreatic cancer. Besides the effort to achieve R0 resection, surgeons must pay great attention to decrease surgical morbidity by avoiding unnecessary extended surgery for early systemic therapy, which is generally performed to increase survival in pancreatic cancer.

References

1. Slidell MB, Chang DC, Cameron JL, et al. Impact of total lymph node count and lymph node ratio on staging and survival after pancreatectomy for pancreatic adenocarcinoma: a large, population-based analysis. Ann Surg Oncol. 2008;15:165–74.
2. D'Angelo FA, Antolino L, La Rocca M, Petrucciani N, Magistri P, Aurello P, Ramacciato G. Adjuvant and neoadjuvant therapies in resectable pancreatic cancer: a systematic review of randomized controlled trials. Med Oncol. 2016;33:28.
3. Richter A, Niedergethmann M, Sturm JW, Lorenz D, Post S, Trede M. Long-term results of partial pancreaticoduodenectomy for ductal adenocarcinoma of the pancreatic head: 25-year experience. World J Surg. 2003;27:324–9.
4. Fortner JG. Regional resection of cancer of the pancreas: a new surgical approach. Surgery. 1973;73:307–20.
5. Takahashi S, Ogata Y, Miyazaki H, et al. Aggressive surgery for pancreatic duct cell cancer: feasibility, validity, limitations. World J Surg. 1995;19:653–9.
6. Nakao A, Takagi H. Isolated pancreatectomy for pancreatic head carcinoma using catheter bypass of the portal vein. Hepato-Gastroenterology. 1993;40:426–9.
7. Reber HA, Ashley SW, McFadden D. Curative treatment for pancreatic neoplasms. Radical resection. Surg Clin North Am. 1995;75:905–12.
8. Kang MJ, Jang JY, Kim SW. Surgical resection of pancreatic head cancer: what is the optimal extent of surgery? Cancer Lett. 2016;382:259–65. Epub ahead of print
9. Cameron JL, Pitt HA, Yeo CJ, Lillemoe KD, Kaufman HS, Coleman J. One hundred and forty-five consecutive pancreaticoduodenectomies without mortality. Ann Surg. 1993;217(5): 430–5.
10. Hirata K, Sato T, Mukaiya M, Yamashiro K, Kimura M, Sasaki K, et al. Results of 1001 pancreatic resections for invasive ductal adenocarcinoma of the pancreas. Arch Surg. 1997; 132:771–6.
11. Ishikawa O, Ohigashi H, Sasaki Y, et al. Practical grouping of positive lymph nodes in pancreatic head cancer treated by an extended pancreatectomy. Surgery. 1997;121:244–9.
12. Heinemann V, Reni M, Ychou M, Richel DJ, Macarulla T, Ducreux M. Tumour-stroma interactions in pancreatic ductal adenocarcinoma: rationale and current evidence for new therapeutic strategies. Cancer Treat Rev. 2014;40:118–28.
13. Makino I, Kitagawa H, Ohta T, Nakagawara H, Tajima H, Ohnishi I, Takamura H, Tani T, Kayahara M. Nerve plexus invasion in pancreatic cancer: spread patterns on histopathologic and embryological analyses. Pancreas. 2008;37:358–65.
14. Japan Pancreas Society. Classification of pancreatic carcinoma. 2nd ed. Tokyo: Kanehara; 2003.

15. Kimura W, Watanabe T. Anatomy of the pancreatic nerve plexuses and significance of their dissection. Nihon Geka Gakkai Zasshi. 2011;112:170–6.
16. Fortner JG, Kim DK, Cubilla A, Turnbull A, Pahnke LD, Shils ME, et al. Regional pancreatectomy: en bloc pancreatic, portal vein and lymph node resection. Ann Surg. 1977;186:42–50.
17. Ishikawa O, Ohhigashi H, Sasaki Y, Kabuto T, Fukuda I, Furukawa H, et al. Practical usefulness of lymphatic and connective tissue clearance for the carcinoma of the pancreas head. Ann Surg. 1988;208:215–20.
18. Manabe T, Ohshio G, Baba N, Miyashita T, Asano N, Tamura K, et al. Radical pancreatectomy for ductal cell carcinoma of the head of the pancreas. Cancer. 1989;64:1132–7.
19. Pedrazzoli S, DiCarlo V, Dionigi R, et al. Standard versus extended lymphadenectomy associated with pancreatoduodenectomy in the surgical treatment of adenocarcinoma of the head of the pancreas: a multicenter, prospective, randomized study. Lymphadenectomy study group. Ann Surg. 1998;228:508–17.
20. Yeo CJ, Cameron JL, Lillemoe KD, et al. Pancreaticoduodenectomy with or without distal gastrectomy and extended retroperitoneal lymphadenectomy for periampullary adenocarcinoma, part 2: randomized controlled trial evaluating survival, morbidity, and mortality. Ann Surg. 2002;236:355–66.
21. Farnell MB, Pearson RK, Sarr MG, et al. A prospective randomized trial comparing standard pancreatoduodenectomy with pancreatoduodenectomy with extended lymphadenectomy in resectable pancreatic head adenocarcinoma. Surgery. 2005;138:618–28.
22. Nimura Y, Nagino M, Takao S, et al. Standard versus extended lymphadenectomy in radical pancreatoduodenectomy for ductal adenocarcinoma of the head of the pancreas: long-term results of a Japanese multicenter randomized controlled trial. J Hepatobiliary Pancreat Sci. 2012;19:230–41.
23. Jang JY, Kang MJ, Heo JS, et al. A prospective randomized controlled study comparing outcomes of standard resection and extended resection, including dissection of the nerve plexus and various lymph nodes, in patients with pancreatic head cancer. Ann Surg. 2014;259: 656–64.
24. Neoptolemos JP, Stocken DD, Friess H, et al. A randomized trial of chemoradiotherapy and chemotherapy after resection of pancreatic cancer. N Engl J Med. 2004;350:1200–10.
25. Wagner M, Redaelli C, Lietz M, Seiler CA, Friess H, Buchler MW. Curative resection is the single most important factor determining outcome in patients with pancreatic adenocarcinoma. Br J Surg. 2004;91:586–94.
26. Murakami Y, Satoi S, Motoi F, Sho M, Kawai M, Matsumoto I, Honda G, Multicentre Study Group of Pancreatobiliary Surgery (MSG-PBS). Portal or superior mesenteric vein resection in pancreatoduodenectomy for pancreatic head carcinoma. Br J Surg. 2015;102:837–46.
27. Giovinazzo F, Turri G, Katz MH, Heaton N, Ahmed I. Meta-analysis of benefits of portal-superior mesenteric vein resection in pancreatic resection for ductal adenocarcinoma. Br J Surg. 2016;103:179–91.
28. Siriwardana HP, Siriwardena AK. Systematic review of outcome of synchronous portal-superior mesenteric vein resection during pancreatectomy for cancer. Br J Surg. 2006; 93:662–73.
29. Han SS, Park SJ, Kim SH, et al. Clinical significance of portal-superior mesenteric vein resection in pancreatoduodenectomy for pancreatic head cancer. Pancreas. 2012;41:102–6.

Pylorus-Resecting Pancreaticoduodenectomy

Manabu Kawai and Hiroki Yamaue

7.1 Transition of Pancreaticoduodenectomy

Pancreaticoduodenectomy (PD), in which distal stomach and duodenum were resected, was first performed by the German surgeon Kausch in 1912 [1] and later developed by the American surgeon Whipple for the treatment of carcinoma of the ampulla of Vater in 1941 [2]. Afterward, pylorus-preserving pancreaticoduodenectomy (PpPD), in which the whole stomach and 2.5 cm of duodenum were preserved, was described by Watson in 1944 [3]. Moreover, PpPD was popularized for the treatment of chronic pancreatitis as a modification of conventional PD with antrectomy reported by the American surgeons, Traverso and Longmire, in the late 1970s [4].

PpPD has been reported to reduce postgastrectomy syndromes such as dumping, diarrhea, and bile reflux gastritis or to have a better nutritional status compared to PD with antrectomy [5–9]. Therefore, PpPD has been generally accepted for surgical procedure of periampullary neoplasms such as pancreatic head cancer or bile duct cancer. However, several randomized controlled trials (RCTs) or meta-analysis comparing PD to PpPD have been conducted, and the two procedures are equivalent with regard to morbidity and mortality [10–16]. Moreover, several reports have discussed whether the preservation of the pylorus can provide a better nutritional status and more favorable quality of life (QOL) compared with PD [17–24]. The superiority concerning long-term nutrition or QOL between PD and PpPD remains still controversial.

Delayed gastric emptying (DGE) after PpPD is a persistent and frustrating complication, although DGE is not life-threatening complications. Moreover, it results in a prolonged length of stay that contributes to increase hospital costs and to

M. Kawai, M.D. (✉) • H. Yamaue, M.D.
Second Department of Surgery, School of Medicine, Wakayama Medical University,
811-1 Kimiidera, Wakayama 641-8510, Japan
e-mail: kawai@wakayama-med.ac.jp

© Springer Science+Business Media Singapore 2017
H. Yamaue (ed.), *Innovation of Diagnosis and Treatment for Pancreatic Cancer*,
DOI 10.1007/978-981-10-2486-3_7

decrease quality of life [23, 25–28]. To preserve pylorus ring with denervation or devascularization in PpPD may be a risk factor of DGE. In 2007, subtotal stomach preserving pancreaticoduodenectomy (SSPPD), in which duodenum and the stomach 2–3 cm proximal to the pylorus ring were removed, has been reported for periampullary and pancreas head tumors of malignancy by the Japanese surgeon Hayashibe [29]. However, the definition of SSPPD in resection site of stomach remains unclear. It has reported in 2011 that the new surgical procedure resecting just pylorus ring in pancreaticoduodenectomy was designed as pylorus-resecting pancreaticoduodenectomy (PrPD) [30].

7.2 Procedure of PrPD

In operative method, only the resection site of the stomach in PrPD is different from that in PpPD. The right gastric artery and vagal nerve are transected by the same levels in both PpPD and PrPD. The right gastric artery is dissected by the root, and the first pyloric branch is dissected along the lesser curvature of the stomach. The first pyloric branch of the right gastroepiploic artery is also dissected along the greater curvature of the stomach. The pyloric branch of the vagal nerve is dissected along with lymph nodes around the pylorus ring (Fig. 7.1). In PrPD, the stomach is divided just adjacent the pylorus ring and the nearly total stomach more than 95% is preserved (Fig. 7.2). As the first step in reconstruction during PrPD, the proximal jejunum is brought through the transverse mesocolon by the retrocolic route. Pancreaticojejunostomy after PrPD is performed by duct-to-mucosa using a single layer of interrupted absorbable stitches. In seromuscular-parenchymal anastomosis,

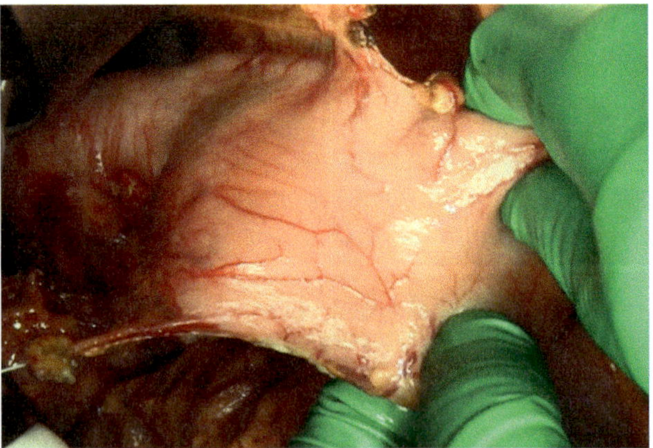

Fig. 7.1 Dissection around the pylorus ring; the right gastric artery is dissected by the root, and the first pyloric branch is dissected along the lesser curvature of the stomach. The first pyloric branch of the right gastroepiploic artery is also dissected along the greater curvature of the stomach

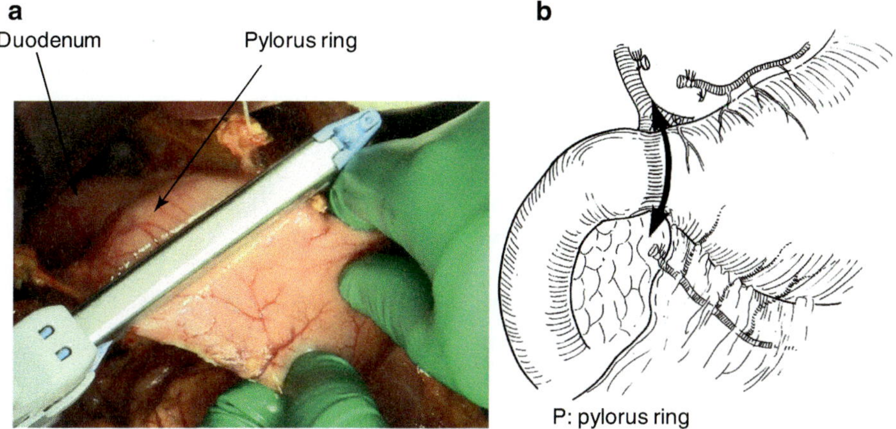

Fig. 7.2 (**a**) Resection site of the stomach in PrPD. (**b**) The stomach is divided just adjacent the pylorus ring

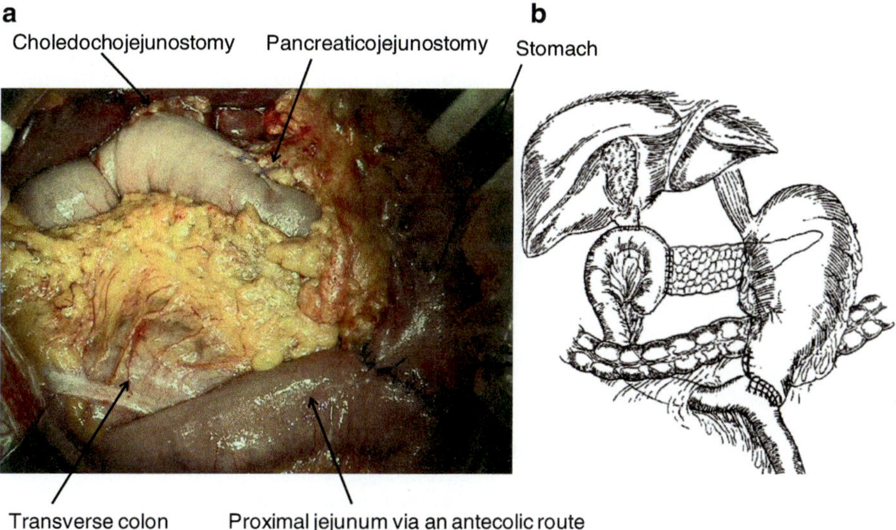

Fig. 7.3 (**a**) Gastrojejunostomy in PrPD is performed by a two layer anastomosis via an antecolic route. (**b**) The reconstruction is performed by conventional Billroth II reconstruction

nonabsorbable interrupted stiches are placed in end-to-side. Then, a single layer choledochojejunostomy is constructed using interrupted stitches without a stent. Gastrojejunostomy in PrPD is performed by a two-layer anastomosis via an antecolic route (Fig. 7.3). The final step is construction of the gastrojejunostomy using a two-layered anastomosis. The inner layer was 4–0 PDS-II and the outer layer used 3–0 silk for seromuscular anastomosis.

7.3   Which Is Better, PD, PpPD, or PrPD?

There are three types of procedures for periampullary tumors or pancreatic head cancer as follows: PD, PpPD, and PrPD. However, it remains still controversial which is better procedure to reduce postoperative complication or improve long-term outcomes among three procedures.

Five RCTs comparing PD with PpPD have been conducted regarding short-term outcomes and long-term outcomes (Table 7.1) [10–14]. These studies have

Table 7.1 Summary of five randomized controlled trials comparing PD to PpPD

Authors	Years	Variable	Sample size	DGE (%)	Definition of DGE[a]	PF[b] (%)	Mortality (%)
Lin et al. [10]	1999	PD	16	7	The nasogastric tube is left in place for 10 days or more plus one of the following: (1) Emesis after removal of nasogastric tube, (2) Reinsertion of nasogastric tube, or (3) Failure to progress with diet	0	7
		PpPD	15	38		13	0
Seiler et al. [11]	2000	PD	40	45	A persistent drainage via the nasogastric tube of more than 500 ml/day for at least 5 days after surgery, or recurrent vomiting in combination with edema of the gastrojejunostomy or duodenojejunostomy and proximal dilatation on contrast radiography	2	5
		PpPD	370	37		3	3
Tran et al. [12]	2004	PD	83	23	Gastric stasis requiring nasogastric intubation for 10 days or more or the inability to tolerate a regular diet on the 14th postoperative day	14	7
		PpPD	87	22		13	3
Seiler et al. [13]	2005	PD	66	45	A persistent drainage via the nasogastric tube of more than 500 ml/day for at least 5 days after surgery, or recurrent vomiting in combination with edema of the gastrojejunostomy or duodenojejunostomy and proximal dilatation on contrast radiography	2	3
		PpPD	64	31		3	2
Lin et al. [14]	2005	PD	19	0	The nasogastric tube is left in place for 10 days or more plus one of the following: (1) Emesis after removal of nasogastric tube, (2) Reinsertion of nasogastric tube, or (3) Failure to progress with diet	5	11
		PpPD	14	43		7	7

[a]*DGE* delayed gastric emptying
[b]*PF* pancreatic fistula

demonstrated that PpPD can facilitate a better nutritional status and more favorable quality of life without differences in mortality, morbidity, or oncologic outcomes, compared to PD. Regarding short-term outcomes, five RCTs revealed no significant differences in the incidence of postoperative complications such as pancreatic fistula, intra-abdominal abscess, or intra-abdominal bleeding between PD and PpPD. Two meta-analyses suggested that there were no significant differences in postoperative complications between PD and PpPD [15, 16]. PD had a mortality range of 0–7%, while the mortality due to PpPD ranged from 3 to 11% in the five RCTs. There were no significant differences between the two procedures regarding mortality. Therefore, the two procedures were equally effective for periampullary tumors in terms of morbidity and mortality.

Regarding long-term outcome between PD and PpPD, two RCTs have reported that body weight change and QOL did not exhibit significant differences between the two procedures [12, 13]. Seiler et al. used the Sickness Impact Profile (SIP), a standard questionnaire that assesses various physical, psychological, and social functions to compare the long-term QOL between PD and PpPD [13]. They reported that the capacity to work at 6 months after surgery was better after PpPD (77%) than after PD (56%), although the postoperative QOL did not significantly differ between the two procedures [13]. Regarding the survival rate between patients treated by PD and PpPD, Seiler et al. and Tran et al. in their RCTs reported that the long-term survival and disease-free survival were not significantly different between the two procedures [12, 13]. The two meta-analyses also suggested that there were also no significant differences in long-term survival between the two procedures. Therefore, the two procedures offered similar survival for periampullary tumors [15, 16].

7.4 The Impact of Pylorus-Resecting Pancreaticoduodenectomy (PrPD)

DGE is a persistent and frustrating complication in pancreaticoduodenectomy. Regarding DGE between PD and PpPD, Lin et al. reported that DGE occurred more frequently with PpPD (6 of 14 patients; 42.8%) than PD (0 of 19 patients; 0%) ($P < 0.05$) [14]. However, the sample size of this RCT was small ($n = 33$) and the RCT was limited to patients with pancreatic head cancer. On the other hand, Tran et al. reported in their RCT that no significant difference between PpPD (19 of 85 patients; 22%) and PD (18 of 80 patients; 23%) regarding the incidence of DGE [12] was observed. Seiler et al. also reported that there was no significant difference between PpPD (30 of 66 patients; 45%) and PD (20 of 64 patients; 31%) regarding the incidence of DGE [13]. The pathogenesis of DGE after PpPD has been thought to include several factors, such as (1) antroduodenal ischemia [31, 32], (2) gastric atony caused by vagotomy [33], (3) pylorospasm [34–36], (4) the absence of gastrointestinal hormones [37], (5) gastric dysrhythmia secondary to other complications such as a pancreatic fistula [38–40], and (6) antroduodenal congestion [41]. In particular, DGE after PpPD has been attributed to denervation and devascularization of the pyloric ring due to pylorospasms caused by surgical injuries of the vagus nerves

Table 7.2 Summary of comparative studies between PpPD and PrPD (SSPPD)

Authors	Study design	Years	Variable	Sample size	Definition of DGE[a]	DGE (%)	P value
Kurahara et al. [42]	Retrospective study	2010	PpPD	48	ISGPS[b]	34.8	NS
			SSPPD	64		13.0	
Kawai et al. [30]	Randomized controlled trial	2011	PpPD	64	ISGPS[b]	17.2	0.024
			PrPD	66		4.5	
Fujii et al. [43]	Retrospective study	2012	PpPD	33	ISGPS[b]	27.3[c]	0.0012
			SSPPD	56		5.8[c]	
Nanashima et al. [44]	Retrospective study	2013	PpPD	28	ISGPS[b]	46[c]	<0.01
			SSPPD	27		7[c]	
Hackert et al. [45]	Retrospective study	2013	PpPD	40	ISGPS[b]	42.5	0.0066
			PrPD	40		15.0	
Matsumoto et al. [46]	Randomized controlled trial	2014	PpPD	50	ISGPS[b]	20	NS
			SSPPD	50		12	

NS not significant, *PpPD* pylorus-preserving pancreaticoduodenectomy, *PrPD* pylorus-resecting pancreaticoduodenectomy, *SSPPD* subtotal stomach preserving pancreaticoduodenectomy
[a]Delayed gastric emptying
[b]Pancreatic fistula is defined according to the International Study Group of Pancreatic Surgery (ISGPS)
[c]The rate of ISGPS grade B/C

innervating the pyloric ring. In PrPD, the stomach is divided adjacent to the pylorus ring and more than 95% of the stomach is preserved, although the pylorus ring is resected. PrPD was designed with expectation in maintaining the favorable stomach pooling ability and reducing the incidence of DGE compared to PpPD [30]. The technical modification of resecting pylorus ring may provide a simple and effective method to prevent the incidence of DGE.

Table 7.2 shows summary for comparative study between PpPD and PrPD (SSPPD) [30, 42–46]. There are two RCTs and five retrospective studies which compared PpPD to PrPD (SSPPD) based on DGE defined by the international study group of pancreatic surgery (ISGPS) [47]. RCT which compared PpPD with PrPD demonstrated that PrPD (4.5%) resulted in a significant reduction in the incidence of DGE compared with PpPD (17.2%) ($P = 0.0244$) [30]. As the objective data for DGE in this study, the ^{13}C-acetate breath test, which is a simple and excellent indirect test to reflect gastric emptying, was examined. T_{max} (the time of peak ^{13}CO$_2$ content after the administration of ^{13}C-acetate) was reported to be a more useful marker reflecting gastric emptying. The time to peak ^{13}CO$_2$ content in the ^{13}C-acetate breath test at 1, 3, and 6 months postoperatively to evaluate gastric emptying was significantly delayed in the PpPD group compared with the PrPD group [30]. On the other hand, another RCT by Matsumoto et al. reported that the incidence of DGE was 20% with PpPD and 12% with SSPPD ($P = 0.414$) [46]. The RCT demonstrated that no significant difference in the incidence of DGE was observed between PpPD and SSPPD. Matsumoto et al. discussed that this discrepancy between two RCTS was due to differences in the study subjects. So, in their study, pancreatic cancer was excluded because patients with pancreatic cancer underwent a more invasive surgery including portal vein resection and regional lymph node dissection than other benign or low-grade malignant lesions. However, Fujii et al. reported that SSPPD offers better perioperative and long-term outcomes for pancreatic cancer compared to PpPD [44]. Two meta-analyses comparing PrPD with PpPD reported that PrPD resulted in a significant reduction of the incidence of DGE compared to PpPD [48, 49]. As a modified anastomosis to prevent occurrence of DGE in SSPPD, Nakamura et al. demonstrated the greater curvature side-to-side anastomosis of gastrojejunostomy [50]. In the side-to-side anastomosis, the jejunal loop is anastomosed to the greater curvature 5–10 cm proximal to the closed gastric stump, and the anastomosis is just the greater curvature, not the anterior nor the posterior wall of the stomach. The study reported that the incidence of DGE in side-to-side anastomosis was 2.5% in side-to-side anastomosis and 21.3% in end-to-side anastomosis ($P = 0.0002$). It was concluded that the greater curvature side-to-side anastomosis of gastrojejunostomy significantly reduced the incidence of DGE compared to the gastric stump-to-jejunal end-to-side anastomosis in SSPPD. Now, PROPP study which compares PrPD to PpPD by RCT with sample size for 89 patients per group has been proceeding by Hackert et al. in Germany [51].

7.5 Long-Term Outcomes in PrPD

Long-term outcomes for survivors have been becoming a great concern because advances in surgical techniques and perioperative management have led to a low mortality rate and long post-PD survival. In particular, nutritional status, body weight change, and late postoperative complications such as dumping syndrome, diarrhea, and marginal ulcer affect quality of life (QOL). The superiority of PrPD compared with PpPD regarding long-term outcomes remains still controversial. PrPD may have an equally favorable pooling ability in the stomach as PpPD. However, PrPD with resection of the pylorus ring may result in the more frequent occurrence of dumping syndrome than PpPD. The study for 2-year follow-up period between PpPD and PrPD has shown that only 1 of 66 patients (1.6%) with PrPD had dumping syndrome during follow-up, and the patients with dumping syndrome could be treated with dietary management alone. The study concluded that PrPD offers similar long-term outcomes with PpPD regarding QOL, nutritional status, and late complications [30]. The RCT by Matsumoto et al. also reported that SSPPD is equally effective in long-term nutritional status comparing to PpPD [46]. The study demonstrated that no significant differences were observed between PpPD and SSPPD regarding postoperative serum albumin levels, serum cholesterol levels, and body mass index during the 3-year follow-up period. On the other hand, Fujii et al. reported that serum albumin concentration and total lymphocyte count at 1 year postoperatively were significantly higher in SSPPD than in PpPD for patients with pancreatic cancer ($P = 0.0303$ and $P = 0.0203$, respectively) [44]. As the reason, they discussed that the gastric outlet diameter was larger after SSPPD than after PPPD, and this may have contributed to improved oral intake followed by more favorable nutritional status in their study.

Conclusion

There are three types of procedures for periampullary neoplasms as follows: PD, PpPD, and PrPD (SSPPD). However, it remains still controversial which is best procedure to improve both short-term outcomes and long-term outcomes. Several RCTs have clarified that PD and PpPD are equally effective for periampullary tumors regarding morbidity, mortality, QOL, and survival. Moreover, two meta-analyses comparing PrPD with PpPD reported that PrPD resulted in a significant reduction of the incidence of DGE compared to PpPD. Further studies are required to clarify the long-term QOL and/or nutritional status resulting after the use of these techniques. However, PrPD is one of the procedures that may be recommended for treatment of periampullary neoplasms including pancreatic adenocarcinoma.

References

1. Kausch W. Das Carnimom der Papilla duodeni und seine radikale Entfernung. Beitr Klin Chir. 1912;78:439–86.
2. Whipple AO, Parsons W, Mullins CR. Treatment of carcinoma of the ampulla of Vater. Ann Surg. 1935;102:763–79.
3. Watson K. Carcinoma of the ampulla of Vater. Successful radical resection. Br J Surg. 1944;31:368–73.
4. Traverso LW, Longmire WJ. Preservation of the pylorus in pancreaticoduodenectomy. Surg Gynecol Obstet. 1978;146:959–62.
5. Traverso LW, Longmire WJ. Preservation of the pylorus in pancreaticoduodenectomy: a follow-up evaluation. Ann Surg. 1980;192:306–10.
6. Jimenez RE, Femandez-del Castillo C, Rattner DW, et al. Outcome of pancreaticoduodenectomy with pylorus preservation or with antrectomy in the treatment of chronic pancreatitis. Ann Surg. 2000;231:293–300.
7. Brasssch JW, Deziel DJ, Rossi RL, et al. Pyloric and gastric preserving pancreatic resection. Experience with 87 patients. Ann Surg. 1986;204:411–8.
8. Hunt DR, McLean R. Pylorus-preserving pancreatectomy: functional results. Br J Surg. 1989;76:173–6.
9. van Berge Henegouwewn MI, van Gulik TM, De Wit LT, et al. Delayed gastric emptying after standard pancreaticoduodenectomy versus pylorus-preserving pancreaticoduodenectomy: an analysis of 200 consecutive patients. J Am Coll Surg. 1997;185:373–9.
10. Lin PW, Lin YJ. Prospective randomized comparison between pylorus preserving and standard pancreaticoduodenectomy. Br J Surg. 1999;86:603–7.
11. Seiler CA, Wagner M, Sadowski C, Kulli C, Büchler MW. Randomized prospective trial of pylorus-preserving vs classic duodenopancreatectomy (Whipple procedure): initial clinical results. J Gastrointest Surg. 2000;4:443–52.
12. Tran KTC, Smeenk HG, van Eijck CHJ, Kazemier G, Hop WC, Greve JWG, et al. Pylorus preserving pancreaticoduodenectomy versus standard Whipple procedure. A prospective, randomized, multicenter analysis of 170 patients with pancreatic and periampullary tumors. Ann Surg. 2004;240:738–45.
13. Seiler CA, Wagner M, Bachmann CA, Schmied RB, Friess UH, Büchler MW. Randomized clinical trial of pylorus-preserving duodenopancreatectomy versus classical Whipple resection-long term results. Br J Surg. 2005;92:547–56.
14. Lin PW, Shan YS, Lin YJ, Hung CJ. Pancreaticoduodenectomy for pancreatic head cancer: PPPD versus Whipple procedure. Hepato-Gastroenterology. 2005;52:1601–4.

15. Diener MK, Knaebel HP, Heukaufer C, Antes G, Büchler MW, Seiler CM. A systematic review and meta-analysis of pylorus-preserving versus classical pancreaticoduodenectomy for surgical treatment of periampullary and pancreatic carcinoma. Ann Surg. 2007;245:187–200.
16. Karanicolas PJ, Davies E, Kunz R, Briel M, Koka HP, Payne DM, et al. The pylorus: take it or leave it? Systematic review and meta-analysis of pylorus-preserving versus standard Whipple pancreaticoduodenectomy for pancreatic or periampullary cancer. Ann Surg Oncol. 2007;14:1825–34.
17. Takada T, Yasuda H, Amano H, Yoshida M, Ando H. Results of a pylorus-preserving pancreatoduodenectomy for pancreatic cancer: a comparison with results of the Whipple procedure. Hepato-Gastroenterology. 1997;44:1536–40.
18. Schniewind B, Bestmann B, Henne-Bruns D, Faendrich F, Kremer B, Kuechler T. Quality of life after pancreaticoduodenectomy for ductal adenocarcinoma of the pancreatic head. Br J Surg. 2006;93:1099–107.
19. Klinkenbejil JH, van der Schelling GP, Hop WC. The advantage of pylorus-preserving pancreatoduodenectomy in malignant disease of the pancreas and periampullary region. Ann Surg. 1992;216:142–5.
20. Di Carlo V, Zerbi A, Balzano G, Corso V. Pylorus-preserving pancreaticoduodenectomy versus conventional whipple operation. World J Surg. 1999;23:920–5.
21. Huang JJ, Yeo CJ, Sohn TA, Lillemoe KD, Sauter PK, Coleman J, et al. Quality of life and outcomes after pancreaticoduodenectomy. Ann Surg. 2000;231:890–8.
22. Ohtsuka T, Yamaguchi K, Ohuchida J, Inoue K, Nagai E, Chijiiwa K, et al. Comparison of quality of life after pylorus-preserving pancreatoduodenectomy and Whipple resection. Hepato-Gastroenterology. 2003;50:846–50.
23. Horstmann O, Markus PM, Ghadimi MB, Becker H. Pylorus preservation has no impact on delayed gastric emptying after pancreatic head resection. Pancreas. 2004;28:69–74.
24. van Berge Henegouwen MI, van Gulik TM, DeWit LT, Allema JH, Rauws EA, Obertop H, et al. Delayed gastric emptying after standard pancreaticoduodenectomy versus pylorus-preserving pancreaticoduodenectomy: an analysis of 200 consecutive patients. J Am Coll Surg. 1997;185:373–9.
25. El Nakeeb A, Askr W, Mahdy Y, et al. Delayed gastric emptying after pancreaticoduodenectomy. Risk factors, predictors of severity and outcome. A single center experience of 588 cases. J Gastrointest Surg. 2015;19:1093–100.
26. Yeo CJ, Cameron JL, Sohn TA, et al. Six hundred fifty consecutive pancreaticoduodenectomy in the 1990s: pathology, complications, and outcomes. Ann Surg. 1997;226:248–57.
27. Akizuki E, Kimura Y, Nobuoka T, et al. Reconsideration of postoperative oral intake tolerance after pancreaticoduodenectomy-prospective consecutive analysis of delayed gastric emptying according to the ISGPS definition and the amount of dietary intake. Ann Surg. 2009;249:986–94.
28. Hashimoto Y, Traverso LW. Incidence of pancreatic anastomotic failure and delayed gastric emptying after pancreatoduodenectomy in 507 consecutive patients: use of a web-based calculator to improve homogeneity of definition. Surgery. 2010;147:503–15.
29. Hayashibe A, Kameyama M, Shinbo M, et al. The surgical procedure and clinical results of subtotal stomach preserving pancreaticoduodenectomy (SSPPD) in comparison with pylorus preserving pancreaticoduodenectomy (PPPD). J Surg Oncol. 2007;95:106–9.
30. Kawai M, Tani M, Hirono S, Miyazawa M, Shimizu A, Uchiyama K, et al. Pylorus ring resection reduces delayed gastric emptying in patients undergoing pancreatoduodenectomy: a prospective randomized controlled trial of pylorus-resecting versus pylorus-preserving pancreatoduodenectomy. Ann Surg. 2011;253:495–501.
31. Ohwada S, Satoh Y, Kawate S, Yamada T, Kawamura O, Koyama T, et al. Low-dose erythromycin reduces delayed gastric emptying and improves gastric motility after Billroth I pylorus-preserving pancreaticoduodenectomy. Ann Surg. 2001;234:668–74.
32. Park JS, Hwang HK, Kim JK, Cho SI, Yoon DS, Lee WJ, et al. Clinical validation and risk factors for delayed gastric emptying based on the International Study Group of Pancreatic Surgery (ISGPS) classification. Surgery. 2009;146:882–7.

33. Itani KM, Coleman RE, Meyers WC, Akwari OE. Pylorus-preserving pancreaticoduodenectomy. A clinical and physiologic appraisal. Ann Surg. 1986;204:655–64.
34. Gauvin JM, Sarmiento JM, Sarr MG. Pylorus-preserving pancreaticoduodenectomy with complete preservation of the pyloroduodenal blood supply and innervation. Arch Surg. 2003;138:1261–3.
35. Fischer CP, Hong JC. Method of pyloric reconstruction and impact upon delayed gastric emptying and hospital stay after pylorus-preserving pancreaticoduodenectomy. J Gastrointest Surg. 2006;10:215–9.
36. Kim DK, Hindenburg AA, Sharma SK, Suk CH, Gress FG, Staszewski H, et al. Is pylorospasm a cause of delayed gastric emptying after pylorus-preserving pancreaticoduodenectomy? Ann Surg Oncol. 2005;12:222–7.
37. Kobayashi I, Miyachi M, Kanai M, Nagino M, Kondo S, Kamiya J, et al. Different gastric emptying of solid and liquid meals after pylorus-preserving pancreaticoduodenectomy. Br J Surg. 1998;85:927–30.
38. Räty S, Sand J, Lantto E, Nordback I. Postoperative acute pancreatitis as a major determinant of postoperative delayed gastric emptying after pancreaticoduodenectomy. J Gastrointest Surg. 2006;10:1131–9.
39. Riediger H, Makowiec F, Schareck WD, Hopt UT, Adam U. Delayed gastric emptying after pylorus-preserving pancreaticoduodenectomy is strongly related to other postoperative complications. J Gastrointest Surg. 2003;7:758–65.
40. Yeo CJ, Barry MK, Sauter PK, Sostre S, Lillemoe KD, Pitt HA, et al. Erythromycin accelerates gastric emptying following pancreaticoduodenectomy: a prospective, randomized placebo-controlled trial. Ann Surg. 1993;218:229–38.
41. Kurosaki I, Hatakeyama K. Preservation of the left gastric vein in delayed gastric emptying after pylorus-preserving pancreaticoduodenectomy. J Gastrointest Surg. 2005;9:846–52.
42. Kurahara H, Takao S, Shinchi H, et al. Subtotal stomach-preserving pancreaticoduodenectomy (SSPPD) prevents postoperative delayed gastric emptying. J Surg Oncol. 2010;102:615–9.
43. Fujii T, Kanda M, Kodera Y, et al. Preservation of the pyloric ring has little value in surgery for pancreatic head cancer: a comparative study comparing three surgical procedures. Ann Surg Oncol. 2012;19:176–83.
44. Nanashima A, Abo T, Sumida Y, et al. Comparison of results between pylorus-preserving pancreaticoduodenectomy and subtotal stomach-preserving pancreaticoduodenectomy: report at a single cancer institute. Hepato-Gastroenterology. 2013;60:1182–8.
45. Hackert T, Hinz U, Hartwig W, et al. Pylorus resection in partial pancreaticoduodenectomy: impact on delayed gastric emptying. Am J Surg. 2013;206:296–9.
46. Matsumoto I, Shinzeki M, Asari S, et al. A prospective randomized comparison between pylorus- and subtotal stomach-preserving pancreatoduodenectomy on postoperative delayed gastric emptying occurrence and long-term nutritional status. J Surg Oncol. 2014;109:690–6.
47. Wente MN, Bassi C, Dervenis C, et al. Delayed gastric emptying (DGE) after pancreatic surgery: a suggested definition by the International Study Group of Pancreatic Surgery (ISGPS). Surgery. 2007;142:761–8.
48. Hanna MM, Gadde R, Tamariz L, et al. Delayed gastric emptying after pancreaticoduodenectomy: is subtotal stomach preserving better or pylorus preserving? J Gastrointest Surg. 2015;19:1542–52.
49. Huang W, Xiong JJ, Wan MH, et al. Meta-analysis of subtotal stomach-preserving pancreaticoduodenectomy vs pylorus preserving pancreaticoduodenectomy. World J Gastroenterol. 2015;21:6361–73.
50. Nakamura T, Ambo Y, Noji T, et al. Reduction of the incidence of delayed gastric emptying in side-to-side gastrojejunostomy in subtotal stomach-preserving pancreaticoduodenectomy. J Gastrointest Surg. 2015;19:1425–32.
51. Hackert T, Bruckner T, Dörr-Harim C, et al. Pylorus resection or pylorus preservation in partial pancreatico-duodenectomy (PROPP study): study protocol for a randomized controlled trial. Trials. 2013;14:44.

Pancreaticoduodenectomy with Portal Vein Resection

8

Thilo Hackert, Jörg Kaiser, and Markus W. Büchler

Abbreviations

BR	Borderline resectable
CA 19-9	Carbohydrate antigen 19-9
CA	Celiac axis
CE-CT	Contrast-enhanced computed tomography
DP	Distal pancreatectomy
HA	Hepatic artery
ISGPS	International Study Group for Pancreatic Surgery
MRI	Magnet resonance imaging
NCCN	National Comprehensive Cancer Network
PD	Pancreato-duodenectomy
PDAC	Pancreatic ductal adenocarcinoma
PV	Portal vein
SMA	Superior mesenteric artery
SMV	Superior mesenteric vein
SV	Splenic vein

8.1 Diagnostic Workup

For the definition of local resectability in PDAC with venous involvement, the extension of the tumor towards the vascular structures, namely the superior mesenteric (SMV) and the portal vein (PV), must be evaluated preoperatively. A valid

T. Hackert • J. Kaiser • M.W. Büchler, M.D. (✉)
Department of General, Visceral and Transplantation Surgery, University of Heidelberg,
Im Neuenheimer Feld 110, 69120 Heidelberg, Germany
e-mail: Markus_Buechler@med.uni-heidelberg.de

© Springer Science+Business Media Singapore 2017
H. Yamaue (ed.), *Innovation of Diagnosis and Treatment for Pancreatic Cancer*,
DOI 10.1007/978-981-10-2486-3_8

evaluation can be done by contrast-enhanced computed tomography (CE-CT) [1]. This diagnostic modality is available in nearly all institutions and has become the standard diagnostic tool with sensitivity and specificity rates of 63–82% and 92–100%, respectively, with regard to PDAC diagnosis [2]. The use of a pancreas-specific CE-CT examination protocol with a 30° right-sided position of the patient and oral water intake to enhance the contrast in the gastroduodenal region is the basis to maximize accuracy in the preoperative diagnostics [3]. In case of contraindications for a CE-CT, magnet resonance imaging (MRI) can be used instead of CE-CT as the accuracy of MRI is comparable to CE-CT regarding diagnosis of PDAC and evaluation of the local tumor extension [2]. With regard to possible vascular involvement, the use of endoscopic ultrasound (EUS) has gained widespread acceptance today. This diagnostic tool shows best rates of sensitivity and specificity compared to CE-CT and MRI as it offers a very high resolution local imaging along the vessels [2]. The possible disadvantages of EUS include that—besides the invasive character of EUS from the patients' perspective—the region of interest is limited, the accuracy of EUS is depending on the examiner's experience, and the results of this dynamic examination can be reproduced only during the procedure itself. Therefore, EUS has to be regarded as a complementary tool to CE-CT or MRI and is not available as a standard procedure in all institutions.

Resectability is defined as (1) primary resectable PDAC, (2) borderline resectable (BR-PDAC), or (3) unresectable PDAC according to the criteria published by the International Study Group for Pancreatic Surgery (ISGPS) in 2014 [4], which are mainly based on the recommendations of the National Comprehensive Cancer Network [5]. Besides these two recently published definitions, two other classifications are in clinical use, namely the definition of the AHPBA/SSO/SSAT published in 2009 [6] and the M. D. Anderson criteria, that were published in 2006 [7].

All of these definitions are similar with regard to resectable PDAC. This implies that the tumor does not involve any vascular structures [no distorsion of SMV or PV and clearly preserved fat planes towards celiac axis (CA) and AMS].

BR-PDAC is characterized by a distorsion/narrowing or occlusion of the respective veins but a technical possibility of reconstruction on the proximal and distal margin of the veins. PV involvement according to the M. D. Anderson definition does not include contact or narrowing of the vein, but gives occlusion as the criterion for BR-PDAC. With regard to the arterial structures, all definitions describe a semi-circumferential abutment (<180°) of the SMA or an attachment at the hepatic artery (HA) without contact towards the CA as borderline resectable.

Unresectable PDAC is defined as a more extended involvement (>180°) of the SMA, CA, aorta, or inferior vena cava as well as a venous (SMV/PV) involvement without a possibility for surgical reconstruction of the venous tract due to the lack of a suitable luminal diameter of the feeding and/or draining vein. This situation is most likely associated with tumor-associated portal cavernous transformation.

The therapeutic recommendations for resectable and unresectable PDAC are clearly defined. While patients with resectable PDAC should undergo surgical exploration and radical resection, in case of unresectable PDAC, the option of neoadjuvant treatment should be considered as the therapy of choice with the chance of a re-evaluation and eventually surgical exploration. In BR-PDAC, therapeutic decisions have to differentiate between venous and arterial vessel involvement. In venous BR-PDAC, upfront surgery should be performed and—if the intraoperative finding matches the presumed borderline situation as defined above—completed as an en bloc tumor removal with venous replacement [8, 9]. In contrast, when suspected arterial BR-PDAC is intraoperatively found to be a true arterial involvement, no general recommendation for resection is given. For these patients, neoadjuvant treatment with a consecutive re-exploration and the option for a secondary resection is possible as well as direct arterial resection in exceptional cases or under study conditions.

8.2 Classification of Venous Involvement

Several groups around the world have proposed to categorize venous involvement preoperatively [10–12]. These scoring systems are mainly based on CE-CT and the extent of tumor contact towards the major venous vessels. A recent study including 98 patients used a four-stage classification (no tumor–vein interface, <180° interface, >180° interface, and complete occlusion of the vein). The analysis showed that the threshold of >180° contact correlates well with the need for venous resection (90% of the patients), the true histopathological involvement of the vein (82.4% of the patients), and the survival prognosis (30.9 months vs. 37.3 months in patients with a <180° interface) [10]. Other score systems with three- or four-staged classifications based on preoperative CE-CT imaging analysis showed comparable correlations [11, 12]. However, none of these systems has been accepted as a routine tool to predict prognosis or stratify patients preoperatively in surgical decision making. From the clinical point of view, resectability depends on the possibility to prepare vein of a suitable diameter on both resection margins. Towards the liver, this is generally possible in most patients; however, the distal venous vessel may be too small to create an anastomosis with a sufficient diameter to drain the small bowel without resulting in congestion or thrombosis. Consequently, the ISGPS has defined unresectability with regard to a venous tumor involvement as an "unreconstructable SMV/portal vein occlusion," regardless of the extent of venous infiltration [4].

Basically, an accurate diagnostic workup and the abovementioned classifications allow a sufficient planning of the surgical procedure. This is essential to avoid unplanned resection for two reasons. First, harvesting a graft may be necessary and should be done before the resection itself. Second, an unplanned resection may result in a prolonged need for clamping of the SMV/PV with a consequent—at least partial—warm ischemia of the small bowel. As this can result in edema and hemorrhage of the bowel, the time of clamping and reconstruction should be kept as short as possible and a synchronous clamping of the AMS may help to avoid these complications.

Despite a most exact preparation, unplanned venous resection can occur and has been reported in a recent publication with regard to its surgical and oncological outcome [13]. In a cohort of 66 patients who underwent PV resection, the proportion of unplanned resections was 41%. Unplanned resections were required for tumors that had been underestimated preoperatively with regard to venous infiltration due to a significantly smaller diameter than tumors in the patients with a planned resection. Regarding surgical morbidity, the unplanned approach was not inferior to predicted resection, and although the rate of R1 resections at the vascular cut margin was higher during unplanned procedures, this had no influence on long-term oncological outcome [13].

8.3 Technical Aspects of Venous Resections

8.3.1 Types of Resections

Historically, major vessel involvement has been a contraindication to PDAC resection. In 1973, Fortner first described and classified a surgical approach of regional pancreatectomy with en bloc resection of peripancreatic soft tissue, regional lymph nodes and PV resection (type I), or resection and reconstruction of a major artery (type II) [14]. These initial extended resections, which were associated with a high morbidity (67%) and mortality (23%) as well as low survival rates (3-year survival rate 3%), discouraged generalized adoption of major vessel resection and reconstruction [14]. However, major advances in radiological and surgical techniques improved preoperative staging and reduced surgical morbidity and mortality [15–17]. A tumor-related complete obstruction of the portal vein must not be regarded as an obstacle for a resection. Although surgical preparation may be more difficult due to the collateral vessels, the restoration of the portal venous flow after resection and anastomosis offers an adequate drainage of the bowel despite the removal of most of the collateral vessels that may be necessary during the preparation. Basically, four types of reconstruction after venous resection can be differentiated (Fig. 8.1, [4, 18]). Type 1 is characterized by a tangential resection if this is possible, considering the localization and length of tumor invasion. Mostly, tumor infiltration

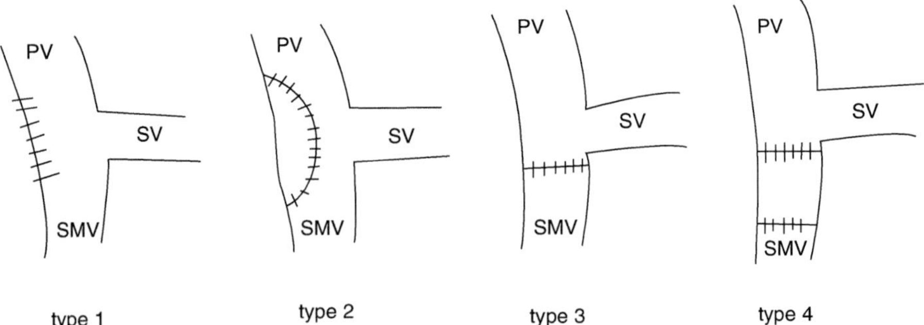

Fig. 8.1 Types of venous reconstruction [4, 18]. *PV* portal vein, *SV* splenic vein, *SMV* superior mesenteric vein

reaches the vein from the right circumference, sometimes allowing the resection of a small patch to directly close the defect without a hemodynamically relevant stenosis. However, the congestion of the venous drainage of the small bowel needs to be ensured. This is certainly possible either by direct flow measurement or by the macroscopic judgement of the experienced surgeon during the remaining operation time, which is usually about 2 h it takes to complete the reconstruction phase with jejunal anastomoses of the pancreas, the bile duct and the duodenum or stomach. In case of a vein stenosis resulting from a direct tangential suture, a type 1 method is not possible and the site of resection can be augmented by a patch (type 2 reconstruction). The patch can be taken from an autologous vein (i.e., saphenous vein), with the disadvantage that an additional preparation is required. To avoid this, a peritoneal patch, which is easily available from the abdominal wall, can alternatively be used [19]. Therefore, a composite of peritoneum and dorsal rectus abdominal muscle fascia is suitable to create an appropriate size without problems. By this method, not only a lateral augmentation (Fig. 8.2) is possible, but it can also be used to produce a tubular graft with the objective to bridge segmental defects.

Type 3 and type 4 of reconstruction imply a segmental resection, resulting in a longer defect of the venous axis. For all attempts of these resections, the mesenteric root should be mobilized completely by resolving the attachment of the right

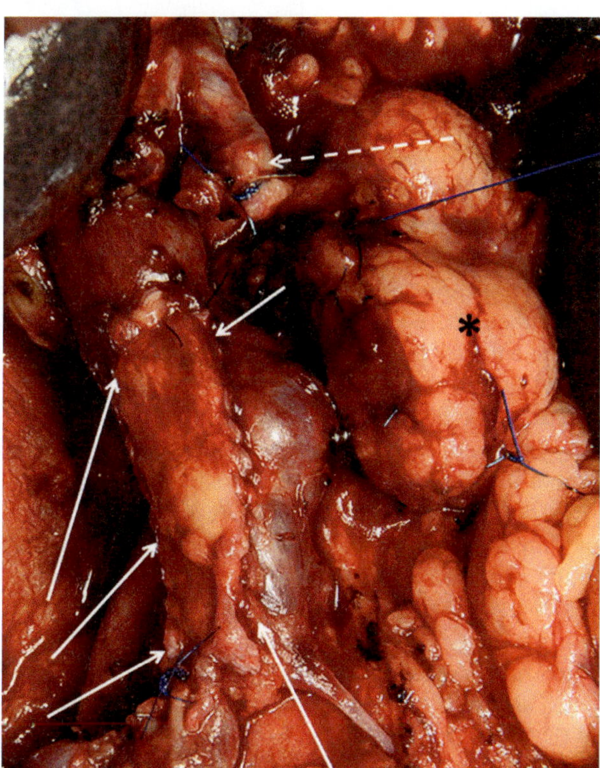

Fig. 8.2 PV reconstruction type 2. Tangential resection and reconstruction by using a peritoneal patch (*white arrows*). Hepatic artery with stump of the gastroduodenal artery (*broken white arrow*), pancreatic remnant (*black star*)

Fig. 8.3 PV/SMV resection during total PD. Type 3 reconstruction without reinsertion of the splenic vein due to concomitant splenectomy. SMV/PV anastomosis (*white circle*), hepatic artery with stump of the gastroduodenal artery (*white arrow*), completely dissected SMA (*black arrow*)

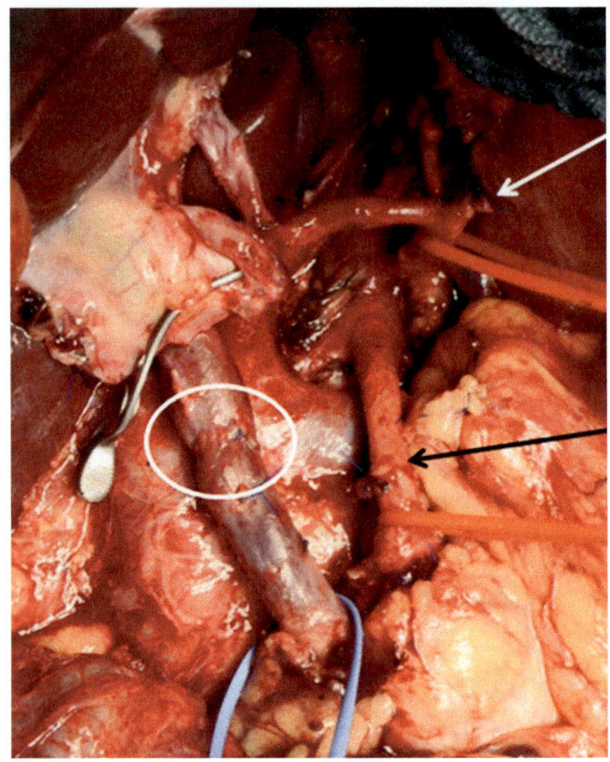

hemicolon to the retroperitoneal adhesions (Cattell-Braasch manoeuver [20]). This allows to bridge even long distances after resection of the vein and graft interposition (type 4) can often be avoided.

In type 3 resections, SMV/PV continuity is restored by a direct end-to-end anastomosis (Fig. 8.3). In case of corresponding diameters of the distal and proximal lumen, there is no obstacle for free venous drainage of the bowel. If it is not possible to bridge the resected length by approximation of the proximal and distal vessel lumen and performing a direct anastomosis, a vascular graft needs to be inserted. For this type 4 reconstruction, autologous as well as allogenous grafts can be used. Regarding autologous grafts, there are various possibilities (Table 8.1). Most commonly, the saphenous vein, the left renal vein (in case of patency of the ipsilateral ovarian/testicular vein to preserve kidney drainage), or the internal jugular vein have been described (Table 8.1, [21–33]). All of these grafts imply that a harvesting procedure must be performed and that the respective vessel is available and suitable with respect to the diameter and to the length which is needed for the reconstruction. As described before, also a peritoneal patch may be harvested and used to create a tubular graft (i.e., by placing the patch around a drainage tube and form the graft by longitudinal suture [19]). All of the described techniques of autologous graft insertion have been reported with good outcomes regarding postoperative morbidity and patency [21–34]. If no

Table 8.1 Methods of reconstruction in type 4 venous resections

• Peritoneal patch
• Left Renal vein
• Gonadal vein
• Saphenous vein
• Internal jugular vein
• External iliacal vein
• Allogenous iliacal vein (deceased donors)
• Bovine patch
• PTFE prosthesis

autologous graft material is available or in case of unplanned venous resection, that requires an "emergency" reconstruction, synthetic material represents a valid option for reconstruction, as well [28, 30]. A ringed polytetrafluoroethylene (PTFE) graft seems preferable as this type of prosthesis offers excellent flow conditions and patency rates [30, 34, 35]. The disadvantage of inserting a synthetic graft lies in the fact that any artificial material may cause problems in case of infection or anastomotic leakage. The in situ situation of a graft in combination with a pancreatic fistula must be regarded as a high-risk constellation for arrosional bleeding or for long-lasting graft infection, which is known difficult to treat. However, in recent clinical studies, no difference in surgical outcome and long-term survival was shown when different types of venous reconstruction (venorrhaphy, end-to-end anastomosis, graft insertion) were compared [30].

An unsolved problem is the confirmation of a R0 situation during PV/SMV resection. As the small bowel does not tolerate warm ischemia due to complete venous congestion (regardless of a synchronous clamping of the SMA) for a long time, the performance of a frozen section of the distal and proximal cut margin of the resected vein segment cannot be routinely performed. From large series, the R1 rate in this position ranges from 13% up to 50% [25, 26, 30]. Despite these considerably high rates in some studies, the oncological outcome may not be compromised and seems to be mostly determined by other factors (i.e., lymphatic spread, lymph node metastases, R1 status in other positions [16]).

Management of the splenic vein is another important issue in segmental resections of the SMV/PV [36]. If the site of resection is located clearly above or below the splenic vein confluence, this can be preserved without any changes in the physiological venous drainage of spleen and stomach. However, as the venous confluence is often the site of tumor infiltration, the proximal splenic vein is often part of the resected specimen. From the technical point of view, the splenic vein can be closed or reinserted during venous resection in PD. In case of lateral reinsertion of the splenic vein, it must be assured that no tangential tension on the venous anastomoses occurs (Fig. 8.4). This may otherwise promote narrowing and thrombosis of the respective vessels. Therefore, a closure of the splenic vein without reinsertion can be advisable in certain situations as long as this does not compromise splenic and gastric drainage which is sustained via left-sided collaterals in many patients.

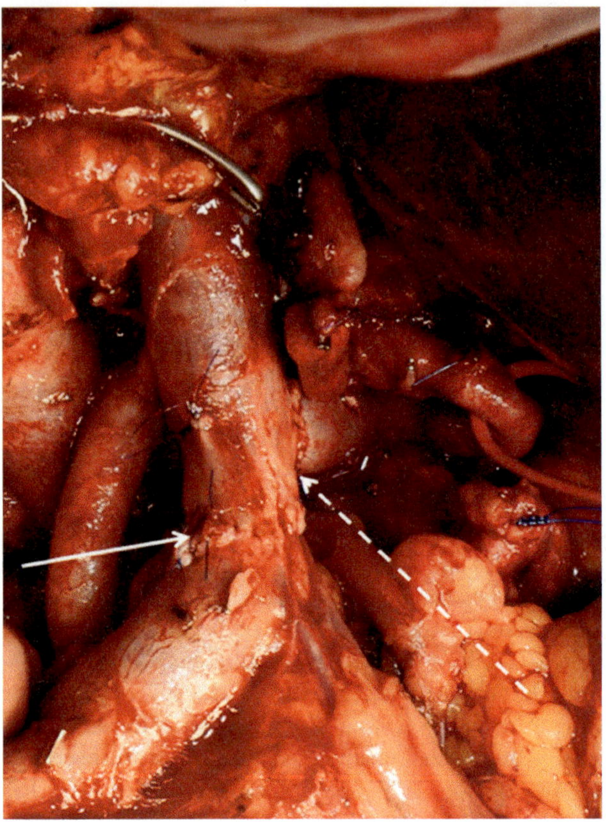

Fig. 8.4 PV/SMV resection during PD with reinsertion of the splenic vein. *White arrow*: SMV/PV anastomosis, *broke white arrow*: reinsertion of the splenic vein

Another aspect that has to be taken into account during venous resections is the perfusion of the right hemicolon. In case of removal of the middle colic vein or the ileocolic vein, which are common locations for lymph node metastases in PDAC [37], a right colectomy may be necessary to avoid colon-associated ischemic complications.

In distal pancreatectomy (DP), venous resections are less frequently performed. The technical challenge during this procedure is the fact that the remaining pancreatic head may block the approximation of the proximal and distal lumen and consequently create tension of both ends when a direct suture is attempted. Furthermore, a lateral compression of the anastomosis with a consequent thrombosis may occur. To avoid both of these situations, a segmental graft insertion is advisable to achieve best rates of patency. Due to the high risk of postoperative pancreatic fistula in DP, autologous graft material should be chosen and a synthetic graft with the inherent risk of fistula-associated infection should be avoided.

Regarding total PD with venous resections, an end-to-end anastomosis with or without graft insertion is possible and the splenic vein is generally removed as most total PDs for oncological indications include splenectomy. In this situation, the venous drainage of the stomach needs to be considered, i.e., by preserving the gastric coronary vein (see Sect. 8.4). Otherwise, an adopted resection of the stomach must be performed to avoid ischemic complications.

8.3.2 Laparoscopic/Robotic PD with Venous Reconstruction

Laparoscopic as well as robotic PD with venous reconstruction has been reported in small case series [38–42]. The respective studies have included between 11 and 34 patients for laparoscopic and robotic approaches, respectively. In all studies, surgical outcome has been proven to be comparable or even superior to open resections, especially with regard to blood loss. The disadvantages, however, include the significantly longer operation times and the excess costs, especially associated with robotic approaches. An Italian publication by Boggi et al. [39] showed that these costs account to app. 6200 Euro per procedure. Furthermore, the authors of all reports confirm that these procedures require a great expertise and are only applicable for highly selected patients. Consequently, the impact of minimally invasive PD with venous resections may increase in the future. To date, these procedures have to be regarded as highly limited approaches that are only available in specialized centers and scientific evidence for their usefulness in terms of surgical or oncological outcomes to justify the burden of excess costs is still lacking.

8.3.3 Venous Resection in Multivisceral Approaches

The resection of adjacent organs during PDAC surgery is an established procedure to achieve a radical tumor removal [43–46]. Although multivisceral resection is associated with an increased morbidity, perioperative mortality and long-term survival are not influenced in these patients. In approximately 20% of the patients, multivisceral resection is performed together with portal or superior mesenteric vein resections [43, 46]. This additional procedure does not increase the risk for complications and should therefore be performed in patients qualifying for an extended approach of complete tumor removal.

8.3.4 Combined Vascular Resections

Resection of the portal or superior mesenteric vein in combination with the celiac axis or mesenteric artery is—comparable to arterial resections alone—not a standard procedure and has only be performed in a small number of patients to date [46–48]. It may be an individual option for selected patients, especially after neoadjuvant treatment. Although it may be technically feasible, oncological outcome of these procedures is determined by the arterial tumor encasement. The oncological value of combined resection of both—portal vein and celiac axis or superior mesenteric artery—has not been proven in larger series. Furthermore, combined resections may be associated with a higher surgical morbidity and impaired postoperative quality of life than standard pancreatic operations, especially with regard to intestinal discomfort and diarrhea due to a higher risk of autonomous denervation of the small bowel during the extensive dissection of perivascular tissue including the respective nerve plexus.

8.4 Special Aspects and Limitations of Venous Resections

8.4.1 Gastric Coronary Vein

During preparation for venous resection, the gastric coronary vein may be injured accidentally or by intention in the case of tumor adherence. The coronary vein, or left gastric vein, drains both the anterior and posterior stomach walls, which results in the relevant physiological importance of this vessel for the perfusion of the stomach [49]. There are two major anatomical variations, as the junction of the coronary and portal vein may be located above or within the confluence of the splenic and portal vein (variant A) or the coronary vein may drain into the splenic vein (variant B) in a situation in which the junction may be located as far left as the junction between the splenic and inferior mesenteric vein [50]. In both situations, the coronary vein may be injured or sacrificed during portal vein resection at the level of the confluence. Especially when total PD is performed in combination with splenectomy, venous drainage of the stomach may be severely compromised, leading to venous congestion and consequent ischemia. A comparable situation can arise, when partial PD is combined with portal vein resection and the splenic vein is not reinserted, which must not be necessarily performed. Acutely compromised venous drainage of the stomach often results in visible intraoperative congestion and ischemia of the stomach. Consecutively, a resection of the stomach has to be performed or the venous drainage needs to be restored. Furthermore, long-term complications, such as left-sided portal hypertension, may occur due to impaired venous drainage of the stomach.

During PD in variant A anatomical situation, the portal vein resection may be performed below the level of the coronary–portal vein junction which preserves sufficient stomach drainage, irrespective of the splenic vein. Second, the coronary vein may be preserved in variant B anatomy when the splenic vein is reinserted into the portal vein after resection. A reinsertion of the splenic vein is not always possible and advisable, as the spleen may put tension on or twist the portal vein anastomosis, resulting in a risk of immediate or postoperative portal vein thrombosis. In this third situation, the spleen can be preserved without reconstruction of the splenic vein, if the coronary vein is reinserted, which can usually be performed without tension and ensures the drainage of both the spleen and the stomach.

In total PD for malignancies, the spleen, including its vessels, is routinely removed. In a variant A anatomical setting, this is not associated with any problems as long as the coronary vein is not injured during dissection or lymphadenectomy, and the stomach may be completely preserved. In the case of portal vein resection, including the coronary and portal vein junction, injury of the coronary vein or in variant B anatomical situations, the coronary vein is cut and the stomach is consecutively drained via the remaining cranial short gastric vessels that are connected to the esophageal drainage. Therefore, the body and fundus of the stomach are subjected to severe venous congestion. In this situation, the remaining part of the coronary vein should be reinserted to avoid intraoperative gastric resection or postoperative complications due to underestimation of this congestion.

Reinsertion of the coronary vein can be performed in an end-to-side fashion. Whenever possible, depending on the extent of resection, a patch of the splenic vein (anatomical variant B) should be preserved during preparation to enable a wider anastomosis and thereby lower the potential risk of thrombosis. The anastomosis is located above the portal vein anastomosis. As the coronary-portal vein anastomosis is the only outlet of venous drainage, the high blood flow will widen the diameter of the vessel and a thrombosis is unlikely to occur. When performing the coronary vein anastomosis, it is of utmost importance to ensure that no twisting of the vein or tension occurs. As the stomach is completely mobile, the coronary vein can always be approximated easily, even when a segment has been removed during the resection phase [51].

Restoration of stomach drainage has to be evaluated intraoperatively after completion of the reinsertion before completing the gastrointestinal reconstruction. In the postoperative period, a direct control of patency of the coronary vein is not possible. In case of suspected occlusion and consecutive gastric perfusion problems, an endoscopic control of the stomach is the examination of choice to evaluate potential ischemia.

Impairment of gastric drainage can result in two postoperative clinical scenarios, either an immediate intraoperative ischemia with the ultimate consequence of a potentially subtotal or even total gastrectomy, or in a delayed postoperative stomach perfusion failure. The latter may lead to either revision with stomach resection or—if less pronounced—to a long-lasting delayed gastric emptying. Both of these problems can be avoided if careful attention is paid to the coronary vein and a reinsertion is performed when necessary.

As subtotal or even total gastrectomy combined with partial or total PD is associated with an impairment of the patients' quality of life and may be associated with increased perioperative morbidity [46], surgical approaches should aim to preserve the stomach, unless a resection is required for oncological reasons. Another aspect besides acute perfusion failure of the stomach is the development of chronic left-sided portal hypertension following splenic vein obstruction or resection [52–55]. This condition may lead to a porto-caval collateral circulation with variceal vessel transformations, especially in the lower esophagus and the cardia. As the coronary vein is a vessel of a rather large diameter, this implies that it has the capacity to drain both the spleen and the stomach, which lowers the risk of the thrombotic occlusion of the coronary-portal vein anastomosis on the one hand and makes the occurrence of left-sided portal hypertension unlikely, on the other hand.

8.4.2 Limitations of Venous Resections

The two major limitations in venous resections are: (1) a tumor infiltration which is located in a peripheral position of the SMV and does not allow to prepare a sufficient diameter of the distal vessel for an adequate anastomosis and (2) a cavernous transformation of the venous system in terms of SMV/PV thrombosis and consecutive collateral perfusion (Fig. 8.5).

The first situation must generally be regarded as a contraindication to resection as no adequate drainage of the small bowel can be achieved or it is associated with a very high risk of postoperative thrombosis of the reconstruction. Neoadjuvant therapy is not useful as it will not lead to a revascularization of the SMV and therefore will not result in resectability.

With regard to venous thrombosis and collateralization, two aspects need to be critically evaluated. On one hand, a resection may solve the problem as the collaterals—which are removed during pancreatic head resection—are replaced by the anastomosis with a free venous drainage of the intestine. Prerequisite for this approach are sufficient diameters of the PV towards the liver hilum and the SMV towards the small bowel. On the other hand, interventional approaches with preoperative stent placement to overcome thrombosis with a consequent decrease of the collateralization have been reported [56]. These attempts include endovascular stenting of the PV/SMV axis which can facilitate resection technically and reduce intraoperative blood loss as the collateral vessels can be controlled [56].

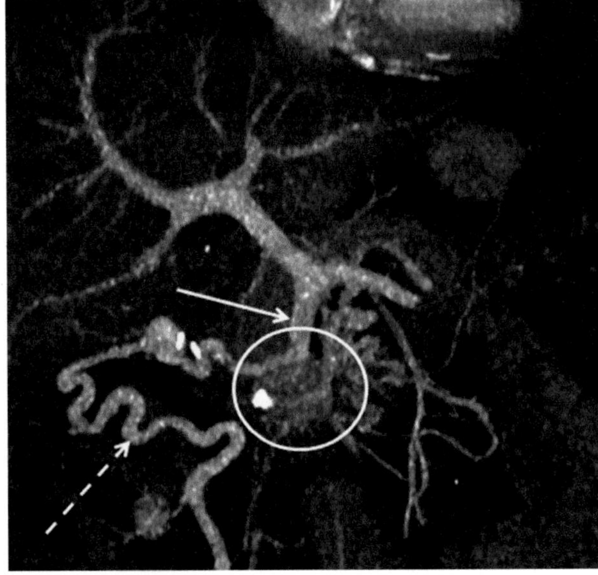

Fig. 8.5 Limitation of portal vein resection. Complete occlusion of the distal SMV by a large PDAC (*white circle*). Collateral vessels and main circulation via the ileocolic vein (*broken white arrow*) to the proximal SMV (*white arrow*)

8.5 Outcome of Venous Resection

Venous resections on PDAC surgery can be performed safely, which has been demonstrated in large series that showed surgical morbidity and mortality rates comparable to pancreatic head resections without vascular involvement [25, 26, 43]. Consequently, the recommendations to perform venous resections to achieve a radical (R0) tumor removal have been implemented in national and international guidelines as well as consensus statements [4, 5, 57]. These recommendations are meanwhile scientifically examined and based not only on large cohort studies but on systematic reviews and meta-analyses [8, 9].

Postoperative patency and thrombosis incidence of PV anastomoses and grafts has been investigated in several trials with regard to short- and long-term outcome [58–64]. In a Korean study on 55 patients undergoing venous resection, a 1-year patency of 80% and 5-year patency of 70% were reported [58]. These results correlated with the underlying pathology and were best for ampullary and bile duct cancer, while PDAC showed a higher risk for venous occlusion. Furthermore, the authors could demonstrate that this observation is associated with decreased survival, certainly also explained by the original tumors themselves. Other studies report 1-year patency rates between 70 and 90% and have shown an association with survival, as well [59, 60]. While chronic SMV/PV occlusion does rarely cause clinically relevant problems and is mainly caused by tumor recurrence, acute postoperative stenosis or thrombosis requires interventional or surgical revision due to the problem of bowel congestion and liver ischemia, which is associated with a high mortality [65]. In case of acute occlusion of the anastomosis of the inserted graft, operative revision with thrombectomy is required in most patients to avoid these complications (Fig. 8.6, [62, 63]). Furthermore, interventional stent placement via

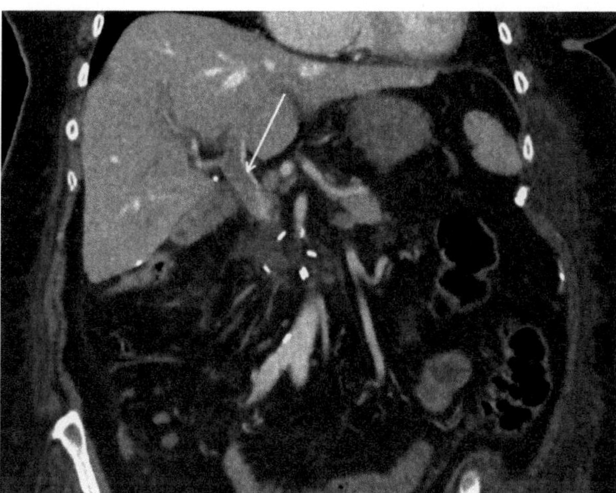

Fig. 8.6 Postoperative CE-CT (coronary formatting) after type 4 PV resection showing a complete venous thrombosis on postoperative day 2 (*white arrow*). Indication for reoperation, surgical thrombectomy, and reanastomosis. Uneventful postoperative course after revision

a transhepatic approach has been described for acute as well as chronic occlusion [61]. This possibility can be considered; however, it requires a high level of radiological expertise and has only been described anecdotally to date. Regarding anticoagulation after venous resection, most authors recommend initial heparin application during the hospital stay, followed by aspirin to improve long-term patency rates [58–60].

Besides the specific complication of venous thrombosis, other perioperative and long-term oncological outcome parameters have been well investigated in systematic reviews and meta-analyses. One systematic review by Siriwardena et al. [8] included 52 publications with 6333 patients in whom pancreatic resection was performed for PDAC. One thousand six hundred and forty six of these patients (26%) underwent synchronous portal–superior mesenteric vein resection mainly together with partial (71%) or total PD (24%). Median operation time was nearly 8.5 h with a median blood loss of 1750 ml, perioperative mortality of 5.9%, and overall morbidity of 42% (9–78%). The long-term survival of 1351 patients after portal–superior mesenteric vein resection was 13 months, with 1-, 3-, and 5-year overall survival rates of 50, 18, and 8%. The wide variations of outcome parameters (e.g., perioperative mortality, operative time, blood loss) reflect the inhomogeneous collective and the wide range of experience within the participating centers included in this review. However, despite these methodological problems, the long-term survival rate demonstrates that resection of the portal or superior mesenteric vein is potentially curative and the involvement of the mesenteric or portal vein seems to be rather a consequence of the tumor located close to these structures than a reflection of an uncommonly aggressive tumor biology. Histologically, portal vein invasion was detected in 64% of the resected specimens, varying between 3 and 86% in the different series. In addition, 67% of all patients with portal–superior mesenteric vein resection had positive lymph nodes detected on histology.

A more recent meta-analysis by Zhou et al. [9] involved 19 studies of pancreatectomies for PDAC, including 661 patients with and 2247 patients without portomesenteric venous resections. Both groups were characterized by comparable surgical outcome. Furthermore, in terms of oncological results, no difference in overall survival between both patient collectives was found, resulting in a 5-year survival rate of 12.3%, which is certainly superior to palliative treatment.

The most recent multicenter study on 406 patients submitted to pancreatectomy with en bloc SMV and/or PV resection for PDAC showed an overall morbidity of 52% and mortality of 7% [26]. Histological invasion of the resected vein was confirmed in 57% of specimens. Compared to the abovementioned studies, oncological outcome was even superior with a median survival of 24 months and 5-year survival of 24%, respectively. In this study, multivariate analysis demonstrated a significant correlation between overall survival and histological venous invasion as well as the administration of adjuvant therapy. These results underline that—although technically feasible—all surgical approaches have to be embedded in a multidisciplinary oncological concept to achieve best results for patient outcome, especially with regard to the common finding of an N1 status in this situation.

In conclusion, PV/SMV resection in BR-PDAC surgery is a valid and accepted procedure to achieve a radical tumor removal. Based on high-level evidence, perioperative and oncological outcomes are comparable to standard resections. Therefore, national and international guidelines and consensus statements recommend this procedure today. Depending on the anatomical situation of tumor infiltration, different types of venous resections can be differentiated, including direct suture techniques as well as graft insertion. Limitations in venous resections may occur due to distal occlusion of the SMV making a safe anastomosis technically impossible due to the small diameter of the distal vessel lumen with a high risk of thrombosis or insufficient drainage of the intestine. Future directions include laparoscopic and robotic approaches to venous resections as well as the emerging paradigm of neoadjuvant treatment for BR-PDAC.

References

1. Klauss M, Mohr A, von Tengg-Kobligk H, et al. A new invasion score for determining the resectability of pancreatic carcinomas with contrast-enhanced multidetector computed tomography. Pancreatology. 2008;8(2):204–10.
2. Shrikhande SV, Barreto SG, Goel M, et al. Multimodality imaging of pancreatic ductal adenocarcinoma: a review of the literature. HPB (Oxford). 2012;14(10):658–68.
3. Grenacher L, Klauss M. Computed tomography of pancreatic tumors. Radiologe. 2009;49(2): 107–23.
4. Bockhorn M, Uzunoglu FG, Adham M, International Study Group of Pancreatic Surgery, et al. Borderline resectable pancreatic cancer: a consensus statement by the International Study Group of Pancreatic Surgery (ISGPS). Surgery. 2014;155(6):977–88.
5. Tempero MA, Malafa MP, Behrman SW, et al. Pancreatic adenocarcinoma, version 2.2014: featured updates to the NCCN guidelines. J Natl Compr Cancer Netw. 2014;12(8):1083–93.
6. Callery MP, Chang KJ, Fishman EK, et al. Pretreatment assessment of resectable and borderline resectable pancreatic cancer: expert consensus statement. Ann Surg Oncol. 2009;16(7):1727–33.
7. Varadhachary GR, Tamm EP, Abbruzzese JL, et al. Borderline resectable pancreatic cancer: definitions, management, and role of preoperative therapy. Ann Surg Oncol. 2006;13(8): 1035–46.
8. Siriwardana H, Siriwardena A. Systematic review of outcome of synchronous portal-superior mesenteric vein resection during pancreatectomy for cancer. Br J Surg. 2006;93:662–73.
9. Zhou Y, Zhang Z, Liu Y, et al. Pancreatectomy combined with superior mesenteric vein-portal vein resection for pancreatic cancer: a meta-analysis. World J Surg. 2012;36(4):884–91.
10. Tran Cao HS, Balachandran A, Wang H, et al. Radiographic tumor-vein interface as a predictor of intraoperative, pathologic, and oncologic outcomes in resectable and borderline resectable pancreatic cancer. J Gastrointest Surg. 2014;18(2):269–78.
11. Marinelli T, Filippone A, Tavano F, et al. A tumour score with multidetector spiral CT for venous infiltration in pancreatic cancer: influence on borderline resectable. Radiol Med. 2014;119(5):334–42.
12. Porembka MR, Hawkins WG, Linehan DC, et al. Radiologic and intraoperative detection of need for mesenteric vein resection in patients with adenocarcinoma of the head of the pancreas. HPB (Oxford). 2011;13(9):633–42.
13. Kim PT, Wei AC, Atenafu EG, et al. Planned versus unplanned portal vein resections during pancreaticoduodenectomy for adenocarcinoma. Br J Surg. 2013;100(10):1349–56.

14. Fortner JG. Regional resection of cancer of the pancreas: a new surgical approach. Surgery. 1973;73:307–20.
15. Hariharan D, Saied A, Kocher HM. Analysis of mortality rates for pancreatic cancer across the world. HPB (Oxford). 2008;10(1):58–62.
16. Hartwig W, Hackert T, Hinz U, et al. Pancreatic cancer surgery in the new millennium: better prediction of outcome. Ann Surg. 2011;254(2):311–9.
17. McPhee JT, Hill JS, Whalen GF, et al. Perioperative mortality for pancreatectomy: a national perspective. Ann Surg. 2007;246(2):246–53.
18. Tseng JF, Raut CP, Lee JE, et al. Pancreaticoduodenectomy with vascular resection: margin status and survival duration. J Gastrointest Surg. 2004;8(8):935–49.
19. Dokmak S, Aussilhou B, Sauvanet A, et al. Parietal peritoneum as an autologous substitute for venous reconstruction in hepatopancreatobiliary surgery. Ann Surg. 2015;262(2):366–71.
20. Del Chiaro M, Segersvärd R, Rangelova E, et al. Cattell-Braasch maneuver combined with artery-first approach for superior mesenteric-portal vein resection during pancreatectomy. J Gastrointest Surg. 2015;19(12):2264–8.
21. Glebova NO, Hicks CW, Piazza KM, et al. Technical risk factors for portal vein reconstruction thrombosis in pancreatic resection. J Vasc Surg. 2015;62(2):424–33.
22. Jara M, Malinowski M, Bahra M, et al. Bovine pericardium for portal vein reconstruction in abdominal surgery: a surgical guide and first experiences in a single center. Dig Surg. 2015;32(2):135–41.
23. Hirono S, Kawai M, Okada K, et al. Pancreatic neck cancer has specific and oncologic characteristics regarding portal vein invasion and lymph node metastasis. Surgery. 2016;159(2):426–40.
24. Kitahata Y, Yamaue H. Indication for the use of an interposed graft during portal vein and/or superior mesenteric vein reconstruction in pancreatic resection based on perioperative outcomes. Langenbeck's Arch Surg. 2014;399(4):461–71.
25. Murakami Y, Satoi S, Motoi F, Multicentre Study Group of Pancreatobiliary Surgery (MSG-PBS), et al. Portal or superior mesenteric vein resection in pancreatoduodenectomy for pancreatic head carcinoma. Br J Surg. 2015;102(7):837–46.
26. Ramacciato G, Nigri G, Petrucciani N, et al. Pancreatectomy with mesenteric and portal vein resection for borderline resectable pancreatic cancer: multicenter study of 406 patients. Ann Surg Oncol. 2016;23:2028–37.
27. Xing-Mao Z, Hua F, Jian-Tao K, et al. Resection of portal and/or superior mesenteric vein and reconstruction by using allogeneic vein for pT3 pancreatic cancer. J Gastroenterol Hepatol. 2016; doi:10.1111/jgh.13299. Epub ahead of print
28. Weitz J, Kienle P, Schmidt J, et al. Portal vein resection for advanced pancreatic head cancer. J Am Coll Surg. 2007;204:712–6.
29. Sasson A, Hoffmann J, Ross E, et al. En bloc resection for locally advanced cancer of the pancreas: is it worthwhile? J Gastrointest Surg. 2002;6:147–58. Discussion 157–8
30. Müller SA, Hartel M, Mehrabi A, et al. Vascular resection in pancreatic cancer surgery: survival determinants. J Gastrointest Surg. 2009;13(4):784–92.
31. Yekebas EF, Bogoevski D, Cataldegirmen G, et al. En bloc vascular resection for locally advanced pancreatic malignancies infiltrating major blood vessels: perioperative outcome and long-term survival in 136 patients. Ann Surg. 2008;247:300–9.
32. Hirono S, Kawai M, Tani M, et al. Indication for the use of an interposed graft during portal vein and/or superior mesenteric vein reconstruction in pancreatic resection based on perioperative outcomes. Langenbeck's Arch Surg. 2014;399(4):461–71.
33. Yamamoto Y, Sakamoto Y, Nara S, et al. Reconstruction of the portal and hepatic veins using venous grafts customized from the bilateral gonadal veins. Langenbeck's Arch Surg. 2009;394(6):1115–21.
34. Chu CK, Farnell MB, Nguyen JH, et al. Prosthetic graft reconstruction after portal vein resection in pancreaticoduodenectomy: a multicenter analysis. J Am Coll Surg. 2010;211(3):316–24.

35. Stauffer JA, Dougherty MK, Kim GP, et al. Interposition graft with polytetrafluoroethylene for mesenteric and portal vein reconstruction after pancreaticoduodenectomy. Br J Surg. 2009;96(3):247–52.
36. Hattori M, Fujii T, Yamada S, et al. Significance of the splenic vein and its branches in pancreatoduodenectomy with resection of the portal vein system. Dig Surg. 2015;32(5):382–8.
37. Okamura Y, Fujii T, Kanzaki A, et al. Clinicopathologic assessment of pancreatic ductal carcinoma located at the head of the pancreas, in relation to embryonic development. Pancreas. 2012;41(4):582–8.
38. Zhan Q, Deng X, Weng Y, et al. Outcomes of robotic surgery for pancreatic ductal adenocarcinoma. Chin J Cancer Res. 2015;27(6):604–10.
39. Boggi U, Signori S, De Lio N, et al. Feasibility of robotic pancreaticoduodenectomy. Br J Surg. 2013;100(7):917–25.
40. Zeh 3rd HJ, Bartlett DL, Moser AJ. Robotic-assisted major pancreatic resection. Adv Surg. 2011;45:323–40.
41. Giulianotti PC, Addeo P, Buchs NC, et al. Robotic extended pancreatectomy with vascular resection for locally advanced pancreatic tumors. Pancreas. 2011;40(8):1264–70.
42. Kendrick ML, Sclabas GM. Major venous resection during total laparoscopic pancreaticoduodenectomy. HPB (Oxford). 2011;13(7):454–8.
43. Hartwig W, Hackert T, Hinz U, et al. Multivisceral resection for pancreatic malignancies: risk-analysis and long-term outcome. Ann Surg. 2009;250:81–7.
44. Shoup M, Conlon KC, Klimstra D, et al. Is extended resection for adenocarcinoma of the body or tail of the pancreas justified? J Gastrointest Surg. 2003;7(8):946–52.
45. Burdelski CM, Reeh M, Bogoevski D, et al. Multivisceral resections in pancreatic cancer: identification of risk factors. World J Surg. 2011;35(12):2756–63.
46. Hartwig W, Gluth A, Hinz U, Koliogiannis D, Strobel O, Hackert T, et al. Outcomes after extended pancreatectomy in patients with borderline resectable and locally advanced pancreatic cancer. Br J Surg. 2016;103:1683–94.
47. Cheung TT, Poon RT, Chok KS, et al. Pancreaticoduodenectomy with vascular reconstruction for adenocarcinoma of the pancreas with borderline resectability. World J Gastroenterol. 2014;20(46):17448–55.
48. Martin RC, Scoggins CR, Egnatashvili V, et al. Arterial and venous resection for pancreatic adenocarcinoma: operative and long-term outcomes. Arch Surg. 2009;144:154–9.
49. Walsham WJ. Observations on the coronary veins of the stomach. J Anatom Phyiol. 1880;14:399–403.
50. Natsume T, Shuto K, Yanagawa N, et al. The classification of anatomic variations in the perigastric vessels by dual-phase CT to reduce intraoperative bleeding during laparoscopic gastrectomy. Surg Endosc. 2011;25(5):1420–4.
51. Hackert T, Weitz J, Büchler MW. Reinsertion of the gastric coronary vein to avoid venous gastric congestion in pancreatic surgery. HPB (Oxford). 2015;17:368–70.
52. Ferreira N, Oussoultzoglou E, Fuchshuber P, et al. Splenic vein-inferior mesenteric vein anastomosis to lessen left-sided portal hypertension after pancreaticoduodenectomy with concomitant vascular resectiono. Arch Surg. 2011;146(12):1375–81.
53. Strasberg SM, Bhalla S, Sanchez LA, et al. Pattern of venous collateral development after splenic vein occlusion in an extended Whipple procedure: comparison with collateral vein pattern in cases of sinistral portal hypertension. J Gastrointest Surg. 2011;15(11):2070–9.
54. Tamura K, Sumi S, Koike M, et al. A splenic-inferior mesenteric venous anastomosis prevents gastric congestion following pylorus preserving pancreatoduodenectomy with extensive portal vein resection for cancer of the head of the pancreas. Int Surg. 1997;82(2):155–9.
55. Evans GR, Yellin AE, Weaver FA, et al. Sinistral (left-sided) portal hypertension. Am Surg. 1990;56(12):758–63.
56. Chua TC, Wang F, Maher R, et al. Endovascular stenting of mesenterico-portal vein stenosis to reduce blood flow through venous collaterals prior to pancreatoduodenectomy. Langenbeck's Arch Surg. 2015;400(5):629–31.

57. Seufferlein T, Bachet JB, Van Cutsem E, ESMO Guidelines Working Group, et al. Pancreatic adenocarcinoma: ESMO-ESDO clinical practice guidelines for diagnosis, treatment and follow-up. Ann Oncol. 2012;23(Suppl 7):vii33–40.
58. Kang MJ, Jang JY, Chang YR, et al. Portal vein patency after pancreatoduodenectomy for periampullary cancer. Br J Surg. 2015;102(1):77–84.
59. Gawlas I, Epelboym I, Winner M, et al. Short-term but not long-term loss of patency of venous reconstruction during pancreatic resection is associated with decreased survival. J Gastrointest Surg. 2014;18(1):75–82.
60. Krepline AN, Christians KK, Duelge K, et al. Patency rates of portal vein/superior mesenteric vein reconstruction after pancreatectomy for pancreatic cancer. J Gastrointest Surg. 2014;18(11):2016–25.
61. Kim KR, Ko GY, Sung KB, et al. Percutaneous transhepatic stent placement in the management of portal venous stenosis after curative surgery for pancreatic and biliary neoplasms. AJR Am J Roentgenol. 2011;196(4):W446–50.
62. Kanda M, Takeda S, Yamada S, et al. Operative treatment of thrombotic occlusion of the portal vein immediately after pancreatectomy with portal vein resection. Pancreas. 2010;39(2): 265–6.
63. Zyromski NJ, Howard TJ. Acute superior mesenteric-portal vein thrombosis after pancreaticoduodenectomy: treatment by operative thrombectomy. Surgery. 2008;143(4):566–7.
64. Smoot RL, Christein JD, Farnell MB. Durability of portal venous reconstruction following resection during pancreaticoduodenectomy. J Gastrointest Surg. 2006;10(10):1371–5.
65. Hackert T, Stampfl U, Schulz H, et al. Clinical significance of liver ischaemia after pancreatic resection. Br J Surg. 2011;98(12):1760–5.

Pancreatoduodenectomy with Concomitant Vascular Resection for Pancreas Cancer

Jordan M. Cloyd and Matthew H.G. Katz

9.1   Introduction

Pancreatic ductal adenocarcinoma (PDAC) is a lethal disease with a 5-year overall survival rate of approximately 7% [1]. This dismal outcome is largely secondary to the fact that nearly 80% of patients present with advanced disease; these patients are expected to live 6–12 months from diagnosis. However, although the 5-year overall survival rates for patients with regionally advanced and distant metastatic disease are 10% and 2%, respectively, that of patients with localized and resectable disease is as high as 27% [1, 2].

The pancreas is anatomically intimately associated with critical vascular structures including the portal vein (PV), superior mesenteric vein (SMV), celiac artery (CA), hepatic artery (HA), and superior mesenteric artery (SMA). Historically, involvement of vascular structures, whether diagnosed radiographically prior to surgery or at the time of laparotomy, was considered a contraindication to surgical resection, so patients with localized cancers that involved major vessels were treated with palliative therapies such as chemotherapy and radiation. Since resection of the primary tumor and regional lymph nodes is a prerequisite for cure, attempts to extend the criteria for surgical resection to patients with vascular involvement have long been of interest.

Individual case reports and small series of PV–SMV resections date back to the 1950s and 1960s [3, 4]. However, the first large series of patients who had undergone pancreatectomy with concomitant vascular resection was reported by Fortner when he introduced the concept of the "regional pancreatectomy" [5, 6]. Although Fortner's original description did demonstrate the technical feasibility of performing concomitant venous and arterial resections, the use of regional pancreatectomy

J.M. Cloyd, M.D. • M.H.G. Katz, M.D. (✉)
Department of Surgical Oncology, University of Texas MD Anderson Cancer Center,
Unit 1484, PO Box 301402, Houston, TX 77230-1402, USA
e-mail: mhgkatz@mdanderson.org

© Springer Science+Business Media Singapore 2017
H. Yamaue (ed.), *Innovation of Diagnosis and Treatment for Pancreatic Cancer*,
DOI 10.1007/978-981-10-2486-3_9

was not associated with improved oncological outcomes relative to a standard pancreatectomy, and therefore the operation was abandoned. Since then, developments in imaging technology, preoperative staging, and emphasis on multimodality therapy (MMT) have prompted surgeons to again consider aggressive resections of tumors with vascular involvement. Today, pancreatectomy with venous resection comprises a substantial proportion of operations for PDAC at high-volume centers [2], and large series have demonstrated that these operations may yield similar oncologic outcomes compared to standard pancreatectomy operations [7, 8]. On the other hand, pancreatectomy with arterial resection has generally been associated with prohibitively high rates of morbidity and performance of these operations has not been universally accepted [9].

In this chapter, we review the indications, technical details, and outcomes of concomitant vascular resection with pancreatoduodenectomy (PD) with a special emphasis on arterial resection and reconstruction.

9.2   Staging

The likelihood of attaining negative surgical margins at the time of pancreatectomy must be assessed critically when evaluating whether or not a patient should undergo resection. Microscopically (R1) and macroscopically (R2) positive margins have generally been associated with both locoregional recurrence (LR) and reduced survival [10, 11]. Traditionally, the American Joint Committee on Cancer (AJCC) staged patients as having either resectable (stage I and II) or locally advanced, unresectable (stage III and IV) disease. However, the ability to safely perform complex resection of tumors with vascular involvement supports a new clinical categorization based on the anatomic relationship of the tumor to its nearby vascular structures, broadly termed resectable, borderline resectable (BR), and locally advanced (LA). Based on high quality preoperative computed tomography (CT), these categories not only predict prognosis but also help guide decisions on delivery of neoadjuvant therapy, ability to undergo surgery, and likely need for vascular resection.

Over the past decade, the University of Texas MD Anderson Cancer Center (MDACC) and the Americas Hepatopancreatobiliary Association (AHPBA)/ Society of Surgical Oncology (SSO)/Society for Surgery of the Alimentary Tract (SSAT) consensus statements have provided detailed imaging criteria that define these groups. These definitions have been used by the National Comprehensive Cancer Network (NCCN) to standardize treatment guidelines and appropriately stratify patients for enrollment in clinical trials. In general, tumors are considered resectable if there is a clear plane of fat or normal pancreas between the tumor and the major arteries and there is no or limited involvement of the SMV–PV. LA tumors are considered unresectable, typically because of $\geq 180°$ involvement of the SMA or complete encasement of other major vessels without reconstruction options. BR represents an intermediate stage of patients that are technically resectable with complex vascular techniques. Such patients are typically offered preoperative

Table 9.1 Current anatomic classification systems for pancreatic ductal adenocarcinoma

	MDACC	AHPBA/SSO/SSAT	NCCN
Resectable			
Celiac axis	No extension	Clear fat plane	No contact
Common hepatic artery	No extension	Clear fat plane	No contact
Superior mesenteric artery	Clear fat plane	Clear fat plane	No contact
Portal-superior mesenteric vein	Abutment or encasement (no occlusion)	No abutment, distortion, encasement, or tumor thrombus	No contact; $\leq 180°$ contact without vein contour irregularity
Borderline resectable			
Celiac axis	Abutment	No abutment or encasement	Contact $\leq 180°$ or contact $>180°$ with uninvolved GDA
Common hepatic artery	Abutment or short segment encasement	Abutment or short segment encasement	Short segment encasement or abutment without extension to CA or HA bifurcation
Superior mesenteric artery	Abutment $<180°$	Abutment $<180°$	Contact $<180°$
Portal-superior mesenteric vein	Short segment occlusion amenable to reconstruction	Abutment $>180°$ or occlusion amenable to reconstruction	Contact $<180°$ or $\geq 180°$ with vein contour irregularity
Locally advanced			
Celiac axis	Encasement	Abutment or encasement	Contact $>180°$
Common hepatic artery	Encasement with no reconstruction option	Encasement with extension to celiac axis	Contact with extension to celiac axis or bifurcation
Superior mesenteric artery	Encasement $>180°$	Encasement $>180°$	Contact $>180°$ or contact with first jejunal branch
Portal-superior mesenteric vein	Occluded with no reconstruction option	Occluded with no reconstruction option	Unreconstructible

MDACC MD Anderson Cancer Center, *AHPBA* Americas Hepato-Pancreato-Biliary Association, *NCCN* National Comprehensive Cancer Network

chemotherapy and/or chemoradiation therapy since they have been shown to be at high risk for margin positive resection and the development of early metastatic disease (Table 9.1).

Accurately identifying patients with BR or LA tumors and predicting who will require vascular resection and reconstruction is essential to the development of appropriate treatment regimens. Currently, pancreas-protocol multiphase CT is the most widely used imaging tool to characterize vascular involvement. In fact, CT evaluation of the tumor–vein interface has been shown to be highly predictive of the need for vascular resection [12]. In general, cross-sectional imaging should be obtained prior to endoscopy, biliary stenting, or tissue biopsy in order to prevent peripancreatic inflammation that can obscure the tumor–tissue interface and decrease the imaging sensitivity [13]. In addition to assessing major vascular involvement, regional arterial and venous anatomy should be thoroughly examined. This review should include inspection of the first order jejunal and ileal branches of the SMV, precise location of IMV insertion, and evaluation of hepatic artery variants that will influence the operative strategy [14, 15].

9.3 Venous Resection

Given its intimate relationship to the PV–SMV, venous involvement by PDAC of the head and uncinate is a frequent occurrence. All pancreas surgeons should be capable of performing standard venous resections and reconstructions given their relative frequency and the inability to accurately predict venous involvement preoperatively. Although initially felt to be associated with a high risk of complications, most contemporary series of PD with concomitant venous resection have shown the procedure to be safe and allow a larger proportion of patients to benefit from a margin-negative resection. Indeed, as many as 50% of PDs performed today at large referral centers require some type of vascular resection. Some investigators have even proposed routine segmental venous resection at the time of PD regardless of venous involvement in order to ensure a wide negative margin; however, such a policy is not supported by existing data [16].

9.3.1 Technical Considerations

The two most important considerations for venous resection and reconstruction are the location and the extent of tumor involvement of the vessel. Broadly, the location of tumor involvement can be one of three locations: PV above the confluence, involving the PV–SMV at the confluence, and SMV below the confluence. Various classification systems exist to describe the extent of tumor involvement as a means of guiding the reconstruction. Tseng et al. have proposed a classification system that takes into account both the extent of tumor involvement and its relation to the portosplenic confluence (Fig. 9.1) [18]. The International Study Group of Pancreatic Surgery (ISGPS) has also proposed a simple classification system [19]. In general, the limits of venous resection extend proximally to the bifurcation of the left and right PV and distally to the first jejunal/ileal branches of the SMV at the root of the mesentery. Technically, one of the principal jejunal or ileal branches may be sacrificed as long as the other can be maintained patent. However, vascular dissection, obtaining vascular control, and creation of anastomoses in the root of the mesentery are both challenging and perilous. Ensuring that safe proximal and distal vascular control is achievable is critical prior to embarking on vascular dissection.

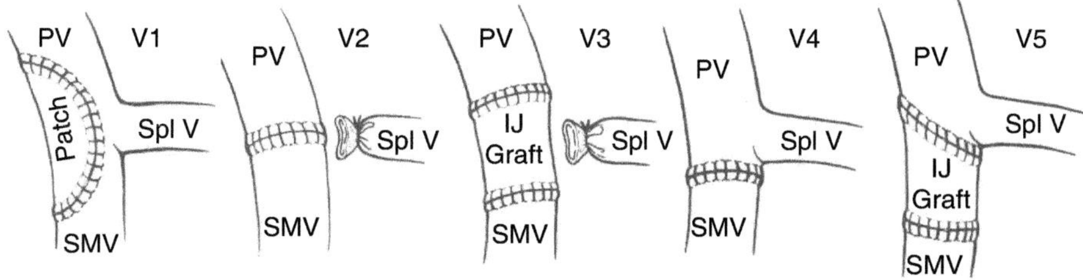

Fig. 9.1 Classification of portal vein–superior mesenteric vein reconstruction according to location and extent of required resection (Used with permission [17])

Although a thorough operative plan should be established prior to entry to the operating room based on a critical examination of cross-sectional imaging, formal assessment of the tumor–vessel interface may be performed following transection of the pancreas and acquisition of complete venous isolation and control. When tumor involves the right lateral wall of the vein, the tumor may be excised with an en bloc segment of vein. Lateral venorrhaphy may be performed with either direct suture closure (if less than approximately 25% of the wall is involved) or patch closure using either autologous vein graft or bovine pericardial patch. For more extensive venous involvement, segmental resection of the vein should be performed. A thorough attempt should be made at primary anastomosis whenever possible. Defects as long as 4 cm or so can often be overcome after removal of the specimen and full mesenteric mobilization. In cases in which primary anastomosis is not possible, an interposition graft should be used. Autologous grafts are preferred over synthetic grafts due to the risk of infection and thrombosis [20]. Our preference is to use the left internal jugular vein for interposition grafts due to its favorable size match to the PV–SMV; however, left renal vein, saphenous vein, and deep femoral vein have also been employed [21]. Alternatively, a customized bovine pericardial tube interposition graft can be fashioned using a vascular stapler.

Since the SMA margin is the margin most frequently found to be positive after PD for PDAC, a fundamental technical principle is to maximize the clearance of cancer cells from the retroperitoneum by meticulous dissection along the periadventitial plane of the SMA. Since tumor involvement of the PV–SMV interferes with straightforward exposure and dissection of the proximal SMA, the conduct of the dissection must be adjusted accordingly to overcome this limitation. For tumors that do not involve the PV–SMV, the vein can typically be reflected to the patient's left after separation from the tumor and pancreas in order to expose the SMA. Since this is not possible when the pancreatic tumor involves the venous confluence, we often recommend division of the splenic vein which permits rightward mobilization of the PV–SMV (Fig. 9.2a). The SMA dissection then begins inferiorly at the level of the first jejunal branch of the SMV and proceeds cephalad. All fat, fibrous tissues, lymphatics, and nerves are dissected towards the right and the inferior pancreaticoduodenal arteries are individually ligated. The pancreatic neck is divided and the dissection of the SMA, avoiding circumferentially skeletonizing the vessel, is

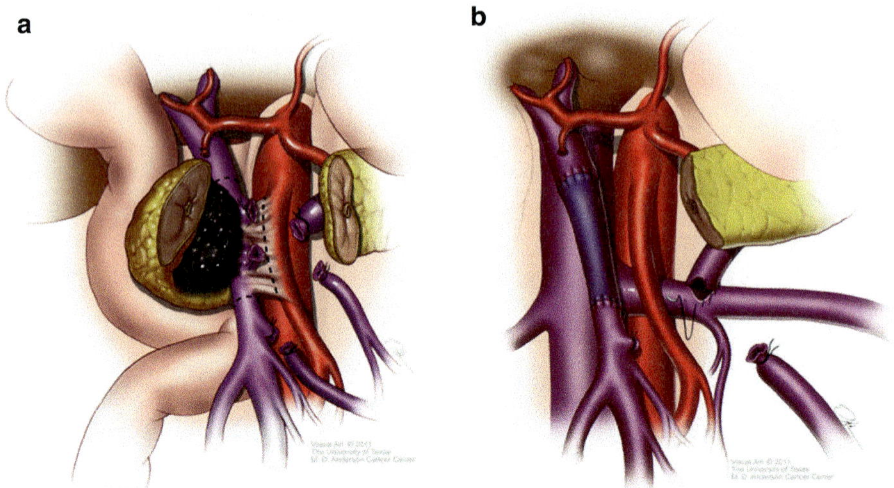

Fig. 9.2 (**a**) Division of the pancreas and splenic vein optimizes exposure of the SMA in cases of tumor involvement of the portosplenic confluence. *Dotted line* demonstrates correct line of dissection adjacent to the SMA. (**b**) Once SMA dissection is complete, venous resection and reconstruction may be performed. Splenorenal shunt (shown here) may or may not be performed depending on the insertion of the IMV and adequate gastrosplenic outflow (Used with permission [22])

continued towards its origin on the aorta. Once the deep retroperitoneal tissues are divided, the tumor will remain attached only to the PV–SMV and venous reconstruction can be performed (Fig. 9.2b).

There are several key physiological issues that should be considered when undertaking venous resection during PD. Although we do not routinely perform superior mesenteric artery (SMA) clamping, others have proposed this practice as a means of preventing intestinal wall congestion and edema that might interfere with subsequent anastomosis. Equally important is the maintenance of hepatopetal flow by minimizing vascular clamping time and ensuring adequate venous patency. An underappreciated issue is the maintenance of gastrosplenic outflow when the splenic vein must be divided during venous segmental resection. In the majority of cases, outflow is maintained through retrograde collaterals such as the inferior mesenteric artery (IMV) or coronary vein. However, while the IMV typically inserts into the splenic vein, it may insert into the SMV below the confluence in up to one-third of patients. In these cases, splenic vein division results in inadequate gastrosplenic outflow, especially if the coronary vein has been divided. In order to prevent sinistral hypertension, a distal splenorenal shunt may be created [23]. Finally, in patients with SMV–PV occlusion and cavernous transformation, pancreatic resection and venous reconstruction are associated with significant venous collateral hemorrhage. In these situations, creation of a temporary mesocaval shunt prior to pancreatic or portal dissection may result in decompressed varices and a safer dissection.

9.3.2 Outcomes

Venous resection and reconstruction is a technically challenging endeavor and one might expect a higher rate of perioperative complications. Indeed, an analysis of the American College of Surgeons National Surgical Quality Improvement Program (NSQIP) found higher postoperative morbidity (39.9% vs 33.3%) and mortality (5.7% vs 2.9%) rates in patients undergoing PD with vascular resection compared to standard PD [24]. However, the dataset is limited in its ability to accurately code these events; for example, operations with inadvertent vascular injury and repair, typically associated with higher postoperative complication rates, were not excluded. Other single institution series [25–27], multi-institutional reports [8], and meta-analyses [7, 28, 29] have demonstrated no statistically significantly different morbidity and mortality rates of patients undergoing concomitant venous resection with PD.

It is now widely accepted that venous involvement should not be a contraindication to resection on the basis of oncologic reasons. In fact, pancreatectomy with venous resection results in improved survival compared to nonoperative therapies. Lygidakis et al. randomized patients with limited vascular involvement to complete surgical resection or double bypass and found 2-year survival rates of 81.8% vs 0%, respectively [30]. In a non-randomized prospective, multi-institutional study comparing pancreatectomy with vascular resection versus chemoradiation alone, median survival in the surgery group was 11.8 months longer [31]. Several contemporary reports have suggested comparable long-term survival for patients undergoing PD with concomitant PV–SMV resection compared to PD alone, especially when neo-adjuvant therapies are utilized [32, 33].

In general, porto-mesenteric venous reconstruction during PD is associated with high patency rates. Primary repair and autologous vein grafts are associated with the lowest rates of thrombosis [34, 35]. Although venous thrombosis can occur any time after surgery, acute thrombosis in the immediate postoperative period is associated with the greatest morbidity. Late thromboses are often related to cancer recurrence [36, 37]. Although the optimal pharmacologic prophylaxis is not well established, we typically recommend aspirin for patients who have undergone venous reconstruction. This is administered on the first postoperative day and patients are encouraged to remain on aspirin life-long. Patients also receive subcutaneous lovenox for 28 postoperative days at a prophylactic dose, as do all patients who undergo pancreatectomy.

9.3.3 Case Example

A 52 yo woman presented with PDAC in the head of the pancreas involving the portosplenic confluence with short segment occlusion (Fig. 9.3a). She underwent preoperative therapy consisting of 2 months of mFOLFIRINOX and 50.4 Gy of external beam radiation. Restaging scans demonstrated no progression of disease and laparoscopy did not reveal peritoneal or hepatic metastases. At the time of surgery, the tumor was found to be involving the anterior pancreas invading through

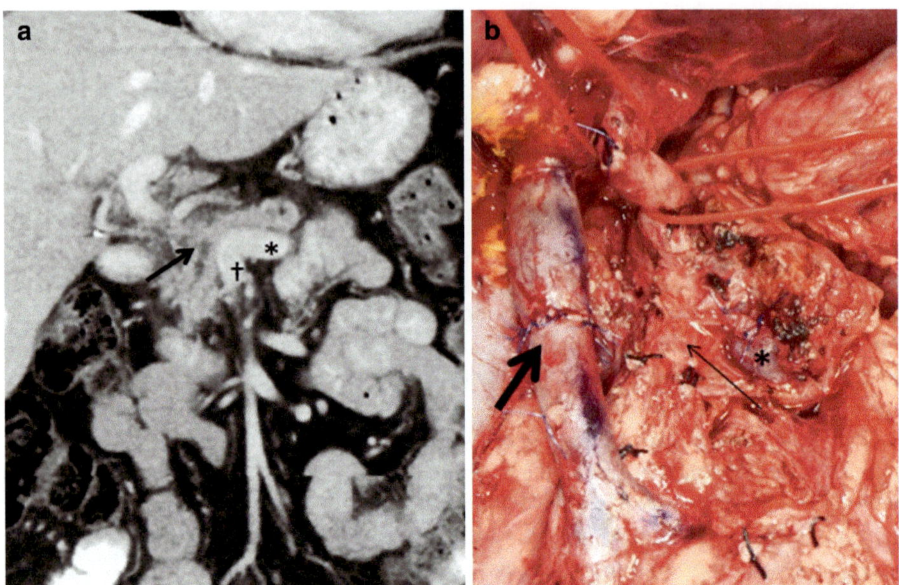

Fig. 9.3 (**a**) Example of pancreatic cancer (*arrow*) with complete encasement of the PV at the portosplenic confluence where the splenic vein (*asterisk*) joins the SMV (*dagger*). (**b**) Division of the splenic vein (*asterisk*) allows adequate exposure of the SMA (*thin arrow*) for complete dissection followed by PV–SMV resection and primary anastomosis (*thick arrow*)

neck into the portosplenic confluence. The neck of the pancreas and the splenic vein were carefully divided. With the tumor and PV–SMV retracted towards the right, a meticulous SMA dissection was performed as described above. Finally, segmental vein resection was performed en bloc with PD; reconstruction was performed with a primary vein anastomosis (Fig. 9.3b). Because the IMV inserted into the splenic vein, thereby providing adequate collateral outflow, a splenorenal shunt was not felt to be necessary.

9.4 Arterial Resection

Traditionally, arterial resections for pancreas cancer have not widely been supported because these operations have been associated with significant perioperative morbidity, high rates of positive resection margins, and an unclear survival benefit [9]. In addition, arterial invasion is generally considered to be a marker of aggressive tumor biology and the presence of occult metastatic disease. However, with improvements in effective preoperative therapy, vascular resection techniques, and perioperative care, aggressive operations with arterial resections are more frequently being performed. In fact, isolated common hepatic artery involvement and SMA abutment both qualify as BR disease (not unresectable) in current staging systems (Table 9.1). Nevertheless, acknowledging significant perioperative risk and uncertain oncologic benefits, all patients with arterial involvement should be strongly considered for preoperative therapy. Using a multimodality approach with induction chemotherapy and local irradiation of the tumor and regional lymph nodes, this strategy treats the micrometastatic disease presumed present in all patients, helps sterilize critical surgical margins and lymph nodes, and provides a critical selection period to ensure favorable tumor biology and personal physiology prior to major surgery. Only after completing aggressive, standardized preoperative therapy, should patients be considered for pancreatectomy with concomitant arterial resection. Given the technical complexity and perioperative risk, these operations should only be offered in highly selected patients at high-volume experienced referral centers.

9.4.1 Technical Considerations

Arterial structures that are risk for local involvement by cancers of the head of the pancreas include the CA, CHA and SMA and variant hepatic artery anatomy, most commonly a replaced right hepatic artery (RRHA) that arises from the SMA posterior to the head of the pancreas. Potential vascular interventions include simple ligation, resection with primary repair, and resection with interposition grafting. Preoperative planning is essential and depends upon high quality thin-cut CT angiography to define the extent of tumor involvement, appropriate reconstruction options, and aberrant arterial anatomy.

With regard to CHA resections, the anatomic limits of potential resection are defined by the bifurcation of the left and right HAs distally and the CA proximally. Reconstruction to distal segments of the left/right HA are technically challenging given their small size and are at high risk for anastomotic failure, the consequences of which include bilioenteric anastomotic leak, hepatic ischemia, and liver abscess. Arterial resections may extend proximally to the root of the CHA as it arises from the CA for tumors in the head of the pancreas. En bloc CA resections almost always occur in conjunction with a left-sided pancreatectomy, also known as the modified Appleby procedure, with hepatic perfusion maintained via collateral circulation through the pancreaticoduodenal and gastroduodenal vessels [38]. For CA resections, retrograde flow through the gastroduodenal should be confirmed prior to committing with the resection; if retrograde flow exists, then ligation of the CHA should have little consequence. Complex resection and vascular reconstructions involving the celiac axis (as well as left gastric and splenic arteries) have also been performed in conjunction with PD or total pancreatectomy but may require mutivisceral resection (e.g., splenectomy, gastrectomy), the degree of which is determined by the resultant arterial insufficiency [39]. After arterial resection, primary anastomosis should be attempted whenever feasible. This is typically possible when short segment CHA resections are performed. When interposition grafting is required, various conduits may be used. Our preference is the reversed saphenous vein graft (rSVG) because of its size compatibility and ease to obtain. Others have reported using superficial femoral artery (with the primary vessel reconstructed with synthetic graft) [40], internal iliac artery [41], or other visceral arteries including the splenic [42], left gastric [43], or gastroduodenal [44]. Occasionally, interposition grafting will be required to reconstruct a RRHA that was involved by tumor and resected en bloc with PD. Alternatively, preoperative embolization of the RRHA may promote collateralization and obviate the need for vascular reconstruction [45].

Resection and reconstruction of the SMA at the time of pancreatectomy, although reported in select series, is typically thought to be associated with prohibitive risk to be justified on a routine basis. Bleeding complications and mesenteric ischemia associated with SMA thrombosis are common and associated with significant perioperative mortality. In addition, most tumors with SMA involvement will also require simultaneous major venous resection and reconstruction, elevating the technical complexity and risk for complications. On the other hand, significant preoperative therapy in patients with pretreatment SMA involvement may result in fibrosis of the soft tissue adjacent to the SMA. Therefore, a planned resection with performance of a meticulous dissection along the periadventitial plane of the SMA may be warranted for highly selected patients who underwent significant preoperative chemotherapy and chemoradiation. Some have advocated an SMA-first approach to patients with suspected SMA involvement in order to evaluate the extent of arterial involvement early in the course of the operation but we strongly believe that decisions like these should generally be made prior to surgery based on a thorough examination of cross-sectional imaging studies [46].

Systemic anticoagulation should be given during arterial reconstruction and reversed once arterial flow is restored. Arterial resections should be performed early in the operation, prior to specimen removal and venous reconstruction, if applicable. Hepatic ischemia time should be minimized in the cases of simultaneous arterial/venous reconstructions and postoperative liver function should be followed closely. Again, we recommended the use of aspirin postoperatively.

9.4.2 Outcomes

Evaluating outcomes of PD with concomitant arterial resection is challenging given the heterogeneity in case selection and surgical technique, small number of patients, and the publication biases that are inherent in retrospective single institution series. In 2011, Mollberg et al. performed a comprehensive systematic review and meta-analysis [9]. Their review included 26 studies encompassing 366 patients with PDAC undergoing a range of procedures (PD, total pancreatectomy or distal pancreatectomy, with or without venous resection), arterial resections (CA, CHA, SMA, others), and reconstruction methods. The meta-analysis found that pancreatectomy with arterial resection was associated with longer operating time, greater estimated blood loss, longer hospital stay, greater perioperative morbidity (OR 2.17, 95% CI 1.26–3.75), reoperation rates (OR 3.28, 95% CI 1.68–6.41), and perioperative mortality (OR 5.04, 95% CI 2.69–9.45). In addition, median 1-, 3-, and 5-year overall survival rates for patients undergoing arterial resection were 49.1%, 8.3%, and 0%, respectively. Oncologic outcomes were inferior in patients undergoing arterial resection compared to both patients undergoing pancreatectomy without vascular resection and also patients undergoing pancreatectomy with venous resection. On the other hand, arterial resection was found to be associated with more favorable survival compared to patients with localized PDAC who did not undergo surgery. One criticism of this meta-analysis is the potential inclusion of unplanned arterial resections that were necessitated after inadvertent arteriotomies during surgery. A recent series of planned arterial resections after significant preoperative therapy demonstrated an R0 resection rate of 85% (11 out of 13), morbidity rate of 20%, perioperative mortality rate of 0 and 62% of patients were alive without evidence of disease with a median follow-up of 21 months [42].

9.4.3 Case Examples

A 71-year-old woman presented with a BR tumor in the head of the pancreas with short segment encasement of the CHA as well as the PV at the portosplenic confluence (Fig. 9.4a). She received preoperative gemcitabine and Xeloda followed by 50.4 Gy external beam radiation with concurrent Xeloda. Restaging scans demonstrated no progression of disease. At the time of surgery, the tumor was found to

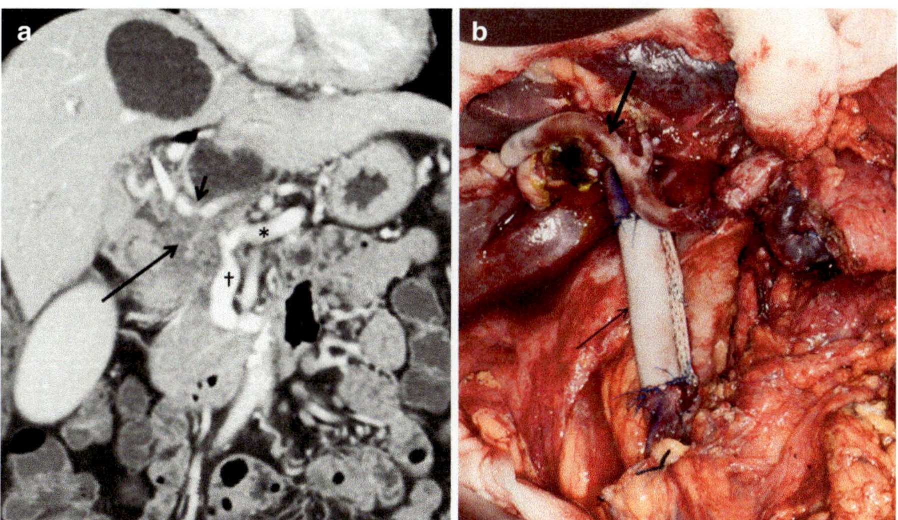

Fig. 9.4 (**a**) Tumor in the head/neck of the pancreas (*long arrow*) involving the common and proper hepatic arteries (*short arrow*) at the gastroduodenal artery as well as the portosplenic confluence where the splenic vein (*asterisk*) joins the SMV (*dagger*). (**b**) Final reconstruction after pancreatoduodenectomy en bloc with hepatic artery and the portosplenic confluence. Common hepatic artery has been reconstructed with reverse saphenous vein graft (*thick arrow*) and portal vein reconstructed with a bovine pericardial interposition graft (*thin arrow*)

involve the CHA at the origin of the GDA. Arterial resection and reconstruction with reverse saphenous vein graft was performed early in the operation after portal dissection. The remainder of the PD ensued in the standard fashion, leaving the PV–SMV resection for last. The PV–SMV was reconstructed using an interposition graft of bovine pericardium fashioned over a 24-Fr chest tube using a vascular stapler (Fig. 9.4b). Since the splenic vein was divided and the IMV inserted inferiorly into the SMV, a splenorenal shunt was created.

A 54-year-old man was found to have pancreatic cancer in the head of the pancreas that was encasing a RRHA (Fig. 9.5a). The patient underwent preoperative chemotherapy with gemcitabine and Abraxane followed by 5.5 weeks of Xeloda-based chemoradiation. Follow-up scans demonstrated no evidence of progression. At the time of surgery, the tumor was found to be adherent to the anterior surface of the inferior vena cava which was dissected free after obtaining vascular control. PD was performed in a standard fashion except the RRHA was controlled proximally at its origin on the SMA and distally in the porta hepatis. After PD with en bloc resection of the RRHA, the artery was reconstructed using reverse saphenous vein graft (Fig. 9.5b).

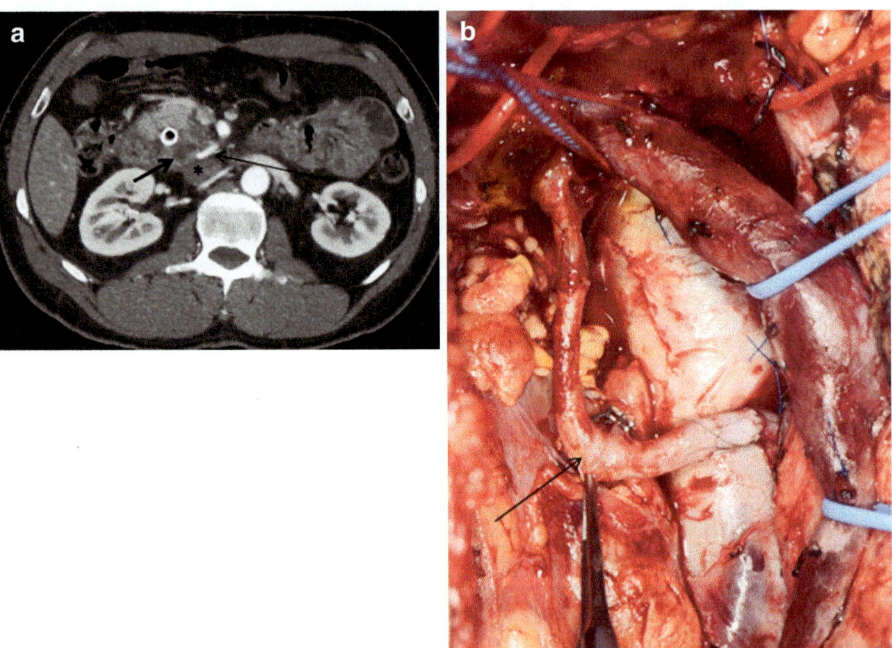

Fig. 9.5 (**a**) Tumor in the uncinate process of the pancreas (*short arrow*) encasing a replaced right hepatic artery (*long arrow*) and involving the anterior wall of the inferior vena cava (*asterisk*). (**b**) Intraoperative photo demonstrating reconstructed replaced right hepatic artery (*arrow*) with reversed saphenous vein graft

9.5   Impact of Preoperative Therapy

All patients with BR/LA cancers of the head of the pancreas should strongly be considered for preoperative multimodality therapy [47], preferably as part of either a clinical trial or prospective registry. The preoperative setting provides a critical window to select for patients who will ultimately benefit from an operation that is necessary (although clearly not sufficient) for cure and to forgo surgery in those patients, because of either unfavorable tumor biology or personal physiology, who are not likely to benefit. Preoperative therapy has many other potential advantages including the ability to guarantee delivery of multimodality therapy to all patients, provide early treatment of micrometastatic disease, and facilitate a successful margin-negative resection. Although randomized, phase III data are lacking, multiple large institutional series [2] and several phase I/II [48–50] studies support this approach.

Several important considerations exist prior to proceeding with surgical resection following extensive preoperative therapy. First, previous studies have found that radiographic evidence of downstaging does not reliably predict resectability [51, 52]. Rather, one should focus on the absence of local progression or development of distant metastatic disease, as well as the stabilization of nutritional and physiologic indices to inform decision-making about undertaking surgery. Second, patients should receive modern chemotherapy and radiotherapy with frequent communication among medical, surgical, and radiation oncologists. Caution should be given to extended regimens of cytotoxic chemotherapy as the risk of treatment-related toxicity increases. On the other hand, the evidence suggests that preoperative therapy does not increase perioperative morbidity rates. In fact, preoperative radiation has the advantage of being associated with reduced rates of postoperative pancreatic fistula [53].

Conclusions

The understanding and management of patients with localized PDAC involving nearby vascular structures continues to evolve. With a multidisciplinary approach utilizing contemporary chemotherapy and radiation, modern vascular techniques, and excellent perioperative care, select patients with limited involvement of the PV, SMV, or CHA may achieve satisfactory survival outcomes. The key to achieving these results is identifying this complex subgroup of patients likely to benefit from aggressive surgical resection and approaching their treatment in a multimodality fashion that consists of preoperative chemotherapy and chemoradiation followed by operative resection with critical attention to surgical technique. Further innovation in systemic therapies and preoperative treatment regimens may continue to expand the role of extended pancreatectomy with vascular resection.

References

1. American Cancer Society. Cancer facts & figures 2015. Atlanta: American Cancer Society; 2015.
2. Katz MHG, Wang H, Fleming JB, Sun CC, Hwang RF, Wolff RA, et al. Long-term survival after multidisciplinary management of resected pancreatic adenocarcinoma. Ann Surg Oncol. 2009;16:836–47.
3. Hubbard TB. Carcinoma of the head of the pancreas: resection of the portal vein and portacaval shunt. Ann Surg. 1958;147:935–44.
4. Sigel B, Bassett JG, Cooper DR, Dunn MR. Resection of the superior mesenteric vein and replacement with a venous autograft during pancreaticoduodenectomy: case report. Ann Surg. 1965;162:941–5.
5. Fortner JG. Regional resection and pancreatic carcinoma. Surgery. 1973;73:799–800.
6. Fortner JG. Regional pancreatectomy for cancer of the pancreas, ampulla, and other related sites. Tumor staging and results. Ann Surg. 1984;199:418–25.
7. Chua TC, Saxena A. Extended pancreaticoduodenectomy with vascular resection for pancreatic cancer: a systematic review. J Gastrointest Surg. 2010;14:1442–52.
8. Ravikumar R, Sabin C, Abu Hilal M, Bramhall S, White S, Wigmore S, et al. Portal vein resection in borderline resectable pancreatic cancer: a United Kingdom multicenter study. J Am Coll Surg. 2014;218:401–11.
9. Mollberg N, Rahbari NN, Koch M, Hartwig W, Hoeger Y, Büchler MW, et al. Arterial resection during pancreatectomy for pancreatic cancer: a systematic review and meta-analysis. Ann Surg. 2011;254:882–93.
10. Raut CP, Tseng JF, Sun CC, Wang H, Wolff RA, Crane CH, et al. Impact of resection status on pattern of failure and survival after pancreaticoduodenectomy for pancreatic adenocarcinoma. Ann Surg. 2007;246:52–60.
11. Verbeke CS, Gladhaug IP. Resection margin involvement and tumour origin in pancreatic head cancer. Br J Surg. 2012;99:1036–49.
12. Tran Cao HS, Balachandran A, Wang H, Nogueras-González GM, Bailey CE, Lee JE, et al. Radiographic tumor-vein interface as a predictor of intraoperative, pathologic, and oncologic outcomes in resectable and borderline resectable pancreatic cancer. J Gastrointest Surg. 2014;18:269–78. Discussion 278
13. Al-Hawary MM, Francis IR, Chari ST, Fishman EK, Hough DM, Lu DS, et al. Pancreatic ductal adenocarcinoma radiology reporting template: consensus statement of the society of abdominal radiology and the American Pancreatic Association. Gastroenterology. 2014;146:291–304.e1.
14. Katz MHG, Fleming JB, Pisters PWT, Lee JE, Evans DB. Anatomy of the superior mesenteric vein with special reference to the surgical management of first-order branch involvement at pancreaticoduodenectomy. Ann Surg. 2008;248:1098–102.
15. Balachandran A, Darden DL, Tamm EP, Faria SC, Evans DB, Charnsangavej C. Arterial variants in pancreatic adenocarcinoma. Abdom Imaging. 2008;33:214–21.
16. Turrini O, Ewald J, Barbier L, Mokart D, Blache JL, Delpero JR. Should the portal vein be routinely resected during pancreaticoduodenectomy for adenocarcinoma? Ann Surg. 2013;257:726–30.
17. Tseng JF, Raut CP, Lee JE, Pisters PWT, Vauthey J-N, Abdalla EK, et al. Pancreaticoduodenectomy with vascular resection: margin status and survival duration. J Gastrointest Surg. 2004;8:935–49. Discussion 949–50
18. Tseng JF, Tamm EP, Lee JE, Pisters PWT, Evans DB. Venous resection in pancreatic cancer surgery. Best Pract Res Clin Gastroenterol. 2006;20:349–64.
19. Bockhorn M, Uzunoglu FG, Adham M, Imrie C, Milicevic M, Sandberg AA, et al. Borderline resectable pancreatic cancer: a consensus statement by the International Study Group of Pancreatic Surgery (ISGPS). Surgery. 2014;155:977–88.

20. Chu CK, Farnell MB, Nguyen JH, Stauffer JA, Kooby DA, Sclabas GM, et al. Prosthetic graft reconstruction after portal vein resection in pancreaticoduodenectomy: a multicenter analysis. J Am Coll Surg. 2010;211:316–24.
21. Lai ECS. Vascular resection and reconstruction at pancreatico-duodenectomy: technical issues. Hepatobiliary Pancreat Dis Int. 2012;11:234–42.
22. Katz MHG, Lee JE, Pisters PWT, Skoracki R, Tamm E, Fleming JB. Retroperitoneal dissection in patients with borderline resectable pancreatic cancer: operative principles and techniques. J Am Coll Surg. 2012;215:e11–8.
23. Christians KK, Riggle K, Keim R, Pappas S, Tsai S, Ritch P, et al. Distal splenorenal and temporary mesocaval shunting at the time of pancreatectomy for cancer: initial experience from the Medical College of Wisconsin. Surgery. 2013;154:123–31.
24. Castleberry AW, White RR, De La Fuente SG, Clary BM, Blazer 3rd DG, McCann RL, et al. The impact of vascular resection on early postoperative outcomes after pancreaticoduodenectomy: an analysis of the American College of Surgeons National Surgical Quality Improvement Program database. Ann Surg Oncol. 2012;19:4068–77.
25. Yekebas EF, Bogoevski D, Cataldegirmen G, Kunze C, Marx A, Vashist YK, et al. En bloc vascular resection for locally advanced pancreatic malignancies infiltrating major blood vessels: perioperative outcome and long-term survival in 136 patients. Ann Surg. 2008;247:300–9.
26. Leach SD, Lee JE, Charnsangavej C, Cleary KR, Lowy AM, Fenoglio CJ, et al. Survival following pancreaticoduodenectomy with resection of the superior mesenteric-portal vein confluence for adenocarcinoma of the pancreatic head. Br J Surg. 1998;85:611–7.
27. Jeong J, Choi DW, Choi SH, Heo JS, Jang K-T. Long-term outcome of portomesenteric vein invasion and prognostic factors in pancreas head adenocarcinoma. ANZ J Surg. 2015;85: 264–9.
28. Zhou Y, Zhang Z, Liu Y, Li B, Xu D. Pancreatectomy combined with superior mesenteric vein-portal vein resection for pancreatic cancer: a meta-analysis. World J Surg. 2012;36:884–91.
29. Murakami M, Aoki T, Kato T. Video-assisted thoracoscopic surgery: hepatectomy for liver neoplasm. World J Surg. 2011;35:1050–4.
30. Lygidakis NJ, Singh G, Bardaxoglou E, Dedemadi G, Sgourakis G, Nestoridis J, et al. Monobloc total spleno-pancreaticoduodenectomy for pancreatic head carcinoma with portal-mesenteric venous invasion. A prospective randomized study. Hepato-Gastroenterology. 2004;51:427–33.
31. Doi R, Imamura M, Hosotani R, Imaizumi T, Hatori T, Takasaki K, et al. Surgery versus radio-chemotherapy for resectable locally invasive pancreatic cancer: final results of a randomized multi-institutional trial. Surg Today. 2008;38:1021–8.
32. Murakami Y, Satoi S, Motoi F, Sho M, Kawai M, Matsumoto I, et al. Portal or superior mesenteric vein resection in pancreatoduodenectomy for pancreatic head carcinoma. Br J Surg. 2015;102:837–46.
33. Giovinazzo F, Turri G, Katz MH, Heaton N, Ahmed I. Meta-analysis of benefits of portal-superior mesenteric vein resection in pancreatic resection for ductal adenocarcinoma. Br J Surg. 2016;103:179–91.
34. Krepline AN, Christians KK, Duelge K, Mahmoud A, Ritch P, George B, et al. Patency rates of portal vein/superior mesenteric vein reconstruction after pancreatectomy for pancreatic cancer. J Gastrointest Surg. 2014;18:2016–25.
35. Dua MM, Tran TB, Klausner J, Hwa KJ, Poultsides GA, Norton JA, et al. Pancreatectomy with vein reconstruction: technique matters. HPB. 2015;17:824–31.
36. Gawlas I, Epelboym I, Winner M, DiNorcia J, Woo Y, Lee JL, et al. Short-term but not long-term loss of patency of venous reconstruction during pancreatic resection is associated with decreased survival. J Gastrointest Surg. 2014;18:75–82.
37. Smoot RL, Christein JD, Farnell MB. Durability of portal venous reconstruction following resection during pancreaticoduodenectomy. J Gastrointest Surg. 2006;10:1371–5.

38. Smoot RL, Donohue JH. Modified Appleby procedure for resection of tumors of the pancreatic body and tail with celiac axis involvement. J Gastrointest Surg. 2012;16:2167–9.
39. Hartwig W, Hackert T, Hinz U, Hassenpflug M, Strobel O, Büchler MW, et al. Multivisceral resection for pancreatic malignancies: risk-analysis and long-term outcome. Ann Surg. 2009;250:81–7.
40. Truty M. The role and techniques of vascular resection. In: Katz MHG, Ahmad SA, editors. Multimodality management of borderline resectable pancreatic cancer. New York: Springer; 2016.
41. Amano H, Miura F, Toyota N, Wada K, Katoh K, Hayano K, et al. Is pancreatectomy with arterial reconstruction a safe and useful procedure for locally advanced pancreatic cancer? J Hepato-Biliary-Pancreat Surg. 2009;16:850–7.
42. Hackert T, Weitz J, Büchler MW. Splenic artery use for arterial reconstruction in pancreatic surgery. Langenbecks Arch Surg. 2014;399:667–71.
43. Amano R, Kimura K, Nakata B, Yamazoe S, Motomura H, Yamamoto A, et al. Pancreatectomy with major arterial resection after neoadjuvant chemoradiotherapy gemcitabine and S-1 and concurrent radiotherapy for locally advanced unresectable pancreatic cancer. Surgery. 2015;158:191–200.
44. Christians KK, Pilgrim CHC, Tsai S, Ritch P, George B, Erickson B, et al. Arterial resection at the time of pancreatectomy for cancer. Surgery. 2014;155:919–26.
45. Cloyd JM, Chandra V, Louie JD, Rao S, Visser BC. Preoperative embolization of replaced right hepatic artery prior to pancreaticoduodenectomy. J Surg Oncol. 2012;106:509–12.
46. Sanjay P, Takaori K, Govil S, Shrikhande SV, Windsor JA. "Artery-first" approaches to pancreatoduodenectomy. Br J Surg. 2012;99:1027–35.
47. National Comprehensive Cancer Network. NCCN practice guidelines for pancreatic cancer [Internet]. 2016. http://www.nccn.org/professionals/physician_gls/pdf/pancreatic.pdf
48. Evans DB, Varadhachary GR, Crane CH, Sun CC, Lee JE, Pisters PWT, et al. Preoperative gemcitabine-based chemoradiation for patients with resectable adenocarcinoma of the pancreatic head. J Clin Oncol Off J Am Soc Clin Oncol. 2008;26:3496–502.
49. Varadhachary GR, Wolff RA, Crane CH, Sun CC, Lee JE, Pisters PWT, et al. Preoperative gemcitabine and cisplatin followed by gemcitabine-based chemoradiation for resectable adenocarcinoma of the pancreatic head. J Clin Oncol Off J Am Soc Clin Oncol. 2008;26:3487–95.
50. Kim EJ, Ben-Josef E, Herman JM, Bekaii-Saab T, Dawson LA, Griffith KA, et al. A multi-institutional phase 2 study of neoadjuvant gemcitabine and oxaliplatin with radiation therapy in patients with pancreatic cancer. Cancer. 2013;119:2692–700.
51. Katz MHG, Fleming JB, Bhosale P, Varadhachary G, Lee JE, Wolff R, et al. Response of borderline resectable pancreatic cancer to neoadjuvant therapy is not reflected by radiographic indicators. Cancer. 2012;118:5749–56.
52. Ferrone CR, Marchegiani G, Hong TS, Ryan DP, Deshpande V, McDonnell EI, et al. Radiological and surgical implications of neoadjuvant treatment with FOLFIRINOX for locally advanced and borderline resectable pancreatic cancer. Ann Surg. 2015;261:12–7.
53. Cooper AB, Parmar AD, Riall TS, Hall BL, Katz MHG, Aloia TA, et al. Does the use of neoadjuvant therapy for pancreatic adenocarcinoma increase postoperative morbidity and mortality rates? J Gastrointest Surg. 2015;19:80–6. Discussion 86–7

Laparoscopic Pancreaticoduodenectomy

10

Ying-Jui Chao and Yan-Shen Shan

10.1 Introduction

Minimal invasive surgery has shown superiority in patient recovery, wound infection, blood loss, length of hospital stay, and complications in many operative procedures when compared to open surgery. Since laparoscopic approach for left pancreatic lesions has become well established and gold standard procedure in experienced surgeons [1], laparoscopic pancreaticoduodenectomy (LPD) remains an uncommon procedure for right pancreatic lesions. The dissemination and evolution of LPD was slow and unpopular. The first LPD was described by Gagner in 1994 [2] but the large study containing more than 30 patients was reported until 2007 by Palanivelu [3]. The complex procedure, long operation time, proximity of major vessels, patient population, and technical demanding of laparoscopic suturing make the surgeons reluctant to LPD. The teamwork and surgical planning have the determinant impact on the LPD program as well as the surgeon's advanced laparoscopic technique. Forty to fifty patients are required to overcome the learning curve of LPD and minimal invasive approach for pancreaticoduodenectomy (MIPD) may not be suitable or require more experience to obtain the same results

Y.-J. Chao
Division of General Surgery, Department of Surgery, National Cheng Kung University Hospital, Institute of Clinical Medicine, College of Medicine, National Cheng Kung University, Tainan City, Taiwan

Y.-S. Shan, M.D., Ph.D. (✉)
Division of General Surgery, Department of Surgery, National Cheng Kung University Hospital, Institute of Clinical Medicine, College of Medicine, National Cheng Kung University, Tainan City, Taiwan

Department of Clinical Medicine Research, National Cheng Kung University Hospital, Institute of Clinical Medicine, College of Medicine, National Cheng Kung University, Tainan City, Taiwan
e-mail: ysshan@mail.ncku.edu.tw

© Springer Science+Business Media Singapore 2017
H. Yamaue (ed.), *Innovation of Diagnosis and Treatment for Pancreatic Cancer*,
DOI 10.1007/978-981-10-2486-3_10

as open pancreaticoduodenectomy (OPD) in smaller and lower-volume hospitals or surgeons performed less than 20 cases per year. Hybrid laparoscopic-assisted pancreaticoduodenectomy is the ideal approach in the beginning and serves as a bridge from OPD to LPD [4]. The hybrid laparoscopic–open approach for pancreaticoduodenectomy includes completion of resection laparoscopically and completion of the reconstruction via minimal midline laparotomy, which has both the advantages of open and laparoscopic surgery and reduces the risk of anastomosis complication within the learning curve. Since the conversion rate of LPD (around 10%) is higher than other laparoscopic abdominal surgeries, the patient selection is important and the surgeon should avoid the elderly, patients with previous abdominal major operation, large tumor, uncinate lesion, malignant involvement of major vessels, and chronic inflammation, especially in the initial cases. Besides, an experienced assistant familiar with both laparoscopic and pancreas surgery is favored to facilitate the operation and reduce unnecessary intraoperative complication. The vascular anatomy of hepatic artery should be well read preoperatively and identified to avoid injury to the replaced right hepatic artery, which may increase the risk of failure of biliary anastomosis and liver abscess. There are three critical procedures in LPD including dissection of the uncinate process, performing hepaticojejunostomy, and pancreaticojejunostomy. It should be standardized to reduce the operation time and minimize the complication. In experienced hands, LPD can be performed with major vein reconstruction in pancreatic cancer with mesentericoportal invasion [5] and provide the oncologic benefits of early initiating chemotherapy and better disease-free survival [6]. Although LPD may provide the advantages of minimal invasive approach in well-selected cases, level 1 evidence of LPD is still lacking and further randomized control trials or prospective studies are warranted to address the benefits and outcome of LPD. In this chapter, we will introduce the detailed procedures of LPD, which was separated into two stages, the resection stage and reconstruction stage. The resection stage contains duodenum resection, biliary system resection, and pancreas resection. The reconstruction stage consists of pancreaticojejunostomy, hepaticojejunostomy, and gastrojejunostomy/duodenojejunostomy.

10.2   Surgical Procedures

10.2.1 Surgeon's Preparation

Due to the complex procedures of pancreaticoduodenectomy (PD), demand of surgeon's advanced technique, acknowledgement of anatomy and experience, surgeon volume and hospital volume are the determinant factors of morbidity and mortality. LPD has a steeper learning curve than other laparoscopic gastrointestinal surgeries. Even in OPD, 20 PDs and 60 PDs were required to achieve an equivalent morbidity and mortality as experienced surgeons to overcome the learning curve [7]. Surgeons who attempt to initiate the LPD program should have a well-established procedure and experience in OPD as well as the delicate intracorporeal suturing technique in laparoscopic surgery to complete the three important reconstructions of pancreaticojejunostomy, hepaticojejunostomy, and gastrojejunostomy/duodenojejunostomy. Besides, a laparoscopic team, advanced laparoscopic instruments, and assistant who is familiar with laparoscopic technique and pancreas surgery are also essential to minimize the obstacles during the development of LPD program. In LPD, 40–50 cases are required to attain the experience and technical competence in surgeons with experience in OPD [8, 9]. At low-volume institution or surgeon (<20 cases per year), more cases and longer time are expected to overcome the learning curve and standardize the procedure. Therefore, minimal invasive approach may not be considered as a routine procedure in PD in low-volume surgeon or hospital.

Hybrid laparoscopic-assisted pancreaticoduodenectomy (HLAPD) is the ideal approach in the beginning and serves as a bridge from OPD to LPD [4]. The hybrid laparoscopic–open approach includes pancreaticoduodenectomy performed laparoscopically and reconstruction completed via upper midline mini-laparotomy. The surgeon can begin the LPD program from the resection stage by laparoscopic approach and complete the three reconstructions with open method through the upper midline mini-laparotomy. After the resection stage is well standardized, pure LPD with intracorporeal anastomosis proceeds. Through this transitional approach, HLAPD can provide the advantages of minimal invasive surgery without increasing the postoperative complication within the learning curve.

10.2.2 Patient Selection

Although the growing surgeon experience in LPD, patient selection is the first issue for LPD and most patients receiving LPD are well selected. There are a variety of diseases indicated for PD including periampullary tumor and chronic pancreatitis, but some patients should be excluded for LPD especially for the initial cases. The suitable cases are the patients with dilated common bile duct (CBD) and pancreatic duct. There are two critical procedures in LPD including uncinated process dissection and reconstruction of pancreatic stump. The conversion rate of LPD (around 10%) was higher than other laparoscopic abdominal surgery. The most common causes of conversion to open surgery were tumor involvement or uncontrollable bleeding during the mesenterico-portal vein dissection. Patients with small CBD, large tumor, prominent uncinate process, severe inflammation around mesentericoportal vein, tumor invasion to major vessels, obesity, vascular anomaly, the elderly or other contraindication for minimal invasive surgery should be carefully selected in LPD. Obstructive jaundice is the common clinical manifestation in periampullary lesion and preoperative biliary drainage may increase the morbidity and mortality in patients receiving PD [10]. However, in patients with obstructive jaundice, preoperative jaundice relief is suggested before LDP because the pneumoperitoneum will increase the abdominal pressure which may cause ascending cholangitis in patients with bile stasis. In these two methods of biliary drainage (percutaneous external drainage or endoscopic internal drainage), external drainage is favored to avoid the inflammation effect of internal stent inserted in CBD. In non-drained obstructive jaundice preoperatively, the CBD was opened in the early stage of LPD to relieve the bile stasis and minimize the risk of ascending cholangitis.

10.2.3 Patient Position and Trocar Placement

After received general anesthesia, intubation, and central venous catheterization, the patient was then placed in the supine position with the legs separated. The camera man stood between the legs of the patient. The operator standing on the right side or left side of the patient depended on the procedure, the assistant on the contrary side to the operator. Five trocars were needed in LPD and the umbilical trocar was used as camera port (Fig. 10.1). The pneumoperitoneum pressure was maintained at 15 mmHg and a 30-degree laparoscope was applied. Most of the time, the patient was placed in a 30–40° reverse Trendelenburg position. Also, a 20-degree left sided tilt down to reveal the superior mesenteric artery and mesenterico-portal vein when the uncinate process dissection was proceeding.

10.2.4 Intraoperative Evaluation

All intra-abdominal viscera were assessed carefully and the ascites was aspirated and sent for cytology if present. All peritoneal cavity, especially around the tumor,

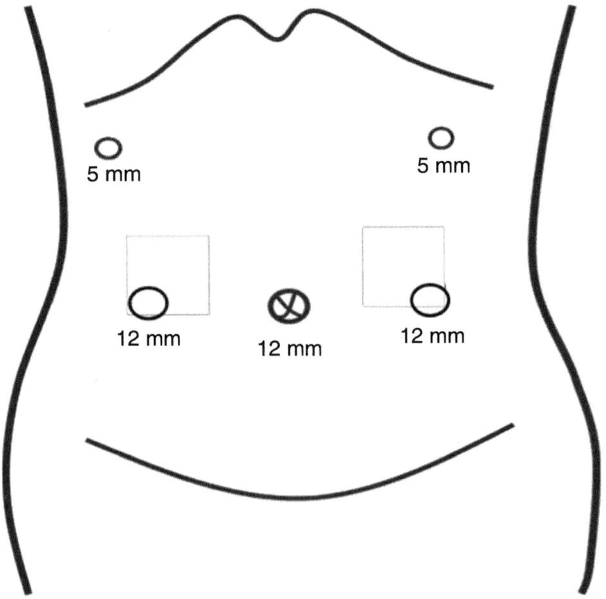

Fig. 10.1 Trocar position for laparoscopic pancreaticoduodenectomy

was carefully inspected and any suspicious lesion was biopsied. The intraoperative sonography was used to detect small and unexpected liver metastasis that might be missed in the abdominal computed tomography. If distant metastasis was proved, pancreaticoduodenectomy procedure should not proceed and prophylactic laparoscopic biliary and gastrointestinal bypass would be considered. The gastrocolic ligament was opened first to evaluate the tumor location and the mesenterico-portal vein. If the mesenterico-portal vein invasion or severe inflammation was noted, conversion to open surgery might be more suitable in initial cases.

10.2.5 Operative Procedures

The operative procedure is divided into two stages: the resection stage and reconstruction stage. The resection stage is composed of three parts of surgery: duodenum resection, biliary system resection, and pancreas resection. The reconstruction stage also includes three parts of surgery to reconstruct the gastrointestinal tract: pancreaticojejunostomy, hepaticojejunostomy, and duodenojejunostomy in pylorus-preserving PD or gastrojejunostomy in conventional PD. Due to the longer operative time and complex procedures in LPD, LPD may be performed by two surgeons or a time-break between the two stages of surgery to reduce fatigue, pressure, and loss of attention of surgeon during this long endoscopic surgery.

10.2.5.1 Resection Stage

Duodenum Resection

In the resection stage, the surgeon initially stood on the left side of the patient and the gastrocolic ligament was opened first and the mesenterico-portal vein was dissected to exclude invasion of major vessels. The right side of transverse colon and ascending colon were mobilized off to provide enough space for dissection of the uncinate process and mesenterico-portal vein (Fig. 10.2a). After the right side of T-colon was mobilized downward, the henle trunk was dissected and the right gastroepiploic vein was clipped and divided (Fig. 10.2b, c). For pylorus-preserving PD, the right gastroepiploic artery was clipped and divided. The duodenum was dissected till the attachment with pancreas and 1–2 cm duodenum distal pylorus was preserved for further reconstruction and divided by endoscopic stapler using 45 mm white cartridge (Fig. 10.2d). The right gastric artery was ligated and divided, and the stomach was put over left upper quadrant. For conventional PD, the antrum was divided using endoscopic stapler with 60 mm blue cartridge. The colon was retracted by the assistant to explore the 4th part of duodenum and the duodenojejunal fold was opened (Fig. 10.2e). The proximal jejunum was divided at 10–15 cm distal to Treitz's ligament by endoscopic stapler using 45 mm white cartridge, then the Treitz's ligament was divided and the mesentery of proximal jejunum was divided by harmonic scalpel (Fig. 10.2f). One gauze was put behind the uncinate process as the landmark of kocherization after the duodenojejunal fold was opened.

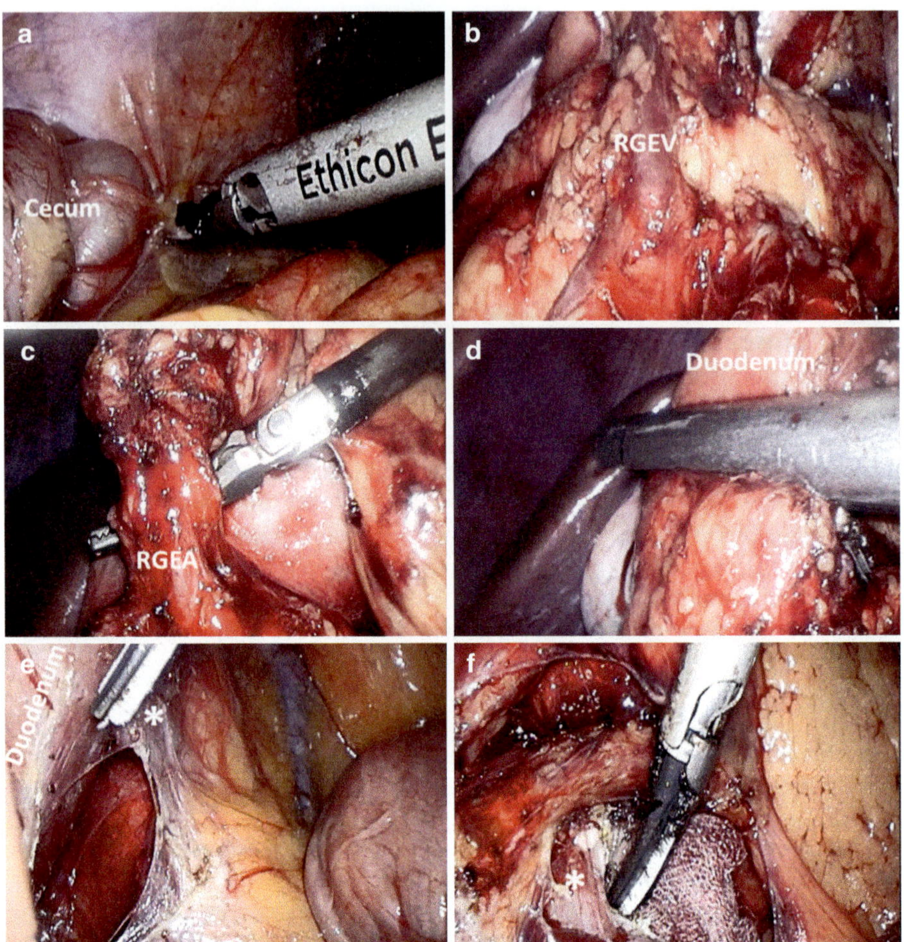

Fig. 10.2 Duodenum transection. (**a**) The ascending colon and cecum was mobilized, (**b**) Right gastroepiploic vein (RGEV) was identified, (**c**) Right gastroepiploic artery (RGEA) was ligated and divided. (**d**) Duodenum was transected using endoscopic stapler with 45 mm white cartridge. (**e**) Duodenocolic fold (*asterisk*) and any adhesion between duodenum and peritoneum were divided. (**f**) The ligamentum of Treitz (*asterisk*) was divided by harmonic scalpel and one gauze was put behind the uncinate process of pancreas as the landmark of kocherization

Biliary System Resection

At this stage, the vascular and biliary tract anatomy should be carefully interpreted before operation, especially the hepatic artery system. The gallbladder was removed after cystic duct and artery were divided. The common hepatic artery was identified and group 8 lymph node was dissected (Fig. 10.3a). The proper hepatic artery and gastroduodenal artery were explored and dissected carefully (Fig. 10.3b). The gastroduodenal artery was double ligated with hemolock and divided. The group 12 lymphatic tissue was dissected to expose the left and

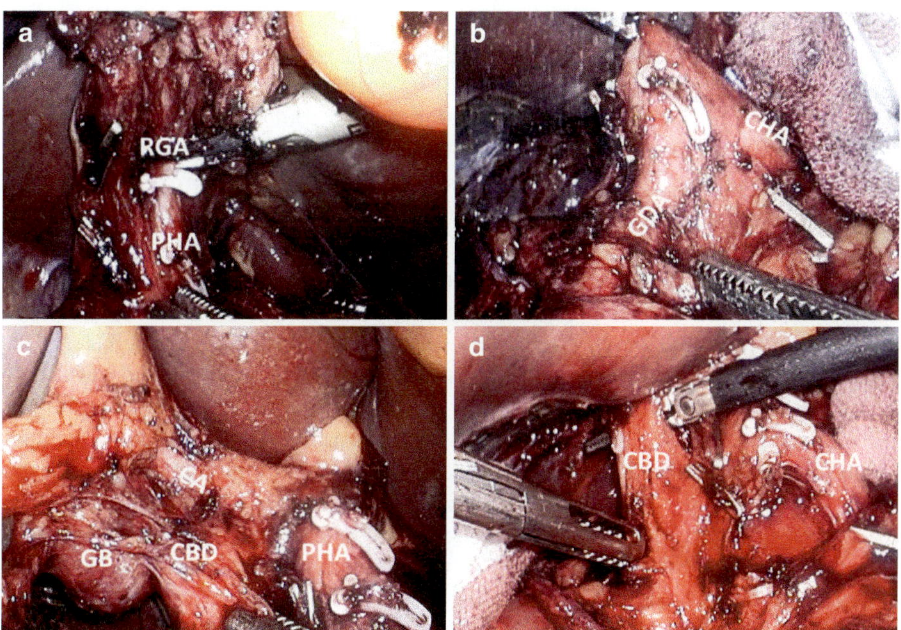

Fig. 10.3 Biliary system resection. (**a**) Right gastric artery (RGA) was clipped and ligated as well as group 12 lymph node dissection; (**b**) Gastroduodenal artery (GDA) was dissected, clipped, and ligated. (**c**) Gallbladder was removed after cystic artery (CA) and cystic duct clipped and divided. (**d**) Common bile duct was encircled and ligated

posterior side of CBD and superior border of the portal vein (Fig. 10.3c). The common bile duct was encircled and clipped or ligated with a thread at the proximal part to avoid bile spillage after CBD transection. In non-drained obstructive jaundice, the CBD was opened and the bile was suctioned to decrease the risk of ascending cholangitis during operation. After the bile stasis was relieved, the CBD was temporally clamped with endoscopic vascular bulldog clamp or hemoclip. Care should be taken to avoid injuring the replaced or the aberrant right hepatic artery during CBD dissection due to the high prevalence of 8.7–11% of aberrant right hepatic artery [11, 12], which usually located at the posterior or right side of the CBD. The replaced or aberrant right hepatic artery should be carefully identified and preserved at this procedure if present (Fig. 10.7d). When the replaced or the aberrant right hepatic artery was transected, the blood flow of biliary duct might be interfered and increased the risk of bile leak of bilioenteric anastomosis or postoperative liver abscess. If the replaced or the aberrant right hepatic artery was transected accidentally, an external drainage stent for bilioenteric anastomosis was suggested to reduce the incidence of postoperative bile leakage. Eletrocautery and harmonic scalpel should not be used for CBD transection when facing normal diameter of CBD and thermal effect may induce long-term stenosis of bilioenteric anastomosis.

Pancreas Resection

The operator could change position to the right side of the patient and the assistant shifted to the contrary side in this phase of operation. Extended Kocher maneuver was performed until the left side renal vein and the route of the superior mesentery artery were revealed (Fig. 10.4). After the retroperitoneum attachment of pancreatic head was lysed, the pancreas neck and uncinated process dissection were performed around the SMA and the mesenterico-portal vein. The henle trunk was double ligated with hemolock and divided, which may cause massive bleeding if the hemolok dislodged. The tunnel of pancreas neck was dissected away from the mesenterico-portal vein (in a caudal to cephalad direction). The pancreas neck was transected by electrocautery slowly to identify the pancreatic duct (Fig. 10.5a, b), which usually located approximately in the middle and lower part of the pancreas and can be correlated to the abdominal computed tomography or the magnetic resonance image. Caution should be noted that the harmonic scalpel should be avoided when approaching the pancreatic duct, which might seal off the pancreatic duct if the duct is small. After the pancreatic neck was transected, the transected jejunum loop can be identified after extended Kocher maneuver and retracted to the right. The mesentery of the duodenum was divided by harmonic scalpel and the assistant gingerly pushed the SMV to the left to expose the attachment of the uncinate process and the SMA. The first jejunal branch to the SMV was the landmark for uncinate process dissection (Fig. 10.7a). The dissection

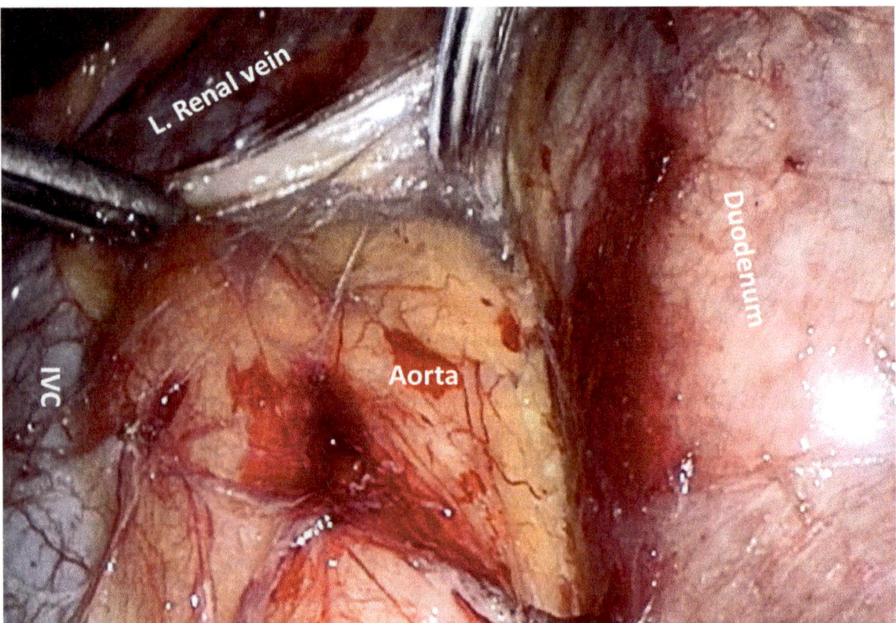

Fig. 10.4 Kocher maneuver. The inferior vena cava (IVC), aorta, and left renal vein were well identified after extended Kocher maneuver

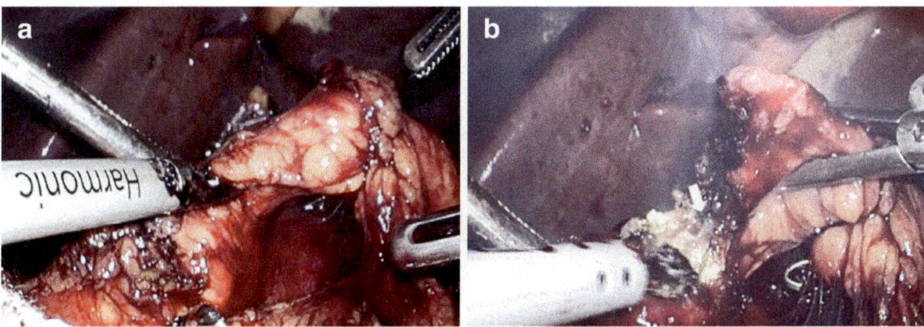

Fig. 10.5 The pancreatic neck transection. (**a**) The retropancreatic neck tunnel was dissected and encircled with a thread. The assistant pulled the thread to the left and the pancreatic transection was performed above the SMV using harmonic scalpel or electrocautery. (**b**) The pancreatic duct (*white arrow*) was identified when performing pancreatic transection

plane just located between the groove of the uncinate process and the first jejunal branch. The jejunal branches should be preserved to prevent proximal jejunum swelling during reconstruction. The meticulous dissection of uncinate process proceeded along the SMA in a caudo-cranial direction. Caution should be noted that all the small tributary veins to mesenterico-portal vein should be well clipped and divided to prevent massive bleeding during dissection, which would be difficult to be controlled.

The uncinate process dissection is the most critical procedure in laparoscopic PD, where is difficult to approach and easily bleeding when the surgical plan is not clear, especially in inflammation status or with large uncinate process. The uncinated process hooks the SMA by three different layers of structure: the anterior supportive adventitial tissue/lymphatic neural plexus, inferior pancreaticoduodenal artery, and the posterior supportive adventitial tissue/lymphatic neural plexus (Fig. 10.6). In open surgery, IPDA was mostly identified through anterior approach (after the anterior layer was opened). However, laparoscopic approach has the advantage of caudal and posterior view and the posterior layer dissection can be first dissected easily, where there were fewer tributary veins to portal vein than the anterior layer. When the anterior layer or posterior layer was dissected, the specimen was retracted upward and the assistant gingerly grasped the SMV, retracting to the left. The inferior pancreaticoduodenal artery (IPDA) was carefully dissected and ligated (Fig. 10.7b), followed by the posterior superior pancreaticoduodenal vein (Fig. 10.7c). In some patients, two IPDAs may be identified. The specimen was inserted into the specimen bag, which was put in the left upper quadrant and was retrieved after all the reconstruction was completed.

10.2.5.2 Reconstruction Stage

In the initial experience of laparoscopic-assisted PD, mini-laparotomy (5–7 cm upper midline incision) was suggested for more competent pancreatic and biliary reconstruction.

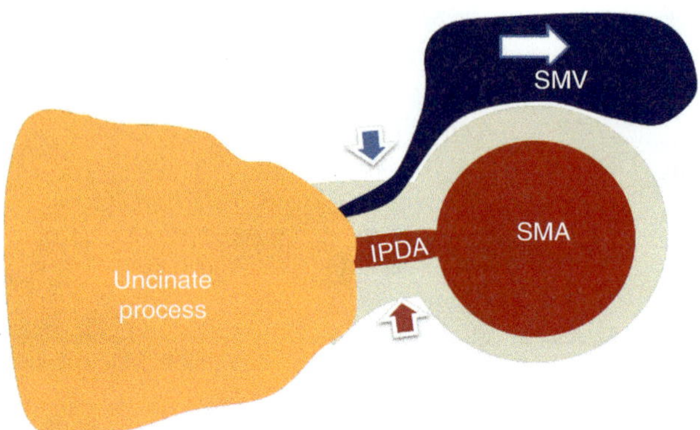

Fig. 10.6 The anatomy and concept of the uncinate process dissection. There are three layers of the attachment between the uncinate process of pancreas and the SMA including the anterior supportive adventitial tissue/lymphatic neural plexus (*blue arrow*), inferior pancreaticoduodenal artery (IPDA), and the posterior supportive adventitial tissue/lymphatic neural plexus (*red arrow*). The drainage vein of the uncinate process usually located at the anterior layers. When performing the uncinate process dissection, the SMV was grasped or pushed to the left (*white arrow*) to expose the attachment

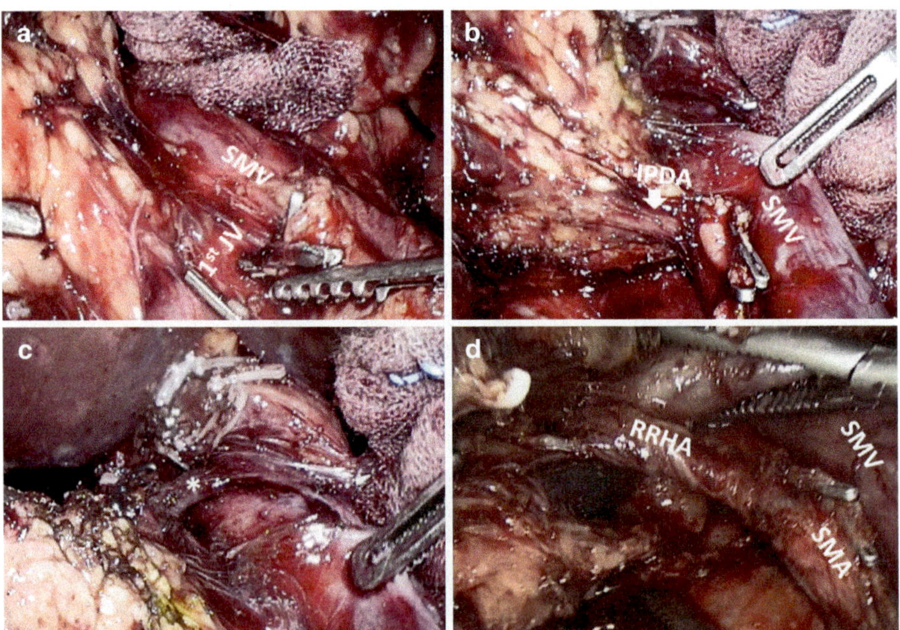

Fig. 10.7 The uncinate process dissection. (**a**) The SMV was pushed to the left to expose the 1st jejunal branch (1st JV) to the SMV and the dissection plane just located between the groove of the 1st JV and the uncinated process. (**b**) The inferior pancreaticoduodenal artery (IPDA; *white arrow*) was identified after the anterior and posterior layer of the attachment of uncinate process was opened. (**c**) Superior pancreaticoduodenal vein (*asterisk*) was visualized at the superior border of pancreatic head. (**d**) The replaced right hepatic artery (RRHA) from SMA was noted during the uncinate process dissection and should be carefully preserved to prevent the risk of leakage of biliary anastomosis

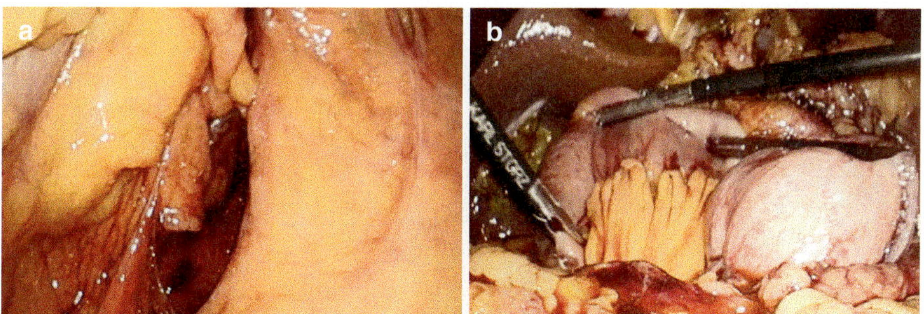

Fig. 10.8 Retrocolic route biliary and pancreatic reconstruction. (**a**) The mesocolon of transverse colon was opened. (**b**) The jejunal loop was delivered across the opening for further reconstruction

The transverse mesocolon near the inferior duodenal flexure was opened (Fig. 10.8a, b) and the proximal jejunal loops were brought across the opening for further reconstruction. The retrocolic pancreaticojejunostomy was performed first, followed by retrocolic hepaticojejunostomy, and antecolic duodenojejunostomy/gastrojejunostomy.

Pancreaticojejunostomy

There were various methods for pancreaticojejunostomy or pancreaticogastrostomy in open surgery. In laparoscopic surgery, the majority of pancreatic reconstruction was completed by pancreaticojejunostomy technique. The pancreaticojejunostomy can be divided into duct-to-mucosa or invagination technique, and the pancreatic fistula rate and overall morbidity were similar in both groups [13]. There was no any comparative study of duct-to-mucosa and invagination technique in LPD currently. It's time consuming to perform duct-to-mucosa anastomosis when the pancreatic duct is smaller than 2 mm. Hence, we preferred two-layer duct-to-mucosa technique in pancreatic duct larger than 1 mm and invagination technique in small pancreatic duct less than 1 mm. The surgeon stood between the legs of the patient, the camera man to the right, and the assistant to the left. The pancreatic stump was mobilized 2 cm away from the splenic vein and elevated for posterior layer suturing, and two-layer duct-to-mucosa pancreaticojejunostomy was performed.

Two-Layer Duct-to-Mucosa Pancreaticojejunostomy

The posterior layer was sutured with 4-0 monofilament horizontal mattress sutures first and usually three horizontal mattress sutures were required. Following the inner layer of duct-to-mucosa layer, one small opening in the jejunal loop near the pancreatic duct with harmonic scalpel or hook, then one 6–10 cm internal stent (6–8 Fr. suction tube) was introduced into the pancreatic duct before anastomosis and 5-0 polydioxanone (PDS) interrupted sutures for small pancreatic duct or continuous suture for large pancreatic duct was performed. Besides, 3 mm laparoscopic needle

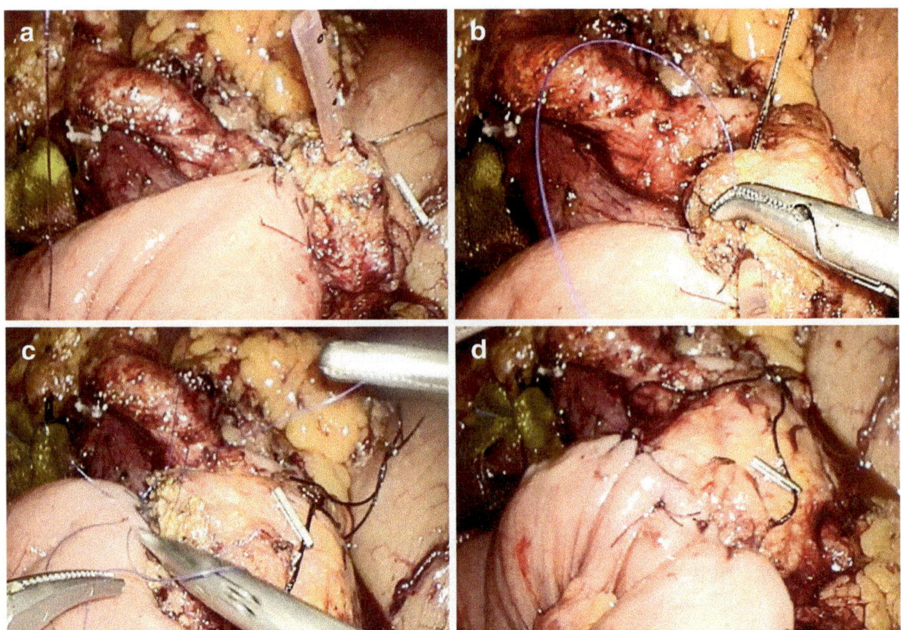

Fig. 10.9 Two-layer duct-to-mucosa pancreaticojejunostomy. (**a**) The posterior outer row was performed with horizontal mattress sutures using 4-0 monofilament suture. (**b**) The posterior layer of duct-to-mucosa was anastomosed with 5-0 PDS after one small opening of the jejunum was created opposite to the pancreatic duct. (**c**) The internal stent was delivered into the jejunum after the posterior layer of duct-to-mucosa anastomosis was completed. Three interrupted preset sutures were placed over anterior layer of duct-to-mucosa anastomosis. (**d**) Completion of pancreaticojejunostomy after the anterior outer row with three horizontal mattress sutures

holder might be used for better manipulation of the delicate duct-to-mucosa sutures. Finally, three anterior layer of 4-0 monofilament horizontal mattress sutures was done to complete pancreaticojejunostomy (Fig. 10.9).

Hepaticojejunostomy

The surgeon stood on the left side of the patient and the assistant changed to the right side of patient. End-to-side hepaticojejunostomy was performed 5 cm away from the pancreaticojejunostomy. One small opening was made at the jejunal loop according to the size of common hepatic duct. One-layer continuous suture with 4-0 or 5-0 prolene or PDS was performed (Fig. 10.10). The traction of CBD should be gentle in normal size and thin wall of CBD, and the thread might cut the CBD if inappropriate force or direction of traction by the assistant. After the biliary anastomosis was completed, the jejunal loop was fixed to the liver to decrease the tension of hepaticojejunostomy. For small common bile duct or preventing anastomosis stricture or leakage, an external stent for hepaticojejunostomy may be considered. If there was evidence of intraoperative bile leak, an external stent was also useful to decrease the postoperative bile leak (Fig. 10.11).

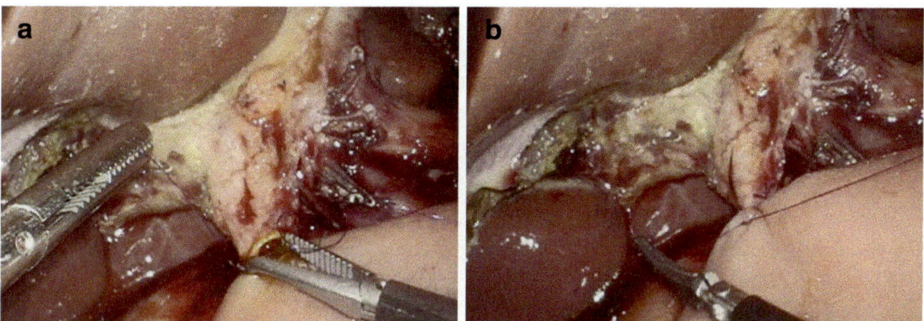

Fig. 10.10 Hepaticojejunostomy (**a**) The posterior layer was anastomosed with 5-0 PDS continuous suture and the openings of common hepatic duct and jejunum were dilated. (**b**) The anterior layer was completed with 5-0 PDS continuous suture

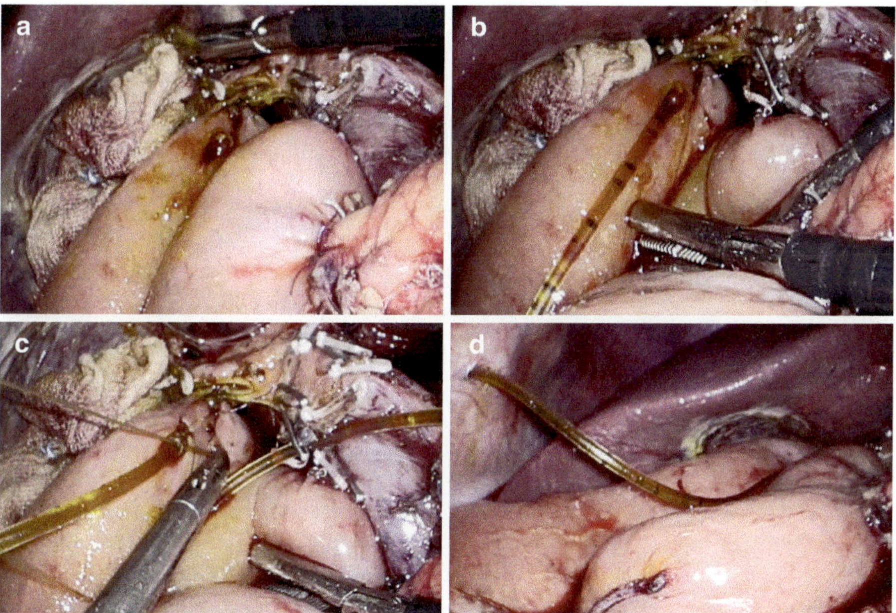

Fig. 10.11 The external stent of hepaticojejunostomy. (**a**) One small opening was created over 1 cm near the hepaticojejunostomy. (**b**) One 8–10 French suction tube was delivered through the anastomosis to the right hepatic duct and bile stain could be identified in the suction tube if the tube was put into the biliary system. (**c**) After the tube was put into the biliary system, the stenting tube was secured at the exit with 3-0 chromic suture and the exit was strengthened with a purse-string suture of 4-0 monocryl. (**d**) The stenting tube was brought out extraabdominally

Gastrojejunostomy or Duodenojejunostomy

The gastrojejunostomy or duodenojejunostomy was made 40–60 cm distal to biliary anastomosis by antecolic route. For classical Whipple procedure, the gastrojejunostomy was performed intracorporeally by linear stapler with 60 mm blue cartridge and the common entry hole was closed with two-layer continuous suture (Fig. 10.12a, b). For pylorus-preserving PD, to save time, the reconstruction was completed extracorporeally through the umbilical incision (3–5 cm) after the *Alexis wound retractor* (Applied Medical, Rancho Santa Margarita, CA) was placed and the specimen was retrieved.

10.2.6 Fibrin Glue Application

Fibrin glue was routinely applied externally topical to pancreaticojejunostomy and hepaticojejunostomy in LPD (Fig. 10.13a, b). Biological fibrin glue not only has the hemostasis effect but might reinforce the physical barrier of anastomoses. Although there was no evidence of preventing the incidence of pancreatic leak or overall

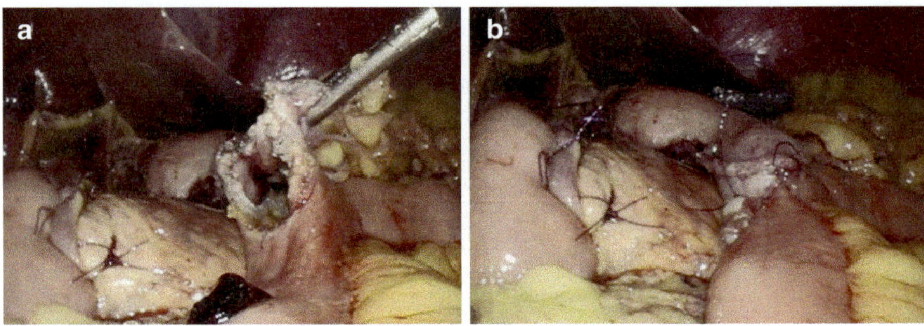

Fig. 10.12 Gastrojejunostomy. (**a**) The side-to-side gastrojejunostomy was performed by linear staple with 60 mm blue cartridge. (**b**) The common entry hole was closed with two-layer continuous sutures

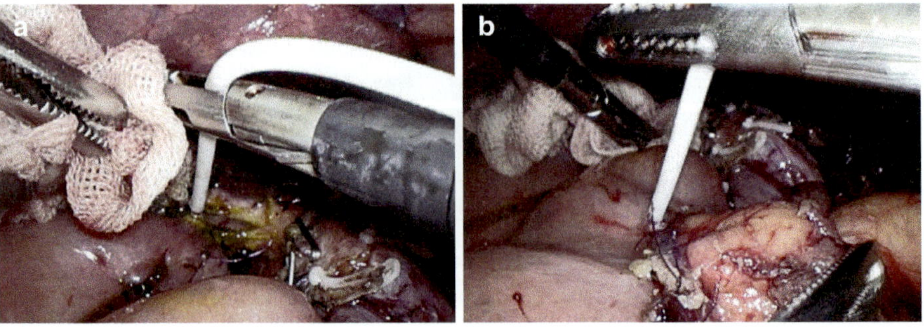

Fig. 10.13 Topical application of fibrin glue to the hepaticojejunostomy (**a**) and pancreaticojejunostomy (**b**)

complications in open pancreaticoduodenectomy [14, 15], some studies reported that fibrin glue augmentation might decrease the risk of pancreatic leakage in pancreaticogastrostomy [16]. However, the result of fibrin glue application in LPD was still lacking.

10.2.7 Drain Placement

The pneumoperitoneum was recreated and the abdomen was lavaged with warm normal saline. Two Jackson–Pratt drains were placed under the biliary and pancreatic anastomosis. If the external stent for biliary anastomosis was planned, it was created after the drains were placed.

10.3 Postoperative Care

The patient was usually extubated at the end of operation and was transferred to general ward for postoperative care. However, the patient might be transferred to intensive care unit if longer operation time in the elderly (age >70), or high-risk patients. Prophylactic somatostatin or octreotide was not routinely used to reduce the incidence of pancreatic leak. Partial parental nutrient would be given on postoperative day 1, sipping water on postoperative day 2, and oral soft diet if the patient got flatus. The nasogastric tube was left until the patient got flatus and early ambulation was commenced on the first postoperative day. The amylase level of the drainage was measured on postoperative day 3 and the development of pancreatic fistula was defined according to the definition of ISGPF (International Study Group on Pancreatic Fistula) [17]. The drainage was removed if no evidence of pancreatic fistula and smooth oral intake.

10.4 Results and Outcome

Since the first laparoscopic PD was described by Gagner in 1994 [2], the large study recruited more than 30 patients was reported until 2007 by Palanivelu [3]. Unlike other abdominal surgeries, the dissemination and evolution of LPD was slow and unpopular. In the early development of minimal invasive surgery, LPD was only performed in selected centers and the number of patients was small and well-selected. There were only few reports before 2010. Due to the development of instrument, standardization of the procedure, and the knowledge of surgical anatomy, LPD has gradually adopted after 2010 and the indication of LPD also expanded. Tumor involvement of the portal vein or SMV was not uncommon in pancreatic cancer. PD associated with major venous resection was the most challenge procedure of pancreatic surgery and was considered relatively contraindicated for laparoscopic approach. However, in experienced hands, LPD with vascular resection was also considered safe and feasible in specialized centers [5, 18]. In the National

Inpatient Database of the United States (a sample of approximately 20% of all hospital discharge), 4.4% of all PD (15,574 patients) was performed laparoscopically between 2000 and 2010, and the proportion of LPD increased from 3.2% in 2000 to 6% in 2010 [19] during the study period. The majority of LPD (67%) were performed in high-volume hospitals (more than 20 PD per year). In the recent review study, more than 2000 cases of MIPD including laparoscopic or robotic PD were reported in English literature, which carried an overall severe morbidity of 14.3% (the Clavien-Dindo classification $\geq$3) and an overall postoperative mortality of 2.3% [20]. Although LPD is a technically feasible and safe procedure, randomized controlled trial to compare the short-term or long-term outcome between LPD and open PD is still lacking. The meta-analysis comparing MIPD and OPD (six retrospective reports) showed that MIPD could provide less blood loss, more harvested lymph nodes, and shorter hospital stay, though smaller tumor size and longer operative time in MIPD group [21]. The overall complication rate and other pancreatic specific complications (pancreatic fistula, delayed gastric emptying, postpancreatectomy hemorrhage, and wound infection) were similar in both groups. However, the conversion rate of LPD (around 10%) is higher than other laparoscopic abdominal surgery and the majority of these were due to uncontrollable bleeding, major vessel invasion, inflammation, etc. postpancreatectomy complications may have a direct impact on the survival of pancreatic cancer patients [22]. LPD may provide fewer complications, fast recovery, and less hospital stay, leading to the willing of patients and earlier schedule of initiating adjuvant chemotherapy than the patients undergoing OPD. Kendrick et al. reported that the time until adjuvant chemotherapy was reduced in LPD group (LPD: 48 days versus OPD: 59 days, $p < 0.001$) and the delayed adjuvant chemotherapy beyond 8 or 12 weeks was also reduced in LPD group [6]. Although the overall survival of pancreatic cancer patients was similar in LPD and OPD groups, the disease-free survival was superior in LPD group. Caution should be noted that LPD may provide short-term or long-term benefit in pancreatic cancer patient but the current reports were all retrospective studies with selection bias and small number of patients. However, the patients receiving LPD were well-selected and less comorbidity. Further randomized or well-designed prospective cohort studies are still warranted to provide more evidence and address the short-term and long-term outcomes of LPD.

References

1. Ammori BJ, Ayiomamitis GD. Laparoscopic pancreaticoduodenectomy and distal pancreatectomy: a UK experience and a systematic review of the literature. Surg Endosc. 2011;25(7): 2084–99.
2. Gagner M, Pomp A. Laparoscopic pylorus-preserving pancreatoduodenectomy. Surg Endosc. 1994;8(5):408–10.
3. Palanivelu C, Jani K, Senthilnathan P, Parthasarathi R, Rajapandian S, Madhankumar MV. Laparoscopic pancreaticoduodenectomy: technique and outcomes. J Am Coll Surg. 2007;205(2):222–30.
4. Wang Y, Bergman S, Piedimonte S, Vanounou T. Bridging the gap between open and minimally invasive pancreaticoduodenectomy: the hybrid approach. Can J Surg. 2014;57(4): 263–70.

5. Kendrick ML, Sclabas GM. Major venous resection during total laparoscopic pancreaticoduodenectomy. HPB (Oxford). 2011;13(7):454–8.

6. Croome KP, Farnell MB, Que FG, Reid-Lombardo KM, Truty MJ, Nagorney DM, et al. Total laparoscopic pancreaticoduodenectomy for pancreatic ductal adenocarcinoma: oncologic advantages over open approaches? Ann Surg. 2014;260(4):633–8. Discussion 8–40

7. Schmidt CM, Turrini O, Parikh P, House MG, Zyromski NJ, Nakeeb A, et al. Effect of hospital volume, surgeon experience, and surgeon volume on patient outcomes after pancreaticoduodenectomy: a single-institution experience. Arch Surg. 2010;145(7):634–40.

8. Speicher PJ, Nussbaum DP, White RR, Zani S, Mosca PJ, Blazer 3rd DG, et al. Defining the learning curve for team-based laparoscopic pancreaticoduodenectomy. Ann Surg Oncol. 2014;21(12):4014–9.

9. Wang M, Meng L, Cai Y, Li Y, Wang X, Zhang Z, et al. Learning curve for laparoscopic pancreaticoduodenectomy: a CUSUM analysis. J Gastrointest Surg. 2016;20(5):924–35.

10. Povoski SP, Karpeh Jr MS, Conlon KC, Blumgart LH, Brennan MF. Association of preoperative biliary drainage with postoperative outcome following pancreaticoduodenectomy. Ann Surg. 1999;230(2):131–42.

11. Michels NA. Newer anatomy of the liver and its variant blood supply and collateral circulation. Am J Surg. 1966;112(3):337–47.

12. Hiatt JR, Gabbay J, Busuttil RW. Surgical anatomy of the hepatic arteries in 1000 cases. Ann Surg. 1994;220(1):50–2.

13. Hua J, He Z, Qian D, Meng H, Zhou B, Song Z. Duct-to-mucosa versus invagination pancreaticojejunostomy following pancreaticoduodenectomy: a systematic review and meta-analysis. J Gastrointest Surg. 2015;19(10):1900–9.

14. Martin I, Au K. Does fibrin glue sealant decrease the rate of anastomotic leak after a pancreaticoduodenectomy? Results of a prospective randomized trial. HPB (Oxford). 2013;15(8): 561–6.

15. Lillemoe KD, Cameron JL, Kim MP, Campbell KA, Sauter PK, Coleman JA, et al. Does fibrin glue sealant decrease the rate of pancreatic fistula after pancreaticoduodenectomy? Results of a prospective randomized trial. J Gastrointest Surg. 2004;8(7):766–72. Discussion 72–4

16. Conaglen PJ, Collier NA. Augmenting pancreatic anastomosis during Whipple operation with fibrin glue: a beneficial technical modification? ANZ J Surg. 2014;84(4):266–9.

17. Bassi C, Dervenis C, Butturini G, Fingerhut A, Yeo C, Izbicki J, et al. Postoperative pancreatic fistula: an international study group (ISGPF) definition. Surgery. 2005;138(1):8–13.

18. Khatkov IE, Izrailov RE, Khisamov AA, Tyutyunnik PS, Fingerhut A. Superior mesenteric-portal vein resection during laparoscopic pancreatoduodenectomy. Surg Endosc. 2017;31(3): 1488–95.

19. Tran TB, Dua MM, Worhunsky DJ, Poultsides GA, Norton JA, Visser BC. The first decade of laparoscopic pancreaticoduodenectomy in the United States: costs and outcomes using the nationwide inpatient sample. Surg Endosc. 2016;30(5):1778–83.

20. Wang M, Cai H, Meng L, Cai Y, Wang X, Li Y, et al. Minimally invasive pancreaticoduodenectomy: a comprehensive review. Int J Surg. 2016;35:139–46.

21. Correa-Gallego C, Dinkelspiel HE, Sulimanoff I, Fisher S, Vinuela EF, Kingham TP, et al. Minimally-invasive vs open pancreaticoduodenectomy: systematic review and meta-analysis. J Am Coll Surg. 2014;218(1):129–39.

22. Howard TJ, Krug JE, Yu J, Zyromski NJ, Schmidt CM, Jacobson LE, et al. A margin-negative R0 resection accomplished with minimal postoperative complications is the surgeon's contribution to long-term survival in pancreatic cancer. J Gastrointest Surg. 2006;10(10):1338–45. Discussion 45–6

Robotic Pancreaticoduodenectomy: Technical Approaches and Outcomes

11

Stacy J. Kowalsky, Amer H. Zureikat, Herbert J. Zeh III, and Melissa E. Hogg

11.1 Robotic Pancreaticoduodenectomy: Technical Approaches and Outcomes

11.1.1 Introduction

Pancreatic resections for both benign and malignant disease remain one of the most complex and challenging procedures for surgeons today. The retroperitoneal location of the gland, the complexities of the different gland textures, and its close proximity to major vascular structures all contribute to the intricacy of pancreatic resections. The pancreaticoduodenectomy (PD) has added complexity inherent in the necessity of reconstruction of gastrointestinal, biliary, and pancreatic continuity, requiring the construction of three separate anastomoses. As such, perioperative morbidity and mortality remained almost prohibitively high for many decades following the description of the PD by Allen O. Whipple in 1935 [1]. Improvements in mortality have been achieved at high volume centers with postoperative mortality rates as low as 1–2%, compared to mortality rates of 30% at the same center in the 1970s [2]. These improvements in postoperative PD mortality with increasing operative volume were demonstrated across many studies within the United States [3, 4], as well as other multiple European and Asian countries, as illustrated in a meta-analysis by Hata and others [5]. This drastic improvement in mortality rates in hospitals with increased

S.J. Kowalsky, M.D.
Division of GI Surgical Oncology, University of Pittsburgh Medical Center, Pittsburgh, PA, USA

A.H. Zureikat, M.D. • H.J. Zeh III, M.D. • M.E. Hogg, M.D. (✉)
Division of GI Surgical Oncology, University of Pittsburgh Medical Center, Pittsburgh, PA, USA

Department of Surgery, University of Pittsburgh Medical Center, Pittsburgh, PA, USA
e-mail: hoggme@upmc.edu

© Springer Science+Business Media Singapore 2017
H. Yamaue (ed.), *Innovation of Diagnosis and Treatment for Pancreatic Cancer*,
DOI 10.1007/978-981-10-2486-3_11

PD volume has led to centralization of the procedure to these high volume centers [3, 4]. However, improvements in morbidity have not been as encouraging.

Over the course of approximately 30 years of evolving PD experience, postoperative morbidity rates have largely remained unchanged. In one series of 1175 PDs from 1970 to 2006 at a single institution, morbidity rates remained elevated in the 30–40% range over more than three decades [2]. Another retrospective review of 17,761 PDs from multiple states in the Unites States from 2002 to 2011 shows significant trends towards decreased complication rates in high volume centers. Decreases in infectious, bleeding, respiratory, and gastrointestinal tract complications were noted. However, complication rates by organ systems individually remained in the range of 5–17%, even among high volume centers [4]. As improvements in perioperative morbidity have been realized with minimally invasive operative approaches for a myriad of other procedures, recent interest has been towards optimizing minimally invasive PD.

The first laparoscopic PD was described by Gagner and Pomp in 1994 [6]. However, widespread adoption of this technique did not follow. The technique has been performed by multiple surgical teams throughout the world [7–11], with most series showing decreased intraoperative estimated blood loss (EBL) [8–10], increased median lymph node harvest [8, 9], decreased length of postoperative stay, and R1 resection rates better than or equal to open PD [8–11]. Multiple series have shown increased operative time for this minimally invasive approach [8, 9, 11]. However, some groups have found improvements in operative time, even approaching open PD, with increased operative experience [9, 11] and equal operative time at one higher volume center [10]. A meta-analysis of series published before 2010 revealed only 285 laparoscopic PDs in the literature, with only 225 completed from start to finish in a minimally invasive fashion. Weighted analysis of these studies showed complication and mortality rates similar to published rates for open approaches, at 48% and 2%, respectively. Similarly, lymph node harvest (weighted average 15) and margin positivity rates (0.4%) were within range for open procedures, and EBL was significantly lower [12]. A retrospective review of the National Cancer Center database of patients undergoing PD for pancreatic ductal adenocarcinoma in the United States between 2010 and 2011 found that laparoscopic PD is associated with decreased postoperative length of stay, as well as increased lymph node harvest and decreased R1 resections, suggesting benefits for the approach. However, this analysis also showed increased 30-day postoperative mortality in hospitals performing less than ten laparoscopic PDs, suggesting the steep learning curve associated with implementation of the approach [13]. While laparoscopic PD has been shown to have some benefits over traditional open PD in terms of decreased EBL, decreased postoperative length of stay and possibly increased lymph node yield, the technical challenges of the approach and steep learning curve have prevented widespread adoption.

Following the introduction of robotic-assisted surgical systems in the late 1990s, there has been increasing application across varying surgical specialties. The benefits of robotic-assisted surgery, including 20–30x field magnification with stereotactic binocular vision, improved surgical instrument dexterity with nearly 540 degrees of range of motion, elimination of surgeon tremor, and improved ergonomics for operating surgeons, provide the ability to overcome some of the obstacles of laparoscopic pancreatic surgery [14]. As such, interest has grown in applying the robotic surgical platform to advanced pancreatic resections. The first robotic-assisted PD was described by Giulianotti and others in Italy in 2003, in a series of eight cases [15]. This very early robotic-assisted PD experience showed that the procedure was feasible with this minimally invasive approach, and soon the technique began to increase in popularity, with our institution beginning robotic pancreatic surgery in 2008 [16].

11.1.1.1 Preoperative Evaluation and Operative Technique

Upon initiation of the robotic-assisted pancreatic surgery program at this institution, care was taken to ensure that the principles of open pancreatic surgery were followed meticulously. Early cases were performed by two experienced pancreatic surgeons for safety and logistic surgical volume concerns to gain momentum and shared experience. Selection of early patients was for patients with ampullary cancers, pancreatic neuro-endocrine tumors, and purely resectable pancreatic adenocarcinomas. This had the added benefit of a more favorable resection, but soft glands and small ducts could also lead to more difficult reconstruction and increased risk for perioperative morbidity from postoperative pancreatic fistulae [17, 18]. Another important aspect of our robotic surgical application, to ensure patient safety, is diligent preoperative evaluation. Over the course of our experience, the inclusion criteria have expanded considerably and the numbers of PDs being performed via the robotic approach has increased substantially (Fig. 11.1). Currently, approximately 80% of PDs are performed robotically, even for borderline resectable pancreatic adenocarcinomas (PDA). The only absolute contraindication to robotic PD is vascular encasement of a long segment of the portal vein (PV) or superior mesenteric vein (SMV), which will likely need an interposition graft. To evaluate for resectability, all patients undergo preoperative triphasic CT scan imaging,

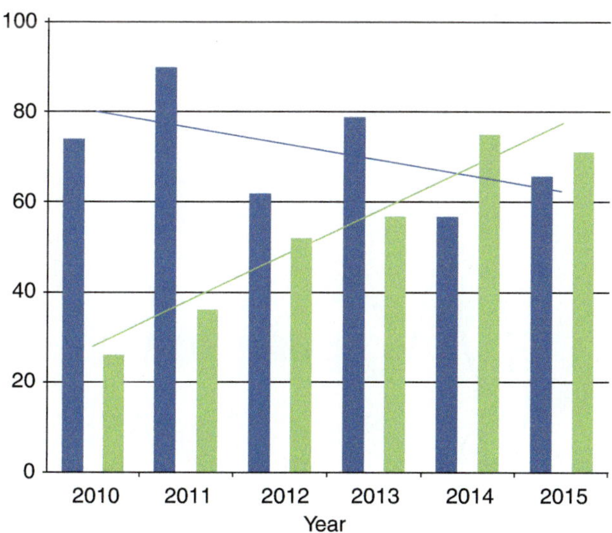

Fig. 11.1 Open vs robotic PD trends between 2010 and 2015. Percentages of total PD completed via open (*blue*) and robotic (*green*) approach at the University of Pittsburgh Medical Center, Pittsburgh, PA, USA, between 2010 and 2015. The overall trend is towards increasing utilization of the robotic surgical platform for performance of PD procedures

as well as endoscopic ultrasound evaluation, which in combination, have been shown to better predict successful margin negative resection [19]. Our current bias is for neo-adjuvant therapy for all borderline resectable PDAs, and most resectable PDAs on clinical trial, as well. On average, 70% of our patients with PDA undergo neoadjuvant chemotherapy or chemoradiation. In the past year, 60.6% of our robotic PDs were performed for PDA, while the remaining cases were for ampullary cancer (9.9%), IPMN (9.9%), neuroendocrine tumors (5.6%), duodenal adenocarcinoma (4.2%), cholangiocarcinoma (4.2%), and other benign lesions (5.6%).

Our operative approach has previously been described [14, 20, 21] and utilizes the daVinci Robotic Surgical System (Intuitive Surgical, Sunny Valley, CA, USA). At the beginning of our experience, the S console system was utilized. Once the company upgraded to the Si, the computer interface and wrist capabilities of the robotic platform were better suited for this complex operation. We also have a Xi system and have performed robotic PDs on this system, as well; however, our preference remains use of the Si system. The procedure begins with laparoscopic evaluation. The configuration of port placements begins with placement of a 5 mm access port placed in the left subcostal region, utilizing an optical separator. This port will later be converted to a robotic 8 mm port. For malignant pathologies, once we confirm there is no metastatic disease, we place the remaining ports under direct visualization in the following fashion (Fig. 11.2):

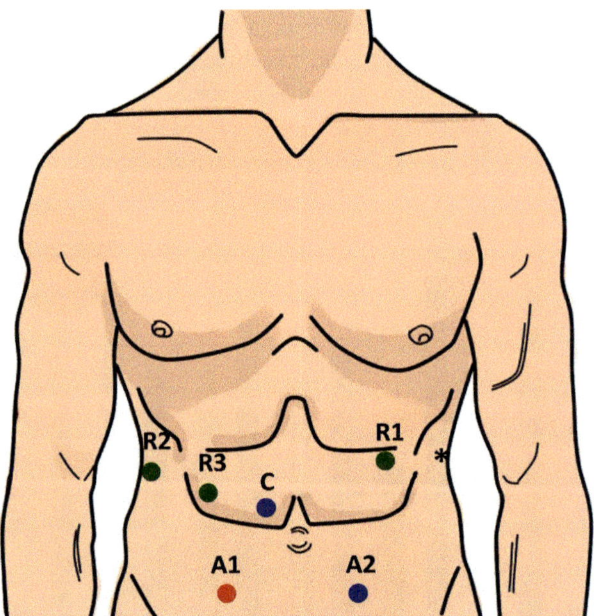

Fig. 11.2 Port placement configuration for robotic-assisted pancreaticoduodenectomy. Robotic 8 mm ports (R1, R2, R3) are used for the robotic arms. The 12 mm camera port (C) is placed above and to the right of the umbilicus. Assistant ports include a 5 mm port in the right lower quadrant (A1) and a 12 mm port in the left lower quadrant (A2), which then serves as specimen extraction site. The *asterisk* indicates a 5 mm self-retaining liver retractor

12 mm camera port 2–3 cm above and to the right of the umbilicus in a patient with an average body habitus, and two additional 8 mm ports for the robotic arms in the right midclavicular line and the right anterior axillary line. A 12 mm port is placed in the left lower quadrant, which serves as a port for the assistant and later for specimen extraction, and a 5 mm port is also placed in the right lower quadrant for the assistant. These are situated between the camera port and its neighboring port on either side. Additionally, a self-retaining liver retractor is placed in the left upper quadrant. When placing these ports, care is taken to ensure that at least a hands-breath, or 5–6 cm, is between ports to allow for free movement of instruments. For the first 6 years, the beginning of the procedure was performed laparoscopically; however, in the past 2 years, we have converted to an almost entirely robotic approach, where we dock the robot after port placement. One key maneuver is to close the camera 12 mm port with a "figure of 8" stitch using a suture passer prior to docking the robot (Fig. 11.2).

The robot is then docked directly over the head of the patient using the Si or at the patient's right shoulder using the Xi. Our primary instruments for a majority of the resection include the hook monopolar in the right hand, the fenestrated bipolar in the left hand, and the cadiere or prograsp in the 3rd hand. The resection begins after entering the lesser sac through the gastrocolic omentum, followed by mobilization of the right colon then the duodenum by means of a Kocher maneuver. One trick to the operation is delivering the jejunum into the right upper quadrant by dissecting the ligament of Treitz until it is freed up about 40 cm, and then it is divided approximately 10 cm from the uncinate process. Then, the right gastric artery is taken with an energy device on the lesser curve, followed by the gastroepiploic artery along the greater curve. The stomach or proximal duodenum is transected. We favor a classic PD, but will occasionally perform a pylorus-preserving PD.

Once the stomach is divided, we move to the next step, which is dissection of the porta hepatis (Fig. 11.3). We start this dissection with removal of the hepatic artery lymph node. We think this is an important step for identification of the hepatic artery, portal vein (PV), and gastroduodenal artery (GDA). Once these structures are identified, we move lateral on the porta hepatis and identify the lateral aspect of the common bile duct (CBD), and then the lateral and posterior portal lymph nodes are dissected off the CBD and left attached to the specimen. Once this area is clear, we try to identify the PV and create a plane between it and the CBD. Then, we go back to the GDA and test clamp to make sure there is still adequate hepatic artery flow once clamped. If any question, we perform an ultrasound of the artery and test clamp under Doppler and ultrasound flow. We ligate the GDA with a vascular stapler and leave a clip on the staple line to mark the stump. Then, we dissect the CBD medially off the PV and once encircled, staple with a vascular load, as well. The benefit to dissecting laterally prior to stapling the GDA and CBD is to assure that there are no replaced or accessory hepatic vessels that need to be preserved (Fig. 11.3).

Next, we dissect the inferior border of the pancreas, locate the SMV, and create a retro-pancreatic tunnel (Fig. 11.4). The pancreas is then divided with hot scissor electrocautery half way from anterior to posterior and inferior to superior. Then, care is taken to divide the pancreatic duct with "cold" scissor transection. Attention is then

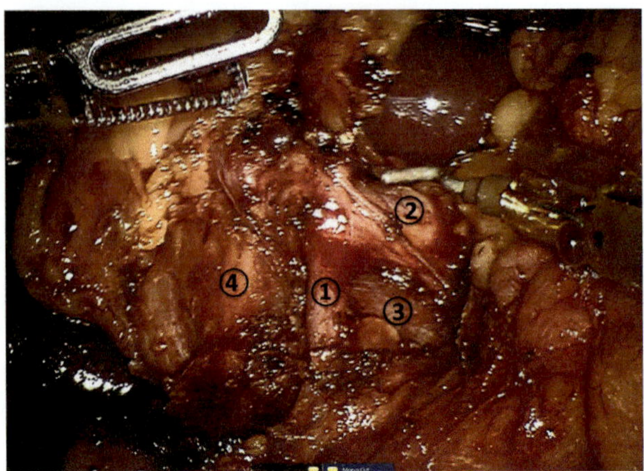

Fig. 11.3 Detailed view of portal dissection. The gastroduodenal artery (1) is isolated for ligation, typically via a vascular stapler and the stump is further reinforced with a clip. The common hepatic artery (2) and portal vein (3) can also be identified. The common bile duct (4) will also be transected using a stapler

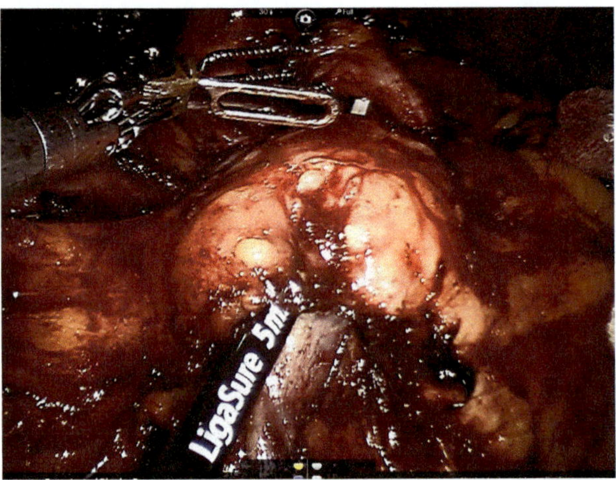

Fig. 11.4 Creation of the retro-pancreatic tunnel. Dissection proceeds along the inferior and superior borders of the pancreas, at the level of the pancreatic neck, and allows for creation of a tunnel beneath the pancreas and above the mesenteric vasculature

turned towards identifying the gastroepiploic and middle colic veins in relation to the SMV. The SMV is dissected fully to reveal the origin of these vessels prior to ligation. When possible, depending on the presence of a common trunk, the middle colic vein is preserved. The gastroepiploic vein is taken at its origin on the SMV. Once this is complete, we roll the SMV off the uncinate process and identify the first jejunal branches. We preserve these where possible; however, there are often numerous recurrent branches to the uncinate process requiring delicate dissection. Once the first

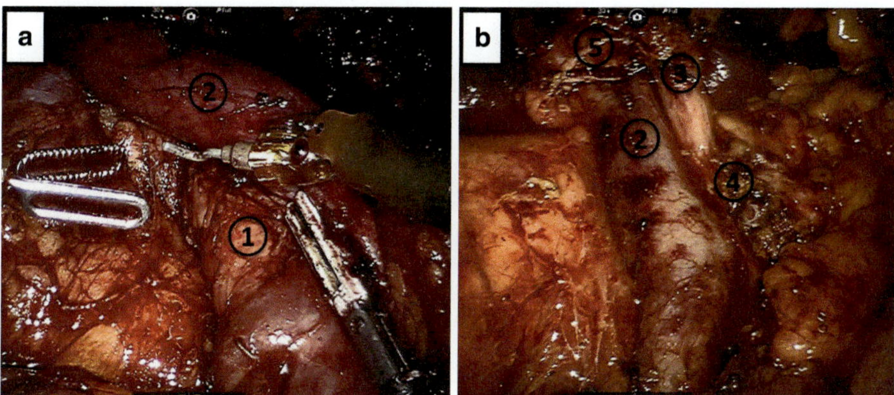

Fig. 11.5 Completed pancreaticoduodenectomy resection view. (**a**) The resection bed, with retraction of the superior mesenteric vein, shows careful dissection and removal of all the perivascular tissue along the plane of Leriche, clearing the superior mesenteric artery (1) and portal vein (2) margins. (**b**) After removal of the specimen, the view prior to reconstruction shows the dissected portal vein margin (2), the gastroduodenal artery stump (3), which is reinforced with a surgical clip, the cut edge of the pancreas (4), with a readily identifiable pancreatic duct, and the divided common bile duct (5)

jejunal is dissected off the uncinate, we identify the superior mesenteric artery (SMA). The magnified field of vision and articulating instruments of the robotic platform allow for both careful identification and management of the GDA and inferior and superior pancreaticoduodenal arteries, as well as smaller jejunal branches, which are often taken with an energy device. Where possible, a clip is placed on the staying side of the pancreaticoduodenals on the SMA. Furthermore, the visualization of the robotic system also allows for thorough resection of perivascular and peripancreatic tissue on the plane of Leriche (Fig. 11.5), allowing for thorough oncologic resection. The approach of the vascular groove and retroperitoneal margin varies based on gland texture and vascular involvement. A soft gland allows for a "back and forth" approach from anterior to posterior utilizing primarily an energy device. Anything with SMV involvement or a very firm gland may necessitate an "artery first" approach from inferior to posterior. If there is SMA involvement, we prefer a "hanging maneuver," where the SMV is dissected above and below the first jejunal, which is then taken with a stapler or energy device. The SMA is then dissected under the SMV from medial to lateral. The advantages of the robotic approach assist in meticulous resection, but further aid in reconstruction (Figs. 11.4 and 11.5).

The reconstructive process of PD is of utmost importance given the morbidity and mortality associated with anastomotic leakage and failure. We utilize a duct-to-mucosa fashion modified Blumgart pancreaticojejunostomy technique (Fig. 11.6) [22]. This two-layer anastomosis is typically constructed over a pancreatic duct stent (4, 5, or 7 French, Hobbs Medical, Stafford Springs, CT, USA). We use three 2-0 silk stitches on a V-20 needle for the outer layers and 5-0 monofilament sutures for the duct to mucosa stitches. We usually place 2 posterior and 2–5 anterior stitches depending on duct size. The hepaticojejunostomy or choledochojejustomy

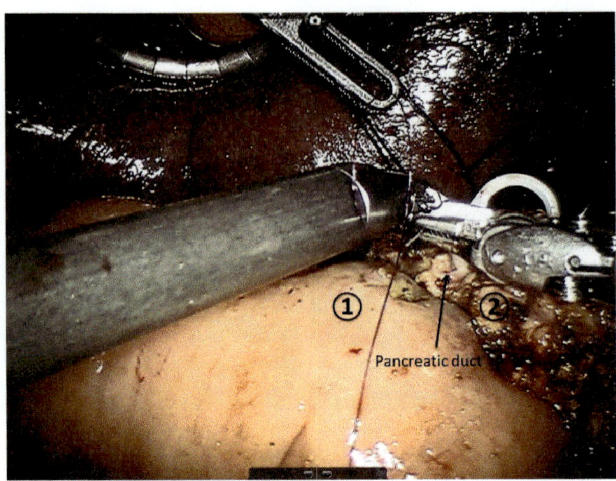

Fig. 11.6 Creation of pancreaticojejunostomy in modified Blumgart technique. The jejunum (1) is approximated to the pancreatic parenchyma (2) with 2-0 silk horizontal mattress sutures through the seromuscular layer of jejunum. Electrocautery is utilized to create a small enterotomy in the jejunum. Then, a duct-to-mucosa pancreaticojejunostomy is created using 5-0 PDS sutures over a Hobbs pancreatic stent (Hobbs Medical, Inc., Stafford Springs, CT, USA) to ensure duct patency. Finally, the anterior layer is created using 2-0 silk sutures to approximate the seromuscular layer of the jejunum to the pancreatic parenchyma

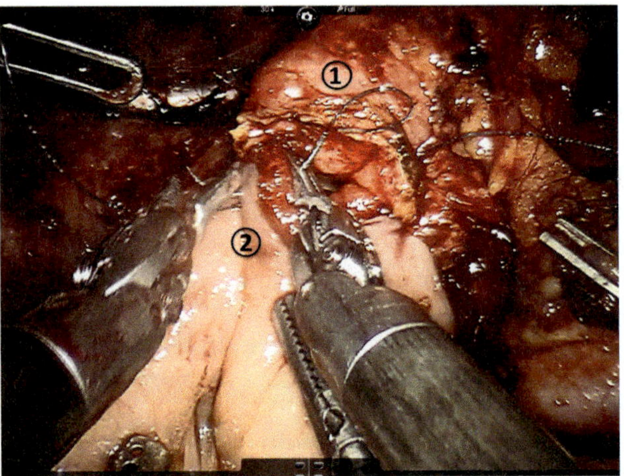

Fig. 11.7 Creation of the choledochojejunostomy. The common hepatic duct (1) is sutured to the jejunum (2) using interrupted absorbable 5-0 sutures for small ducts with or without a stent or running 4-0 V-LOC suture (Covidien, New Haven, CT, USA) for larger, thicker ducts (shown here)

is then created, and bile duct texture and size are considered in determining the technique employed: a running technique is used with larger, thicker bile ducts and an interrupted technique is utilized with smaller, softer ducts (Fig. 11.7). Next, the gastrojejunostomy or duodenojejunostomy is created. For the past year, we have used a stapled technique where we sew the common enterotomy in two layers. Previously, we had performed a two-layer gastrojejunostomy or duodenojejunostomy. The advantages of the robotic surgical platform allow for complete minimally invasive reconstruction, as the magnified view allows for identification of even the smallest pancreatic duct, and the articulating instruments allow for dexterity and precision of suture placement. Following creation of the anastomoses, a 19 French round surgical drain is placed anterior to the pancreaticojejunostomy and the hepaticojejunostomy and posterior to the gastrojejunostomy. We use the falciform to create a pedicled tissue flap to cover the GDA stump. We hope this creates a tissue barrier to protect the artery from pancreatic secretions in the setting of a leak.

Early Experience and Outcomes

Early experience with robotic-assisted PD, as with laparoscopic PD, began slowly with small case series (Table 11.1). As previously discussed, Giulianotti performed and reported the first series of eight robotic PD in 2003. This robotic group had a longer mean operative time compared to open PD (490 vs 250 min), but roughly equivalent morbidity and length of stay (37.5% vs 32.1% and 20 vs 18 days, respectively) [15]. Continued experience by the same surgeon, at hospitals both in Italy and Chicago, IL, USA, was reported as a series of 50 robotic PD, 30 in Italy and 20 in the United States. In this series, mean operative time was 421 min with a conversion rate of 18.3%. Notably, a pancreatic fistula rate of 31.3% was reported. However, this elevated fistula rate includes patients who had sclerosis of the pancreatic duct performed in place of an anastomosis. The fistula rate in patients who had a pancreatic duct anastomosis performed was equivalent to reported rates for open procedures at 21% [23]. The first series of 24 robotic-assisted PD performed at this institution similarly had a postoperative pancreatic fistula rate of 21%, with 8% clinically significant fistula (International Study Group on Pancreatic Fistula grade B/C) and 29% Clavien-Dindo grade 3–5 complication rate [16]. Another series of 44 robotic PD at the University of Illinois at Chicago published in 2011 [24] showed decreased EBL (387 vs 827 ml), as well as increased lymph node retrieval (16.8 vs 11) compared to the open group. Overall, complication rates, including pancreatic fistula were similar between groups, as was the R0 resection rate. Notably, in this series, patients undergoing robotic PD were significantly older (63 vs 56 years), had higher ASA classifications (2.5 vs 2.15) and had higher BMI (27.7 vs 24.8). Despite this seemingly more complicated patient population, operative time in the robotic group was significantly shorter, with a mean of 444 min compared to a mean time of 559 min in the open PD group [24]. These first series of robotic PD showed overall trends towards prolonged operative times with equivalent rates of postoperative pancreatic fistula, but were encouraging enough to continue perfecting the approach.

As experience with the robotic platform developed, larger operative series were reported. Another single surgeon series of 34 robotic PD in Italy showed prolonged mean operative time (597 min) and an excess cost of 55,400 USD (€6193) per patient [25]. This trend of increased operative time was seen in multiple studies, with mean operative times ranging from 431 to 718 min [26, 27, 29, 30]. Multiple series also

Table 11.1 Outcomes of early robotic-assisted pancreaticoduodenectomy (PD)

Study	Time frame	Patients (n)	Operative time (min)	EBL (ml)	Lymph node (n)	R0 rate (%)	POPF[a] (%)	Morbidity (%)	LOS (days)	30-Day mortality (%)
Giulianotti et al. [15]	10/00–11/02	8	490	–	–	–	–	37.5	20	12.5
Giulianotti et al. [23]	10/00–01/09	50 –30 Italy –20 USA	421 –312 (Italy) –351 (USA)	394 –261 (Italy) –323 (USA)	–21 (Italy) –14 (USA)	–100 (Italy) –79 (USA)	31.3 –21 (PJ)	–	22 –28.7 (Italy) –12.5 (USA)	1.5
Buchs et al. [24]	01/02–05/10	44	444	387	16.8	90.9	18.2	36.4	13	4.5
Zureikat et al. [16]	10/08–02/10	24	512	320	–	–	21	–33 Clavien 1–2 –25 Clavien 3–4	9	4.2
Boggi et al. [25]	10/08–12/11	34	597	220	32	100	38.2	55.8 –41.2 Clavien 1–2 –14.7 Clavien 3–4	23	0
Zhou et al. [26]	01/09–12/09	8	718	153	–	100	50	25	16.4	0
Chalikonda et al. [27]	03/09–12/10	30	476	485	13.2	100	6.7	30	9.79	3.3
Chan et al. [28]	05/09–12/10	8	478	200	–	–	33.3	33	12	0
Lai et al. [29]	05/09–02/12	20	491.5	247	10	73.3	35	50	13.7	–
Bao et al. [30]	11/09–07/11	28	431	100	15	63	29	–	7.4	7 (90 days)

[a]POPF: postoperative pancreatic fistula

showed decreased EBL compared to classic open PD [26, 27, 29]. Oncologic parameters, such as R0 resection rate and lymph node harvest varied across series; most studies showed equivalent lymph node harvest (10 in both groups) [29] or greater yield (13.2 vs 11.76) [27], while a single series reported significantly lower lymph node retrieval (15 vs 20) [30]. Similarly, R0 resection rates were excellent with the robotic approach [26, 29]. A series of 50 patients undergoing robotic PD for periampullary lesions at our institution found that 73.3% of patients who met criteria for adjuvant chemotherapy were able to be treated within a mean of 11.5 weeks from surgery [31]. Most notably, postoperative complications were found to be equivalent [29] or decreased [26, 27] and most studies showed decreased length of postoperative length of stay, with mean hospital stays ranging from 9.7 to 16.4 days compared to 13.26–25.8 days [26, 27, 29].

Though these early small number series had variability in measured outcomes, overall trends suggested that robotic-assisted PD is at least equivalent to open PD in regard to oncologic outcomes, R0 resection rates, and lymph node harvest, as well as perioperative morbidity and mortality. Overall, complication rates, including postoperative pancreatic fistula rates similarly were typically equivalent to established open rates. Similar to other minimally invasive approaches, robotic PD was associated with decreased EBL. Though operative times were most often significantly increased, length of stay was generally shorter. Given early promising outcomes, robotic pancreatic resections, and PD in particular, have continued to expand in popularity.

Evolution of Experience: How Far Have We Come?

Initial approaches to robotic PD often began with smaller tumors with no evidence of vascular involvement so that techniques could be honed and skills could be developed. However, the success of these early surgeries allowed for further development of the procedure and application of the technique to a larger number of patients. The first reported robotic PD with vascular resection was described by Giulianotti and others in 2011, with two robotic-assisted PD with portal vein resections between 2007 and 2010: one with tangential vein resection and another with resection and reconstruction with a PTFE patch. These procedures were able to be completed in entirety utilizing a minimally invasive approach, with R0 resection in both and minimal EBL (150–200 ml), as well as no perioperative mortality. Furthermore, the operative time averaged 430 min (400–460 min), reflecting operative times for other robotic PD around the same time period [32]. Similarly, our group completed a series of 30 robotic PD in patients with aberrant or anomalous hepatic arterial anatomy diagnosed on preoperative triphasic computed tomography (CT) scans. Despite the anomalous arteries, all procedures were completed in a minimally invasive fashion, with a mean operative time of 501 min and a median EBL of 250 ml, which did not differ significantly from a robotic group with normal arterial anatomy during the same time period. Similarly, complications, including pancreatic fistula and 90-day mortality, were equal [33]. These studies showed that robotic-assisted PD was both feasible and also safe in the setting of vascular involvement and hepatic artery anomalies, leading to increased utilization of the approach.

Recently, larger series of robotic PD have been performed, and in some cases, matched to classic open PD to compare operative outcomes and cost (Table 11.2). A matched study of patients undergoing PD in Shanghai, China between 2010 and 2013 again found that patients undergoing robotic PD had decreased EBL (400 vs 500 ml) and shorter postoperative hospital stay (20 vs 25 days), with similar R0 resection rates, lymph node harvest, and postoperative morbidity and mortality rates. Oncological outcomes were also similar with no difference in disease-free survival (DFS) and overall survival (OS) between the approaches (DFS 14 vs 13 months, OS 23 vs 22 months). Again, this series did show prolonged operative times (410 vs 323 min); however, operative times decreased with building robotic operative experience: mean operative time from 2010 to 2012 was 445 min, but decreased to 340 min in 2013 for the robotic approach group. This study also further highlighted benefits of a minimally invasive operative approach, with

Table 11.2 Outcomes of recent robot-assisted pancreaticoduodenectomy (PD)

Study	Time frame	Patients (n)	Operative time (min)	EBL (ml)	Lymph node (n)	R0 rate (%)	POPF[a] (%)	Morbidity (%)	LOS (days)	30-Day mortality (%)
Zureikat et al. [34]	08/08–11/12	132	527	300	19	87.7	17	62.8 21% Clavien grade 3–4	10	1.5
Chen et al. [35]	01/10–12/13	60	410	400	13.6	97.8	13.3	35	20	1.7
Baker et al. [36]	08/12–07/13	22	454	425	–	77.8	4.6	40.9	7	0

[a]POPF: postoperative pancreatic fistula

earlier postoperative ambulation (3.2 vs 4.8 days), faster return of bowel function (3.6 vs 5.2 days), and less pronounced negative impact on postoperative nutritional laboratory studies [35].

The potential benefits of minimally invasive PD in terms of faster postoperative recovery have been demonstrated multiple times, but the prolonged operative times and the increased cost of the robotic operating platform, the robotic instruments, and increased operative time have led to questions about the cost-effectiveness of the approach. The financial impact of robotic-assisted PD was evaluated in a series of open and robotic PD by Baker and others in 2015 [36]. In comparing operative, postoperative and financial variables of 71 PD (22 robotic PD, 49 open PD), it was again found that robotic PD was associated with increased median operative time (454 vs 364 min), as well as increased operative costs (50,535 vs 32,309 USD). This was, however, offset by roughly equivalent postoperative inpatient costs (141,581 vs 136,246 USD) and decreased postoperative outpatient follow-up costs (283 vs 519 USD) in the robotic surgical groups, adding up to equivalent total costs with each surgical approach (142,149 vs 150,473 USD). The equivalency in total costs is likely reflective of the decreased overall complication rates (40.9% vs 67.4%) and decreased total number of complications per patient in the robotic group, as well as decreased need for ICU care in the robotic PD patients [36]. A similar trend in total operative cost was seen in the Shanghai series, with decreased postoperative costs (8529 vs 10,559 USD), but increased overall cost (19,755 vs 12,111 USD), likely reflecting the increased operating room cost for the robotic approach [35]. Though the robotic surgical platform itself and its instruments do lend to higher operative costs, the operative costs can be decreased as operating times decrease with increased experience.

The increased operative time of robotic PD has been shown in many series [15, 26, 27, 29, 30, 35, 36], but multiple studies have evaluated whether operative times decrease with increased experience on the robotic platform. As previously described, the Shanghai cohort saw a decrease in mean operative time from 445 to 340 min after their first 40 robotic PD cases, at which time the mean operative time approached the open PD time of 322–324 min. This improvement after the initial 40 procedures was also reflected in median EBL, which decreased from 500 to 200 ml

(500 ml for open PD group) [35]. Our group evaluated our first 200 consecutive robotic PD to determine if the learning curve for the technique could be identified. After the initial 20 robotic PD, there was significant improvement in both rates of conversion to open PD (35–3%) and EBL (600–250 ml). Postoperative pancreatic fistula rates decreased from 27.5 to 14.4% after the first 40 procedures, and the median number of lymph nodes harvested improved after 80 cases (17–26). Most notably, the mean operative time decreased significantly after the initial 80 cases (581–417 min) [37]. In analysis of 80 of our recent cases, median operating time is now 362 min, despite integration of surgical fellow trainees in performance of the procedure. Thorough quality analysis of our early robotic pancreatic experience identified significant improvements in most operative measures after the initial 80 cases, suggesting that benchmark as the number of procedures required to reach proficiency. This is similar to reports in open surgery showing a learning curve in excess of >60 cases before perioperative outcomes are improved. However, this robotic program was developed and implemented through an "on-the-job-training" model by innovative early adopting surgeons. Once our learning curve was met, emphasis focused on the necessary training to safely adopt the platform. A regimented "mastery learning" robotic hepatobiliary training program has been developed utilizing simulation, deliberate practice with inanimate modules, and operative coaching. We have seen tremendous success after 2 years of full integration, where novice hepatobiliary surgeons are able to reach their learning curve after 1 year of training followed by 3 months on service.

As has been described, multiple single center series have published promising outcomes of robotic PD over the last decade. A review of studies published before 2012 included 5 series of robotic PD, with 131 patients. The weighted mean operative time was 510 min and complications occurred in 38.9% of patients, with 26% postoperative pancreatic fistula and 2.3% mortality [38]. This review of the earliest reported robotic PD shows complication and mortality rates within established ranges for open PD with higher operative time. A meta-analysis of seven studies comparing robotic and open PD, including studies highlighted here [24, 26, 27], showed increased mean operation length in all robotic procedures, but significant heterogeneity (I^2 96%). Similarly, EBL and postoperative length of stay were decreased in all robotic groups compared to open, but data was again heterogeneous (I^2 92% and 47%, respectively). Significant risk reduction with robotic approach was found for multiple variables, including reoperation with 12% risk reduction (I^2 0%), positive margins with 18% risk reduction (I^2 0%), and overall complication rates with risk reduction of 12% (I^2 0%). These risk reductions in reoperation, R1 resections, and postoperative complications were seen without significant differences in postoperative pancreatic fistula and postoperative mortality rates [39].

The one variable that has consistently shown to be improved with robotic PD compared to the classical open approach is decreased intraoperative blood loss. This is likely due to the magnified binocular view that allows for easy identification and ligation of the small blood vessels around the uncinate process and retroperitoneal margin, which often account for significant operative blood loss. A multi-institutional study reviewing 700 open PDs for patients with pancreatic adenocarcinoma found that patients receiving any transfusion had decreased median disease-free (13.8 vs 18.3 months) and overall survival (14 vs 21 months). The effect of perioperative transfusion requirements on overall survival was further illustrated with a dose-dependent effect: median survival without blood transfusion, 1–2 units of blood, and >2 units of blood transfused was 21, 16, and 11.1 months, respectively. Also notably, intraoperative blood transfusion greater than 2 units and postoperative transfusions (1–2 units and >2 units) were both independent risk factors for decreased disease-free survival (HR 1.92, HR 1.55, and HR 2.06, respectively) [40]. Though blood transfusion requirements with robotic PD have been varied, most series show trends towards decreased perioperative transfusion rates when compared to the open approach [24, 30]. Decreased intraoperative blood loss with the robotic approach [24, 26, 27, 29, 30, 35, 36], combined with trends towards decreased blood transfusion requirements postoperatively may afford protection against the deleterious effects of transfusion.

These most recent series of robotic PD have shown that the procedure can be performed utilizing a robotic surgical platform and that acceptable oncologic outcomes can be achieved, with lymph node retrieval and R0 resection rates comparable to standard open approach. Similarly, rates of postoperative pancreatic fistula are also comparable. Some studies also show trends towards decreased postoperative complication rates with equivalent postoperative mortality. While median operative times remain longer than those of open PD, decreasing operative times, approaching open PD have been observed with higher volume centers. Similarly, operative costs associated with robotic approach tend to be higher; however, decreased length of postoperative stay and decreasing overall complications may allow for equivalent total costs for the procedure and subsequent hospitalization.

Conclusions

The robotic surgical platform offers unique advantages to the minimally invasive surgical approach with magnified binocular vision, articulating instruments, and elimination of surgeon tremor. These benefits help to overcome the challenges of laparoscopic pancreaticoduodenectomy, allowing for wide application of the minimally invasive approach. Robotic-assisted pancreaticoduodenectomy experience thus far has shown that the approach can be performed with equivalent oncologic measures, including lymph node retrieval and R0 resection rates. Similarly, postoperative morbidity, including pancreatic fistula rates, is equivalent or decreased compared to the classic open approach. Intraoperative blood loss is also decreased when robotic-assistance is employed. Though median operative times and operative costs are higher, operative times have decreased with increased experience with the approach, and decreased duration of postoperative hospitalization and decreasing complication rates may lead to equivalent overall costs. As minimally invasive surgery gains popularities in all surgical fields, especially in pancreatic surgery, it is paramount to ensure a structured training so that new generations of surgeons will master skills of minimally invasive pancreas surgery while still maintaining the tenets of open surgery. Furthermore, as with any new surgical technology, it is imperative to continue rigorous analysis of operative measures, postoperative morbidity and mortality, and oncologic measures of disease-free and overall survival.

References

1. Whipple AO, Parsons WB, Mullins CR. Treatment of the carcinoma of the ampulla of Vater. Ann Surg. 1935;102(4):763–79.
2. Winter JM, Cameron JL, Campbell KA, Arnold MA, Chang DC, Coleman J, Hodgin MB, Sauter PK, Hruban RH, Riall TS, Schulick RD, Choti MA, Lillemoe KD, Yeo CJ. 1423 Pancreaticoduodenectomies for pancreatic cancer: a single institution experience. J Gastrointest Surg. 2006;10(9):1199–210. doi:10.1016/j.gassur.2006.08.018.
3. Sosa JA, Bowman HM, Gordon TA, Bass EB, Yeo CJ, Lillemoe KD, Pitt HA, Tielsch JM, Cameron JL. Importance of hospital volume in the overall management of pancreatic cancer. Ann Surg. 1998;228(3):429–38.
4. O'Mahoney PRA, Yeo HL, Sedrakyan A, Trencheva K, Mao J, Isaacs AJ, Lieberman MD, Michelassi F. Centralization of pancreatoduodenectomy a decade later: impact of the volume outcome relationship. J Surg. 2016; doi:10.1016/j.surg.2016.01.008.
5. Hata T, Motoi F, Ishida M, Naitoh T, Katayose Y, Egawa S, Unno M. Effect of hospital volume on surgical outcomes after pancreaticoduodenectomy. Ann Surg. 2015; doi:10.1097/SLA.0000000000001437.
6. Gagner M, Pomp A. Laparoscopic pylorus-preserving pancreatoduodenectomy. Surg Endosc. 1994;8(5):408–10.
7. Kendrick ML, Cusati D. Total laparoscopic pancreaticoduodenectomy: feasibility and outcome in early experience. Arch Surg. 2010;145(1):19–23.
8. Asburn HJ, Stauffer JA. Laparoscopic vs open pancreaticoduodenectomy: overall outcomes and severity of complications using the accordion severity grading system. J Am Coll Surg. 2012;215(6):810–9. doi:10.1016/j.jamcollsurg.2012.08.006.
9. Speicher PJ, Nussbaum DP, White RR, Zani S, Mosca PJ, Blazer III DG, Clary BM, Pappas TN, Tyler DS, Perez A. Defining the learning curve for team-based laparoscopic pancreaticoduodenectomy. Ann Surg Oncol. 2014;21:4014–9. doi:10.1245/s10434-014-3839-7.
10. Croome KP, Farnell MB, Que FG, Reid-Lombardo KM, Truty MJ, Nagorney DM, Kendrick ML. Total laparoscopic pancreaticoduodenectomy for pancreatic ductal adenocarcinoma: oncologic advantages over open approaches? Ann Surg. 2014;260(4):633–40. doi:10.1097/SLA.0000000000000937.
11. Song KB, Kim SC, Hwang DW, Lee JH, Lee DJ, Lee JW, Park KM, Lee YJ. Matched case-control analysis comparing laparoscopic and open pylorus-preserving pancreaticoduodenectomy in patients with periampullary tumors. Ann Surg. 2015;262(1):146–55. doi:10.1097/SLA.0000000000001079.
12. Gumbs AA, Rodriguez Rivera AM, Milone L, Hoffman JP. Laparoscopic pancreatoduodenectomy: a review of 285 published cases. Ann Surg Oncol. 2011;18:1335–41. doi:10.1245/s10434-010-1503-4.
13. Sharpe SM, Talamonti MS, Wang CE, Prinz RA, Roggin KK, Bentrem DJ, Winchester DJ, Marsh RDW, Stocker SJ, Baker MS. Early national experience with laparoscopic pancreaticoduodenectomy for ductal adenocarcinoma: a comparison of laparoscopic pancreaticoduodenectomy and open pancreaticoduodenectomy from the National Cancer Data Base. J Am Coll Surg. 2015;221(1):175–84. doi:10.1016/j.jamcollsurg.2015.04.021.
14. Ongchin M, Hogg ME, Zeh III HJ, Zureikat AZ. Essential and future directions of robotic pancreatic surgery. In: Kroh M, Chalikonda S, editors. Essentials of robotic surgery. Cham: Springer; 2015. p. 131–48.

15. Giulianotti PC, Coratti A, Angelini M, Sbrana F, Cecconi S, Balestracci T, Caravaglios G. Robotics in general surgery: personal experience in a large community hospital. Arch Surg. 2003;138:777–84.
16. Zureikat AH, Nguyen KT, Bartlett DL, Zeh HJ, Moser AJ. Robotic-assisted major pancreatic resection and reconstruction. Arch Surg. 2011;146(3):256–61.
17. Callery MP, Pratt WB, Kent TS, Chaikof EL, Vollmer Jr CM. A prospectively validated clinical risk score accurately predicts pancreatic fistula after pancreatoduodenectomy. J Am Coll Surg. 2013;216(1):1–14. doi:10.1016/j.jamcollsurg.2012.09.002.
18. Shubert CR, Wagie AE, Farnell MB, Nagorney DM, Que FG, Lombardo R, Truty MJ, Smoot RL, Kendrick ML. Clinical risk score to predict pancreatic fistula after pancreatoduodenectomy: independent external validation for open and laparoscopic approaches. J Am Coll Surg. 2015;221(3):689–98. doi:10.1016/j.jamcollsurg.2015.05.011.
19. Bao P, Potter D, Eisenberg DP, Lenzner D, Zeh HJ, Lee III KKW, Hughes SJ, Sanders MK, Young JL, Moser AJ. Validation of a prediction rule to maximize curative (R0) resection of early-stage pancreatic adenocarcinoma. HPB. 2009;11:606–11. doi:10.1111/j.1477-2574.2009.00110.x.
20. Nguyen KT, Zureikat AZ, Chalikonda S, Bartlett DL, Moser AJ, Zeh HJ. Technical aspects of robotic-assisted pancreaticoduodenectomy (RAPD). J Gastrointest Surg. 2011;15:870–5. doi:10.1007/s11605-010-1362-0.
21. Winer J, Can MF, Bartlett DL, Zeh HJ, Zureikat AZ. The current state of robotic-assisted pancreatic surgery. Nat Rev Gastroenterol Hepatol. 2012;9(8):468–76. doi:10.1038/nrgastro.2012.120.
22. Grobmyer SR, Kooby D, Blumgart LH, Hochwald SN. Novel pancreaticojejunostomy with a low rate of anastomotic failure-related complications. J Am Coll Surg. 2010;210(1):54–9. doi:10.1016/j.jamcollsurg.2009.09.020.
23. Giulianotti PC, Sbrana F, Bianco FM, Elli EF, Shah G, Addeo P, Caravaglios G, Coratti A. Robot-assisted laparoscopic pancreatic surgery: single surgeon experience. Surg Endosc. 2010;24:1646–57. doi:10.1007/s00464-009-0825-4.
24. Buchs NC, Addeo P, Bianco FM, Ayloo S, Benedetti E, Giulianotti PC. Robotic versus open pancreaticoduodenectomy: a comparative study at a single institution. World J Surg. 2011;35:2739–46. doi:10.1007/s00268-011-1276-3.
25. Boggi U, Signori S, Lio ND, Perrone VG, Vistoli F, Belluomini M, Cappelli C, Amorese G, Mosca F. Feasibility of robotic pancreaticoduodenectomy. BJS. 2013;100:917–25.
26. Zhou NX, Chen JZ, Liu Q, Zhang X, Wang Z, Ren S, Chen XF. Outcomes of pancreatoduodenectomy with robotic surgery versus open surgery. Int J Med Rob Comput Assist Surg. 2011;7:131–7. doi:10.1002/rcs.380.
27. Chalikonda S, Aguilar-Saavedrea JR, Walsh RM. Laparoscopic robotic-assisted pancreaticoduodenectomy: a case-matched comparison with open resection. Surg Endosc. 2012;26:2397–402. doi:10.1007/s00464-012-2207-6.
28. Chan OCY, Tang CN, Lai ECH, Yang GPC, Li MKW. Robotic hepatobiliary and pancreatic surgery: a cohort study. J Hepatobiliary Pancreat Sci. 2011;18:471–80. doi:10.1007/s00534-011-0389-2.
29. Lai ECH, Yang GPC, Tang CN. Robot-assisted laparoscopic pancreaticoduodenectomy versus open pancreaticoduodenectomy: a comparative study. IJS. 2012;10:475–9. doi:10.1016/j.ijsu.2012.06.003.
30. Bao PQ, Mazirka PO, Watkins KT. Retrospective comparison of robot-assisted minimally invasive versus open pancreaticoduodenectomy for periampullary neoplasms. J Gastrointest Surg. 2014;18:682–9. doi:10.1007/s11605-013-2410-3.
31. Zeh HJ, Zureikat AH, Secrest A, Dauoudi M, Bartlett D, Moser AJ. Outcomes after robot-assisted pancreaticoduodenectomy for periampullary lesions. Ann Surg Oncol. 2012;19:864–70. doi:10.1245/s10434-011-2045-0.
32. Giulianotti PC, Addeo P, Buchs NC, Ayloo SM, Bianco FM. Robotic extended pancreatectomy with vascular resection for locally advanced pancreatic tumors. Pancreas. 2011;40(8):1264–70.

33. Nguyen TK, Zenati MS, Boone BA, Steve J, Hogg ME, Bartlett DL, Zeh III HJ, Zureikat AH. Robotic pancreaticoduodenectomy in the presence of aberrant or anomalous hepatic arterial anatomy: safety and oncologic outcomes. HPB. 2015;17:594–9. doi:10.1111/hpb.12414.
34. Zureikat AH, Moser AJ, Boone BA, Bartlett DL, Zenati M, Zeh III HJ. 250 robotic pancreatic resections: safety and feasibility. Ann Surg. 2013;258(4):554–62. doi:10.1079/SLA.0b013e3182a4e87c.
35. Chen S, Chen JZ, Zhan Q, Deng XX, Shen BY, Peng CH, Li HW. Robot-assisted laparoscopic versus open pancreaticoduodenectomy: a prospective, matched, mid-term follow-up study. Surg Endosc. 2015;29:3698–711. doi:10.1007/s00464-015-4140-y.
36. Baker EH, Ross SW, Seshadri R, Swan RZ, Iannitti DA, Vrochides D, Martinie JB. Robotic pancreaticoduodenectomy: comparison of complications and cost to the open approach. Int J Med Rob Comput Assist Surg. 2015; doi:10.1002/rcs.1688.
37. Boone BA, Zenati M, Hogg ME, Steve J, Moser AJ, Bartlett DL, Zeh HJ, Zureikat AH. Assessment of quality outcomes for robotics pancreaticoduodenectomy: identification of the learning curve. JAMA Surg. 2015;150(5):416–22. doi:10.1001/jamasurg.2015.17.
38. Strijker M, van Santvoort HC, Besselink MG, van Hillegersberg R, Borel Rinkes IHM, Vriens MR, Molenaar IQ. Robot-assisted pancreatic surgery: a systemic review of the literature. HPB. 2013;15:1–10. doi:10.1111/j.1477-2574.2012.00589.x.
39. Zhang J, Wu WM, You L, Zhao YP. Robotic versus open pancreatectomy: a systematic review and meta-analysis. Ann Surg Oncol. 2013;20:1774–80. doi:10.1245/s10434-012-2823-3.
40. Sutton JM, Kooby DA, Wilson GC, Squires III MH, Hanseman DJ, Maithel SK, Bentrem DJ, Weber SM, Cho CC, Winslow ER, Scoggins CR, Martin II RCG, Kim HJ, Baker JJ, Merchant NB, Parikh AA, Abbott DE, Edwards MJ, Ahmad SA. Perioperative blood transfusion is associated with decreased survival in patients undergoing pancreaticoduodenectomy for pancreatic adenocarcinoma: a multi-institutional study. J Gastrointest Surg. 2014;18:1575–87. doi:10.1007/s11605-014-2567-4.

Part III

Distal Pancreatectomy: Indications and Procedure

Distal Pancreatectomy for Pancreatic Carcinoma

12

Masayuki Sho and Shoichi Kinoshita

12.1 Introduction

Distal pancreatectomy (DP) has been widely used as the standard treatment for carcinoma of the pancreatic body and tail. However, due to the position of the body and tail of the pancreas within the anatomy, tumors in this area may develop before the appearance of clinical symptoms such as pain, weight loss, diarrhea, and appetite loss. Furthermore, once these symptoms appear the cancer is usually at an advanced stage, often with distant metastases including the liver and peritoneal metastases. Therefore, most patients with carcinoma of the pancreatic body or tail are often not operable.

The first left-sided pancreatectomies, namely, DP, were performed in the late 19th century in Europe and the United States [1]. DP entails the removal of the portion of the pancreas extending to the left of the midline and not including the duodenum and distal bile duct. The pancreas is usually divided into the left of the superior mesenteric vein or portal vein trunk, with the exact line of transection depending on the location of the tumor. Regional lymphadenectomy is usually performed concomitantly. Spleen-preserving DP is generally contraindicated for carcinoma of the distal pancreas. DP for pancreatic carcinoma aims to achieve negative surgical margin.

12.2 Postoperative Complication and Pancreatic Fistula After Distal Pancreatectomy

There are distinct differences in the postoperative course of DP, compared to pancreatoduodenectomy (PD). In a cohort of 2322 DP patients from the American College of Surgeons National Surgical Quality Improvement Program, 28.1%

M. Sho (✉) • S. Kinoshita
Department of Surgery, Nara Medical University,
840 Shijo-cho, Kashihara, Nara 634-8522, Japan
e-mail: m-sho@naramed-u.ac.jp

© Springer Science+Business Media Singapore 2017
H. Yamaue (ed.), *Innovation of Diagnosis and Treatment for Pancreatic Cancer*,
DOI 10.1007/978-981-10-2486-3_12

experienced postoperative complications, and 30-day mortality was 1.2% [2]. In a cohort of 11,559 patients reported by the Pancreatic Surgery Mortality Study Group, 218 (1.9%) mortalities followed pancreatectomy. Eighteen (8.3%) of all mortalities followed DP. Among the cause of death, operation-related complications were fewer (5.5% vs. 28.3%), and postoperative pancreatic fistulas (PF) was comparable (11% vs. 15.2%) to PD. In contrast, disease progression (11% vs. 4.4%), pulmonary embolism (11% vs. 0.5%), and medical conditions (11% vs. 1.6%) contributed more frequently [3]. In a cohort of 2360 patients of the Pancreatectomy Readmission Assessment Group Study, 464 (19.7%) patients, including 317 PD and 147 other pancreatectomies, readmitted within 90 days. Many medical conditions and postoperative variables predicted readmission; however, there were no differences in intraoperative variables between the readmission group and no readmission group [4].

Among a number of postoperative complications including intra-abdominal abscess, wound infection, sepsis, malabsorption, and hemorrhage, PF is still the main cause of postoperative morbidity after pancreatectomy. A recent study assessed the clinical impact of PF using a complication severity grading system, and then compared PF after PD and DP [5]. In 2370 pancreatic resections, PF (34.5 vs. 27.2%, $P < 0.001$), as well as clinically significant PF (14.7 vs. 11.4, $P = 0.019$) was more frequent in DP than PD. Furthermore, in DP, PF consisted 31.2% of the overall complication burden, compared to 17.5% in PD. Shown from the data above, although operation-related mortality was less experienced in DP, the postoperative course was characterized by the high incidence and burden of PF.

Many large-scale, multi-institutional studies show the negative effect of postoperative complications following pancreatectomy to the long-term survival [6, 7]. In 761 distal pancreatectomies for pancreatic adenocarcinoma with a median survival of 17 months by the Dutch Pancreatic Cancer Group [6], the 33% of patients who developed major postoperative complications had a significant risk of worse survival (HR 1.67, $P = 0.02$). In 1397 pancreatectomies for pancreatic cancer by the Multicenter Study Group of Pancreatobiliary Surgery [7], there were more distal lesions in Grade B and C compared to Grade A (54.4% vs. 43% vs. 27.6%, $P < 0.001$), and PF Grade C, but not Grade B, was an independent risk factor for overall survival (HR 1.59, $P = 0.035$). Although it is generally thought that reducing morbidity and prompting early postoperative recovery is important in the surgical management of malignant disease, early induction of adjuvant therapy for pancreatic cancer may not be associated with long-term survival [8]. Therefore, the main objective of early recovery from surgery would not necessarily be the early initiation of adjuvant therapy. However, severe complication could hinder the completion of the planned postoperative adjuvant therapy, as well as worsen the overall survival [7]. Kawai et al. report the rate of postoperative therapy was 38% in PF C, in comparison to 81.5% in PF A, and 84.6% in PF B. The mechanisms that cause poor prognosis after severe complication are not fully elucidated. However, it is assumed that an immunosuppressive effect by inflammatory cytokines has a role in tumor progression [9]. It may also be speculated that physical deterioration leads to intolerance of adjuvant therapy administration [7]. Nonetheless, the sustaining effect from postoperative complications may interfere with the sequencing of multimodal therapy, which is vital for the long-term survival of pancreatic cancer. Taken together, especially in DP for pancreatic cancer, all efforts to pursue lower morbidity, namely, PF, may lead to the improvement of the oncological outcomes as well. This highlights the importance of high surgical technique, as well as collective experience of the attending team, in the surgical management of pancreatic cancer.

Hospital volume, as well as surgeon volume has been reported to be associated with lower morbidity and mortality after pancreatectomy in many large studies with heterogeneous backgrounds [10–12]. Volume–outcome relationships are well investigated in PD. On the other hand, the direct impact of volume to postoperative complications in DP is largely unknown. Therefore, it is still unclear whether higher surgeon volume or superior surgical technique will contribute to decrease morbidity, as well as PF, in DP. Regarding the impact of hospital volume to prognosis after pancreatectomy for malignant disease, Derogar et al. showed the tendency of longer prognosis in high volume centers [10]. Moreover, they show the significant difference of prognosis between educational and noneducational institutes. The advantage of centralizing patients is, high-volume centers may be able to provide more robust, diversified therapy including multimodal therapy, greater lymph node harvesting, higher margin-negative resections, and detailed histological evaluation. Furthermore, educational institutes may have advantages such as better adherence to clinical guidelines, improved patient selection, multidisciplinary team management, availability to novel technologies, and concentration of high-volume surgeons [10]. Many high-volume centers report the improvement of short-term, as well as long-term outcomes over the period of time [13].

Taken from above, for the improvement of outcome for pancreatic cancer, equally important to the role of surgeons, is the total quality of high experienced institutions. Furthermore, treatment strategies that are unique to pancreatic cancer may effect postoperative complication after pancreatectomy. Multimodal therapy is becoming recognized as an important treatment strategy for pancreatic cancer. Although it is presumably regarded that preoperative therapy is associated with increased morbidity, in fact, PF as well as morbidity, has been reported to be fewer in neoadjuvant radiotherapy patients [14, 15]. Preoperative radiation has been reported to be associated with significantly lower incidence of PF after DP, possibly due to the induction of atrophy and the distortion of lobular structure with acinar cell dropout [16].

12.3 Management of Pancreatic Stump: Suture, Instrumental, Anastomosis

Surgical techniques and methods are the primary and most important factors that influence postoperative morbidity. In DP, leakage from the stump of the remnant pancreas is the direct cause of PF and leads to severe complications such as intra-abdominal abscess and postoperative hemorrhage. Therefore, it is reasonable that pancreatic surgeons have always devoted much effort to evaluating the optimal pancreatic stump closure method. However, in spite of much inspection, the optimal closure method for DP is not yet determined.

The conventional method for pancreatic parenchyma dissection and remnant pancreatic stump closure is scalpel dissection, followed by ligation of the main pancreatic duct, and then hand-sewn closure. Surgeons have since applied numerous developed novel surgical devices and technologies, in attempt to decrease PF. Surgical techniques may be categorized as (1) stump closure method, (2) stump reinforcement method, (3) parenchyma dissection method, and (4) medication administration. Many unique explorations have been made, but the many of these practices are single institute, observational studies. Several randomized control trials could be identified in the literature. Two evaluated stump closure [17, 18], six evaluated stump reinforcement [19–24], two evaluated somatostatin analogues [25, 26], and one regarded parenchyma dissection method [27]. Furthermore, one prospective controlled clinical trial sought to determine whether prophylactic transpapillary pancreatic duct stenting reduces PF after DP [28]. Fifty-eight patients were randomized to either DP or DP plus stent. Clinically significant PF (Grade B/C) occurred in 6 DP and 11 DP plus stent patients. The results indicated that prophylactic pancreatic stenting did not reduce PF when performing a standardized resection of the body and tail of the pancreas.

The greatest alternative for the hand-sewn method is closure by stapler. Stapler resection can be a safe, fast method, and moreover, can also be applied to minimally invasive surgery. From the technical point of view, it has become favored and widely used in clinical practice. However, in terms of postoperative complications associated to the device, the rate of PF and mortality did not differ with conventional hand-sewn technique [17]. Increased parenchyma compressing injury in a thick pancreas may be a drawback in the stapling method [29]. Kawai et al. hypothesized that a seromuscular patch of the pancreatic stump concomitant with pancreatic duct anastomosis, namely, pancreaticojejunostomy (PJ), could be effective, compared to the stapler method as control. In their RCT, although the overall PF did not differ between the PJ and stapler groups, in a subgroup analysis of a thick pancreas subset, the PJ group trended to have lower PF [18]. The authors advocated further RCTs with stratification by the pancreas thickness.

Although the optimal stump closure method for lowering morbidity is unresolved, the stapler technique remains to be the mainstream method of choice. Many RCTs have evaluated the efficacy of reinforcing the remnant stump. However, the use of falciform patch [20] (20% vs. 19.6%), fibrin sealant patch [19, 22] (62% vs. 68%, 54.5% vs. 56.6%), or seromuscular patch [23] (8.6% vs. 20%) neither had additive protective effect. One RCT showed the significant reduction of clinically relevant PF by reinforcing the staple line with mesh buttress material [21]. PF B/C was 1.9% with mesh reinforcement versus 20% in the control group. Limitations to the study include, that though the study did not specify any stratification by pancreas thickness or texture hardness, some patients were excluded, on account of inability to safely apply stapler in thick pancreas, and also in proximal lesion.

The only other RCT that showed positive results was the administration of prophylactic pasireotide [25]. This study clearly shows that pasireotide reduces PF associated severe complications in any subset of pancreatectomy, including PD, DP, and dilated or non-dilated duct. Furthermore in DP, PF B/C was 7.9% with pasireotide versus 16.9% in control. Although there were some concerns regarding cost-effectiveness [30], it was useful to reduce any complication, which was 11.2% with pasireotide, and 25% in control. A recent meta-analysis by the Cochrane Upper GI and Pancreatic Disease Group evaluated 19 studies on the efficacy of somatostatin analogue use in pancreatic surgery [31]. As a result, all PF was reduced, but clinically significant PF was not significantly different. Furthermore, although mortality rate was comparative, since total complication rate was lower with somatostatin, it was recommended for routine use in pancreatectomy.

12.4 Standard Distal Pancreatectomy Versus RAMPS Procedure for Pancreatic Carcinoma

Strasberg et al. have established a surgical procedure of left-sided pancreatectomy for pancreatic carcinoma, radical antegrade modular pancreatosplenectomy (RAMPS) [32]. RAMPS was designed to achieve the two goals of pancreatic resection for pancreatic cancer, namely, negative dissection planes and regional lymph node resection. The main concepts of RAMPS are: (1) complete resection of N1 lymph nodes, (2) emphasis on posterior margin, (3) dissection in a right-to-left manner. The lymph nodes that circulate the pancreas body and tail, as well as their drainage nodes in the celiac and superior mesenteric arteries are regarded as N1 nodes. Posterior dissection planes were designed according to the relationship of the retroperitoneal fascia planes between the pancreas posterior and anterior of the left kidney. Depending on whether or not the tumor extends to or past the posterior pancreatic capsule, the dissection plane border is in the perirenal space at the anterior of the adrenal gland (anterior RAMPS), or behind the adrenal gland and Gerota fascia (posterior RAMPS). Right-to-left dissection enables early control of major veins, as well as simplifies the identification of anatomical landmarks that indicate the posterior dissection plane.

The procedure is summarized as follows: After dividing and closing the pancreas neck, celiac and superior mesenteric nodes are dissected posteriorly. The splenic vein and artery are ligated and divided, then dissection of fat is done further down, visualizing the celiac axis, superior mesenteric artery origin, and left anterior of the aorta, while resecting lymph nodes between them. Dissection is then done towards the left, according to the predetermined plane. In anterior RAMPS, the left adrenal vein and adrenal gland surface is visualized at the inferior border of dissection. In posterior RAMPS, the left adrenal vein is divided at the origin at the left renal vein, dissection is continued down until the left renal artery, and then turned leftwards in the plane behind the adrenal gland. The inferior border is the left renal artery, left renal vein, diaphragm, retroperitoneal muscle layers, and left kidney surface.

The Strasberg group have achieved negative tangential margins in 94%, with an overall R0 rate of 85%, and a mean 20 lymph nodes were resected in 78 patients [33]. Other groups report R0 rate as 77–90.5%, and lymph node dissection count median 14–26, or mean 15–28.4 [34–36]. In some single-institute series [34, 36] that compare RAMPS with standard DP, RAMPS is associated with greater lymph node count [28.4 ± 11.6 vs. 20.7 ± 10.1, $P = 0.001$, 14 (5–52) vs. 9 (1–36), $P = 0.002$], as well as higher R0 rate (90.5% vs. 67.5%, $P = 0.005$, 89.4% vs. 85.1%). Blood loss was also lower in RAMPS [485 ± 63 vs. 682 ± 72, $P = 0.04$, 325 (50–3400) vs. 400 (50–3300)]. These data indicate that RAMPS is effectively fulfilling the intended concept of design. Furthermore, it is suggested that the improved local control by RAMPS in combination with multimodal therapy may have prognostic impact, and that RAMPS may have an important role in the treatment strategy for pancreatic carcinoma in the distal pancreas. However, to date, the survival benefit of RAMPS is controversial [34, 36]. Further large-scale studies are warranted to evaluate the role of RAMPS.

The Strasberg group also reports 11 patients by laparoscopic-RAMPS [33]. However, in their experience, satisfactory lymph node cleaning in accordance with the RAMPS concept was hard to achieve, resulting in relatively high conversion rate. Furthermore, the Yonsei group also reported the initial experience with laparoscopic and robotic RAMPS [37]. They concluded that minimally invasive RAMPS is not only technically feasible but also oncologically safe in well-selected patients with left-sided pancreatic cancer. However, the evaluation of feasibility and oncological efficacy of minimally invasive RAMPS is still in an exploratory phase.

12.5 Open Versus Laparoscopic Versus Robotic Distal Pancreatectomy for Pancreatic Carcinoma

Minimally invasive surgery (MIS) for pancreatic cancer has not become widely adapted compared to other gastrointestinal tract malignancies. In general, pancreatic surgery demands high skills, including vascular maneuvers. Therefore, MIS in pancreatic surgery, in exchange for a lower surgical stress, may not seem beneficial if the safety of the resection is deemed to be threatened. Since DP is associated with a relatively high morbidity, it must be evaluated whether minimally invasive approach has benefit even in high-risk subsets. Furthermore, when implicating MIS for malignant diseases, i.e., pancreatic cancer, the oncological efficacy, namely, resection margins and lymph node harvesting, must not be compromised. In evidence based on low malignant and benign tumors, laparoscopic surgery (LS) appeared to be associated with comparable or reduced risk of morbidity and lower hospitalization rates. Morbidity was 30–33% versus 28–47%, and postoperative hospital stay was 5–10 versus 7–14 days for LS versus open, respectively [38, 39].

To date, in pancreatic ductal adenocarcinoma, since there are no RCTs that compare LS versus open DP, there is no clear evidence to show whether LS is oncologically non-inferior, while assuring patient safety. In some retrospective studies on pancreatic ductal adenocarcinoma, a French study group reported that the mortality was 3% versus 6% for LS and open DP, respectively [40]. Furthermore, an American study group reported that R0 rate was 86% versus 81%, and number of harvested lymph nodes were 15 ± 10 versus 13 ± 9 for LS and open DP, respectively [41]. These studies on pancreatic ductal adenocarcinoma showed that results of LS were comparable to open DP. However, many non-randomized observational studies, based on small number cohorts, unclear outcome definition, and biased eligibility criteria make it unable to draw a definitive conclusion. In fact, in the recent meta-analysis by the Cochrane Upper GI and Pancreatic Disease Group that evaluated 12 studies, the difference in almost all short- and long-term variables including mortality, serious adverse events, clinically significant PF, recurrence rates, any complications, and positive resection margins were all concluded as imprecise since all studies were retrospective cohort-like studies or case-control studies at unclear or high risk of bias, and with the very low overall quality of evidence [42]. The only significant difference was the shorter hospital stay in the LS group. Furthermore, in another recent review, the authors suggested that LS was basically not indicated for pancreatic cancer [43]. Mehrabi et al. state that, unless an RCT has been undergone, no further observational explorations will be able to aid clinical decision-making [44]. Furthermore, they also state that, since the technical feasibility is almost undoubted, trials should be focused on the comparison of oncological efficacy. Ongoing randomized controlled trials may provide answers to unsolved clinical questions on laparoscopic DP [43].

The Yonsei group has established criteria for the eligibility of minimally invasive (i.e., laparoscopic and robotic surgery) DP in pancreatic cancer [37]. The criteria limited MIS to relatively small tumors that were located away from the celiac trunk. In detail, the criteria are as follows: (1) tumor confined to the pancreas, (2) intact layer between the distal pancreas and left adrenal gland, kidney, (3) tumor located 1–2 cm or more proximal from celiac axis. Utilizing their criteria, they performed 12 minimally invasive DP. After adjustment, the total complication rate was 20% versus 32.5%, retrieved lymph nodes were 11.7 ± 7.2 versus 12.1 ± 8.1, R0 rate was 100% versus 87.5%, for minimally invasive versus open DP, respectively, with no significant difference. The tumor size however was significantly different; 2.3 ± 0.6 versus 3.2 ± 1.5 cm. Therefore, although it may still be biased, they show that MIS was technically feasible especially in small tumors in DP. From their results of the long-term oncologic outcomes of their cohort of DP for pancreatic cancer, they show that prognosis was comparable in MIS versus open technique, when analyzing a small subset of patients within the criteria. Furthermore, the authors acknowledge the success of the procedure depends on high surgical technique, and in addition, the efficacy of MIS may be difficult to validate due to the potential limitation of the procedure to less-extensive lesions [45].

The validity of robotic-assisted surgery (RS) for pancreatic cancer needs further careful consideration. In general, RS has rapidly spread with the expectations of improved surgical quality, especially from the robotic ergonomic enhancement features. However, as the initial experience has become undergone in some early adapting institutes, more doubt has arisen in respect to the cost-benefit of the procedure [46, 47]. The costs associated with RS include the surgeons involved in the procedure, initial capital expenditure, consumable devices, annual maintenance, operation room renovation cost, and operation room occupation time [48]. Many studies including an RCT that conducted extensive health-economic analysis could not show clear benefits to justify the additive costs related to robotic technology [48]. Although some improved short-term outcomes were associated with RS, many long-term outcomes including oncological as well as organ functional-related factors were not different between RS and LS or open surgery in various diseases [49–51]. In pancreatic surgery, only a few institutes have had experience with RS to some extent [52, 53]. Some oncologic outcomes, such as positive resection margins and lymph node harvesting were reported to be superior in RS compared to LS [53]. Short-term outcomes in RS were almost comparable to LS in institutional experience [52, 53]. In an author's opinion, the improved dexterity in RS enabled improved vascular manipulation, as well as lymph node harvesting [53]. However, patient selection bias and inconsistent histopathological evaluation methods between institutions make it unable to conclude any tendencies associated with RS for pancreatic cancer. Furthermore, since clinically relevant PF and length of stay did not differ between LS and RS [52, 53], it seems unlikely that RS could advantage in terms of cost-effectiveness.

As of 2016, there is insufficient evidence to make recommendations for laparoscopic and robotic DP for pancreatic carcinoma. Furthermore, open DP remains the standard treatment for resectable pancreatic cancer in various aspects including oncologic efficacy, safety, and cost-benefit.

References

1. Strasberg SM, Fields R. Left-sided pancreatic cancer: distal pancreatectomy and its variants: radical antegrade modular pancreatosplenectomy and distal pancreatectomy with celiac axis resection. Cancer J. 2012;18:562–70.
2. Kelly KJ, Greenblatt DY, Wan Y, et al. Risk stratification for distal pancreatectomy utilizing ACS-NSQIP: preoperative factors predict morbidity and mortality. J Gastrointest Surg. 2011;15:250–9.
3. Vollmer Jr CM, Sanchez N, Gondek S, et al. A root-cause analysis of mortality following major pancreatectomy. J Gastrointest Surg. 2012;16:89–102.
4. Valero 3rd V, Grimm JC, Kilic A, et al. A novel risk scoring system reliably predicts readmission after pancreatectomy. J Am Coll Surg. 2015;220:701–13.
5. McMillan MT, Christein JD, Callery MP, et al. Comparing the burden of pancreatic fistulas after pancreatoduodenectomy and distal pancreatectomy. Surgery. 2016;159:1013–22.
6. de Rooij T, Tol JA, van Eijck CH, et al. Outcomes of distal pancreatectomy for pancreatic ductal adenocarcinoma in the netherlands: a nationwide retrospective analysis. Ann Surg Oncol. 2016;23:585–91.
7. Kawai M, Murakami Y, Motoi F, et al. Grade B pancreatic fistulas do not affect survival after pancreatectomy for pancreatic cancer: a multicenter observational study. Surgery. 2016;160:293–305.
8. Valle JW, Palmer D, Jackson R, et al. Optimal duration and timing of adjuvant chemotherapy after definitive surgery for ductal adenocarcinoma of the pancreas: ongoing lessons from the ESPAC-3 study. J Clin Oncol. 2014;32:504–12.
9. Pucher PH, Aggarwal R, Qurashi M, et al. Meta-analysis of the effect of postoperative in-hospital morbidity on long-term patient survival. Br J Surg. 2014;101:1499–508.
10. Derogar M, Blomberg J, Sadr-Azodi O. Hospital teaching status and volume related to mortality after pancreatic cancer surgery in a national cohort. Br J Surg. 2015;102:548–57.
11. Eppsteiner RW, Csikesz NG, McPhee JT, et al. Surgeon volume impacts hospital mortality for pancreatic resection. Ann Surg. 2009;249:635–40.
12. McPhee JT, Hill JS, Whalen GF, et al. Perioperative mortality for pancreatectomy: a national perspective. Ann Surg. 2007;246:246–53.

13. Serrano PE, Cleary SP, Dhani N, et al. Improved long-term outcomes after resection of pancreatic adenocarcinoma: a comparison between two time periods. Ann Surg Oncol. 2015;22:1160–7.
14. Cooper AB, Parmar AD, Riall TS, et al. Does the use of neoadjuvant therapy for pancreatic adenocarcinoma increase postoperative morbidity and mortality rates? J Gastrointest Surg. 2015;19:80–6.
15. Sho M, Akahori T, Tanaka T, et al. Importance of resectability status in neoadjuvant treatment for pancreatic cancer. J Hepatobiliary Pancreat Sci. 2015;22:563–70.
16. Takahashi H, Ogawa H, Ohigashi H, et al. Preoperative chemoradiation reduces the risk of pancreatic fistula after distal pancreatectomy for pancreatic adenocarcinoma. Surgery. 2011;150:547–56.
17. Diener MK, Seiler CM, Rossion I, et al. Efficacy of stapler versus hand-sewn closure after distal pancreatectomy (DISPACT): a randomised, controlled multicentre trial. Lancet. 2011;377:1514–22.
18. Kawai M, Hirono S, Okada K, et al. Randomized controlled trial of pancreaticojejunostomy versus stapler closure of the pancreatic stump during distal pancreatectomy to reduce pancreatic fistula. Ann Surg. 2016;264:180–7.
19. Sa Cunha A, Carrere N, Meunier B, et al. Stump closure reinforcement with absorbable fibrin collagen sealant sponge (TachoSil) does not prevent pancreatic fistula after distal pancreatectomy: the FIABLE multicenter controlled randomized study. Am J Surg. 2015;210:739–48.
20. Carter TI, Fong ZV, Hyslop T, et al. A dual-institution randomized controlled trial of remnant closure after distal pancreatectomy: does the addition of a falciform patch and fibrin glue improve outcomes? J Gastrointest Surg. 2013;17:102–9.
21. Hamilton NA, Porembka MR, Johnston FM, et al. Mesh reinforcement of pancreatic transection decreases incidence of pancreatic occlusion failure for left pancreatectomy: a single-blinded, randomized controlled trial. Ann Surg. 2012;255:1037–42.
22. Montorsi M, Zerbi A, Bassi C, et al. Efficacy of an absorbable fibrin sealant patch (TachoSil) after distal pancreatectomy: a multicenter, randomized, controlled trial. Ann Surg. 2012;256:853–9.
23. Olah A, Issekutz A, Belagyi T, et al. Randomized clinical trial of techniques for closure of the pancreatic remnant following distal pancreatectomy. Br J Surg. 2009;96:602–7.
24. Suc B, Msika S, Fingerhut A, et al. Temporary fibrin glue occlusion of the main pancreatic duct in the prevention of intra-abdominal complications after pancreatic resection: prospective randomized trial. Ann Surg. 2003;237:57–65.
25. Allen PJ, Gonen M, Brennan MF, et al. Pasireotide for postoperative pancreatic fistula. N Engl J Med. 2014;370:2014–22.
26. Sarr MG, Pancreatic Surgery G. The potent somatostatin analogue vapreotide does not decrease pancreas-specific complications after elective pancreatectomy: a prospective, multicenter, double-blinded, randomized, placebo-controlled trial. J Am Coll Surg. 2003;196:556–64.
27. Suzuki Y, Fujino Y, Tanioka Y, et al. Randomized clinical trial of ultrasonic dissector or conventional division in distal pancreatectomy for non-fibrotic pancreas. Br J Surg. 1999;86:608–11.
28. Frozanpor F, Lundell L, Segersvard R, et al. The effect of prophylactic transpapillary pancreatic stent insertion on clinically significant leak rate following distal pancreatectomy: results of a prospective controlled clinical trial. Ann Surg. 2012;255:1032–6.
29. Kawai M, Tani M, Okada K, et al. Stump closure of a thick pancreas using stapler closure increases pancreatic fistula after distal pancreatectomy. Am J Surg. 2013;206:352–9.
30. Abbott DE, Sutton JM, Jernigan PL, et al. Prophylactic pasireotide administration following pancreatic resection reduces cost while improving outcomes. J Surg Oncol. 2016;113:784–8.
31. Gurusamy KS, Koti R, Fusai G, et al. Somatostatin analogues for pancreatic surgery. Cochrane Database Syst Rev. 2013;4:CD008370.
32. Strasberg SM, Drebin JA, Linehan D. Radical antegrade modular pancreatosplenectomy. Surgery. 2003;133:521–7.

33. Grossman JG, Fields RC, Hawkins WG, et al. Single institution results of radical antegrade modular pancreatosplenectomy for adenocarcinoma of the body and tail of pancreas in 78 patients. J Hepatobiliary Pancreat Sci. 2016;23:432–41.
34. Abe T, Ohuchida K, Miyasaka Y, et al. Comparison of surgical outcomes between radical antegrade modular pancreatosplenectomy (RAMPS) and standard retrograde pancreatosplenectomy (SPRS) for left-sided pancreatic cancer. World J Surg. 2016;40:2267–75.
35. Murakawa M, Aoyama T, Asari M, et al. The short- and long-term outcomes of radical antegrade modular pancreatosplenectomy for adenocarcinoma of the body and tail of the pancreas. BMC Surg. 2015;15:120.
36. Park HJ, You DD, Choi DW, et al. Role of radical antegrade modular pancreatosplenectomy for adenocarcinoma of the body and tail of the pancreas. World J Surg. 2014;38:186–93.
37. Lee SH, Kang CM, Hwang HK, et al. Minimally invasive RAMPS in well-selected left-sided pancreatic cancer within Yonsei criteria: long-term (>median 3 years) oncologic outcomes. Surg Endosc. 2014;28:2848–55.
38. Yoon YS, Lee KH, Han HS, et al. Effects of laparoscopic versus open surgery on splenic vessel patency after spleen and splenic vessel-preserving distal pancreatectomy: a retrospective multicenter study. Surg Endosc. 2015;29:583–8.
39. Xourafas D, Tavakkoli A, Clancy TE, et al. Distal pancreatic resection for neuroendocrine tumors: is laparoscopic really better than open? J Gastrointest Surg. 2015;19:831–40.
40. Sulpice L, Farges O, Goutte N, et al. Laparoscopic distal pancreatectomy for pancreatic ductal adenocarcinoma: time for a randomized controlled trial? Results of an all-inclusive national observational study. Ann Surg. 2015;262:868–73.
41. Adam MA, Choudhury K, Goffredo P, et al. Minimally invasive distal pancreatectomy for cancer: short-term oncologic outcomes in 1,733 patients. World J Surg. 2015;39:2564–72.
42. Riviere D, Gurusamy KS, Kooby DA, et al. Laparoscopic versus open distal pancreatectomy for pancreatic cancer. Cochrane Database Syst Rev. 2016;4:CD011391.
43. de Rooij T, Klompmaker S, Abu Hilal M, et al. Laparoscopic pancreatic surgery for benign and malignant disease. Nat Rev Gastroenterol Hepatol. 2016;13:227–38.
44. Mehrabi A, Hafezi M, Arvin J, et al. A systematic review and meta-analysis of laparoscopic versus open distal pancreatectomy for benign and malignant lesions of the pancreas: it's time to randomize. Surgery. 2015;157:45–55.
45. Kang CM, Kim DH, Lee WJ. Ten years of experience with resection of left-sided pancreatic ductal adenocarcinoma: evolution and initial experience to a laparoscopic approach. Surg Endosc. 2010;24:1533–41.
46. Yoo J. The robot has no role in elective colon surgery. JAMA Surg. 2014;149:184.
47. Barbash GI, Glied SA. New technology and health care costs—the case of robot-assisted surgery. N Engl J Med. 2010;363:701–4.
48. Tedesco G, Faggiano FC, Leo E, et al. A comparative cost analysis of robotic-assisted surgery versus laparoscopic surgery and open surgery: the necessity of investing knowledgeably. Surg Endosc. 2016;30:5044–51.
49. Sert BM, Boggess JF, Ahmad S, et al. Robot-assisted versus open radical hysterectomy: a multi-institutional experience for early-stage cervical cancer. Eur J Surg Oncol. 2016;42:513–22.
50. Hu JC, Gu X, Lipsitz SR, et al. Comparative effectiveness of minimally invasive vs open radical prostatectomy. JAMA. 2009;302:1557–64.
51. Park EJ, Cho MS, Baek SJ, et al. Long-term oncologic outcomes of robotic low anterior resection for rectal cancer: a comparative study with laparoscopic surgery. Ann Surg. 2015;261:129–37.
52. Lee SY, Allen PJ, Sadot E, et al. Distal pancreatectomy: a single institution's experience in open, laparoscopic, and robotic approaches. J Am Coll Surg. 2015;220:18–27.
53. Daouadi M, Zureikat AH, Zenati MS, et al. Robot-assisted minimally invasive distal pancreatectomy is superior to the laparoscopic technique. Ann Surg. 2013;257:128–32.

Distal Pancreatectomy with En Bloc Celiac Axis Resection for Advanced Pancreatic Cancer

Satoshi Hirano

13.1 Development of Distal Pancreatectomy with Celiac Axis Resection (DP-CAR)

Locally advanced cancer of the body of the pancreas often involves the common hepatic artery (CHA) and/or the celiac axis (CA), with perineural invasion of the nerve plexuses surrounding these arteries. Distal pancreatectomy with celiac axis resection (DP-CAR) may be the only surgical option for the treatment of such an advanced disease [1]. An advantage of DP-CAR is reduction in the likelihood of a positive retroperitoneal margin by complete en bloc resection of the distal pancreas, together with the entire surrounding structures, especially the CHA, CA, and the circumferential nerve plexus along the superior mesenteric artery (SMA), without the need for either arterial, pancreatobiliary, or gastrointestinal reconstruction (Fig. 13.1).

This procedure was originally designed as en bloc lymphadenectomy combined with total gastrectomy and resection of the celiac axis for advanced gastric cancer by Appleby in 1953 [2]. It was first adopted by Nimura in 1976 [3] for patients with advanced pancreatic body cancer with invasion of the celiac axis. A modification to the procedure with preservation of the entire stomach was primarily reported from Japan, which resulted in better postoperative nutritional status [1, 4, 5]. The first report regarding the long-term outcome of DP-CAR was published in 2007 [6], which included the results of 24 consecutive patients with favorable postoperative survival. Nowadays, several pancreatic surgeons have performed this procedure for carcinoma of the body and tail of the pancreas.

In DP-CAR, the entire alimentary tract, including the stomach and bile duct, which are not invaded by the cancer, is preserved. Especially by preserving the

S. Hirano, M.D., Ph.D.
Department of Gastroenterological Surgery II, Hokkaido University Graduate School of Medicine, North-15, West-7, Kita-Ku, Sapporo 060-8638, Japan
e-mail: satto@med.hokudai.ac.jp

© Springer Science+Business Media Singapore 2017
H. Yamaue (ed.), *Innovation of Diagnosis and Treatment for Pancreatic Cancer*,
DOI 10.1007/978-981-10-2486-3_13

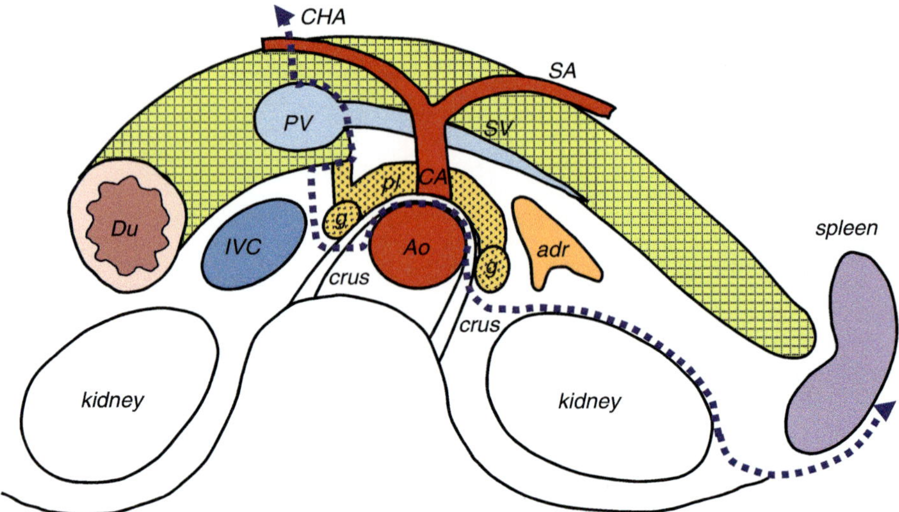

Fig. 13.1 Schematic cross-sectional view demonstrating the resection area of distal pancreatectomy with en bloc celiac axis resection (DP-CAR). The *dotted line* indicates the dissection plane. *Adr* adrenal gland, *Ao* aorta, *CA* celiac axis, *CHA* common hepatic artery, *crus* crus of the diaphragm, *Du* duodenum, *g* celiac ganglion, *IVC* inferior vena cava, *pl* celiac plexus, *PV* portal vein, *SA* splenic artery, *SV* splenic vein

stomach, the patient's nutritional status and tolerance of oral anticancer agents could be maintained. SMA preservation, even with complete eradication of the surrounding plexus, is the key feature of this procedure, which sustains arterial supply to the hepatobiliary system and stomach. Resection of the portal vein and middle colic vessels is an optional procedure.

13.2 Arterial Supply to the Liver and the Stomach After DP-CAR

Although DP-CAR includes en bloc resection of the CA, CHA, and plexus of the SMA, reconstruction of the arterial system is not required because of early development of a collateral arterial circulation via the pancreatoduodenal arcades from the superior mesenteric artery. After division of the CA with the CHA and splenic artery (SA), the hepatic and gastric arterial flow depends on the flow from the gastroduodenal artery (GDA), which should, therefore, definitely be preserved with the pancreatic head during DP-CAR. The collateral pathways via the SMA, pancreatoduodenal arcades, and GDA maintain the arterial blood supply to the hepatobiliary system. Since the collateral pathways also ensure arterial flow to the right gastroepiploic artery, the entire stomach can be preserved (Fig. 13.2).

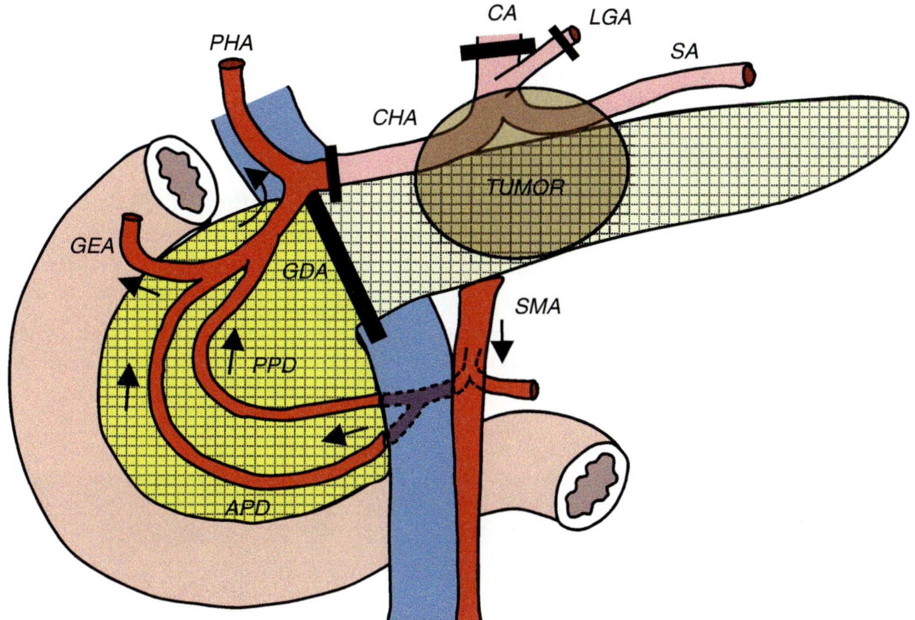

Fig. 13.2 Schematic drawing of collateral arterial pathways via the pancreatoduodenal arcades from the superior mesenteric artery following DP-CAR. The *arrows* show the direction of arterial flow from the superior mesenteric artery to the liver and stomach via the pancreatoduodenal arcades. *APD* anterior pancreatoduodenal arcade, *CA* celiac axis, *CHA* common hepatic artery, *GDA* gastroduodenal artery, *GEA* right gastroepiploic artery, *LGA* left gastric artery, *PHA* proper hepatic artery, *PPD* posterior pancreatoduodenal arcade, *SA* splenic artery, *SMA* superior mesenteric artery

Preoperative coil embolization of the CHA is routinely used to enlarge the collateral arterial pathway in some institutes, so as to reduce ischemia-related complications such as ischemic gastropathy, liver abscess, and perforation of the biliary system [7].

13.3 Selection of Candidates for DP-CAR

Tumor progression is cautiously evaluated mainly with preoperative multidetector row computed tomography (MD-CT), with supplemental use of magnetic resonance imaging (MRI) and endoscopic ultrasonography (EUS). The indication for DP-CAR is locally advanced ductal adenocarcinoma of the body of the pancreas, such as that involving or abutting the CHA, the root of the SA, and/or the CA, without involvement of the GDA, SMA, and inferior pancreatoduodenal artery. Patients with involvement of less than approximately half the circumference of the SMA plexus should be considered candidates for DP-CAR because complete dissection of the SMA plexus without exposing the cancer can be achieved by dividing the plexus on the side opposite to that of the tumor. For oncologically safe ligation and division of the root of the CA in front of the aorta, a 5–7 mm noncancerous length of the CA from the adventitia of the aorta is required (Fig. 13.3).

Even if the tumor of the pancreatic body invades other organs directly, DP-CAR could be completed with concomitant resection of the organs, including the alimentary tract, the left adrenal gland, and/or the left kidney. However, in the case that a tumor has invaded the stomach to a depth that necessitates full-thickness resection, total gastrectomy should be considered because healing of the anastomosis might be disturbed by an insufficient collateral arterial flow.

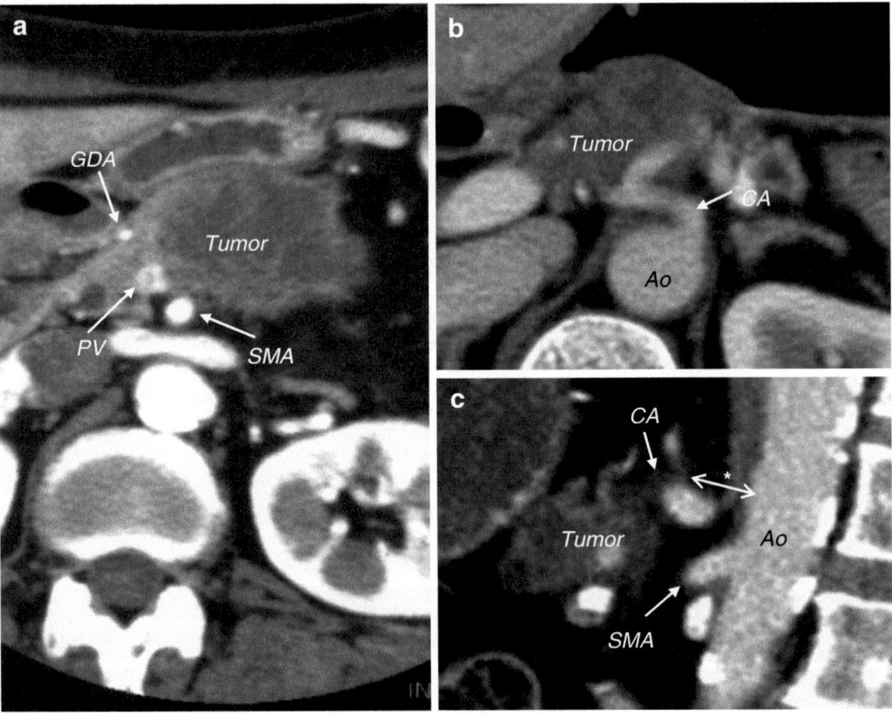

Fig. 13.3 Preoperative diagnosis is obtained by multi-detector row computed tomography (MD-CT). (**a**) The gastroduodenal artery (GDA) is free from the tumor, and invasion of the tumor is limited in the ventral half circumference of the plexus of the superior mesenteric artery (SMA). (**b**) The tumor involvement toward the celiac axis (CA) was estimated in the axial view. (**c**) In the same patient, the sagittal view of MD-CT could show the cancer-free area (*asterisk*) in the root of the CA approximately 7 mm in length. *Ao* Aorta, *CA* celiac axis, *GDA* gastroduodenal artery, *PV* portal vein, *SMA* superior mesenteric artery

13.4   Surgical Procedure of DP-CAR

DP-CAR usually includes resection of the distal pancreas and the spleen, together with en bloc resection of the celiac, common hepatic and left gastric arteries, the celiac plexus and bilateral ganglions, and the circumferential nerve plexus around the SMA. Left perirenal fat tissue, the left adrenal gland, the entire retroperitoneal fat tissue containing lymph nodes cranial to the left renal vein, and the inferior mesenteric vein are also resected. The entire alimentary tract should be preserved; however, cholecystectomy is performed for preventing postoperative ischemic rupture of the gall bladder (Fig. 13.4).

To achieve pathological margin-free (R0) resection, a systematic procedure, which consisted of right and left dorsal approaches to provide sufficient cancer-free margin from the tumor is rather important. In the right dorsal approach, the lower parts of the SMA are exposed following Kocher's maneuver, with complete eradication of the right celiac ganglion and the right para-aortic nodes by exposing the right crus of the diaphragm. The plexus of the SMA is first divided at the dorsal end (opposite to the side of the tumor), and the excision is extended by 4–5 cm in the longitudinal direction. The median arcuate ligament has to be divided to expose just

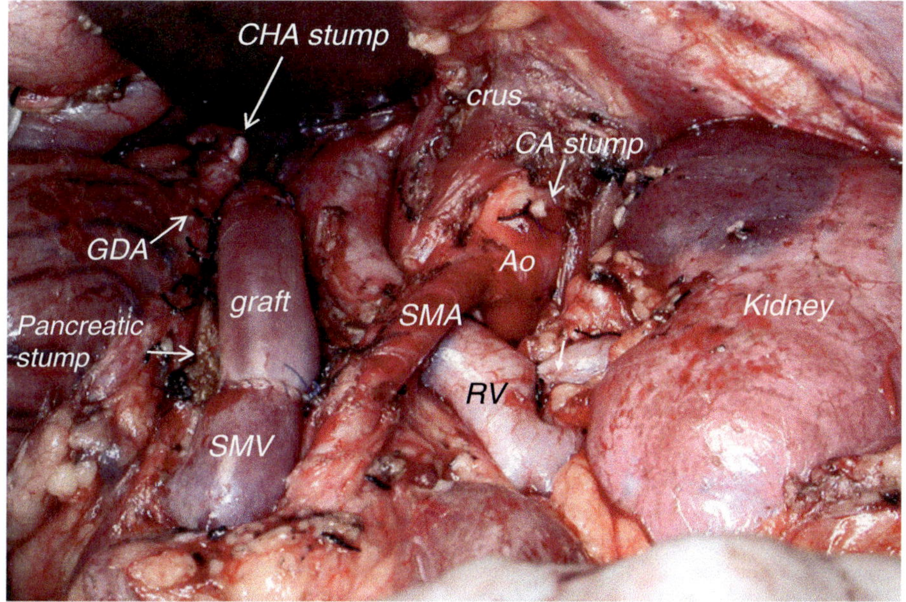

Fig. 13.4 Post-resection view during distal pancreatectomy with en bloc celiac axis resection (DP-CAR). *Ao* aorta, *CA* celiac axis, *CHA* common hepatic artery, *crus* crus of the diaphragm, *GDA* gastroduodenal artery, *graft* interposed iliac vein graft, *IVC* inferior vena cava, *RV* left renal vein, *SMA* superior mesenteric artery, *SMV* superior mesenteric vein

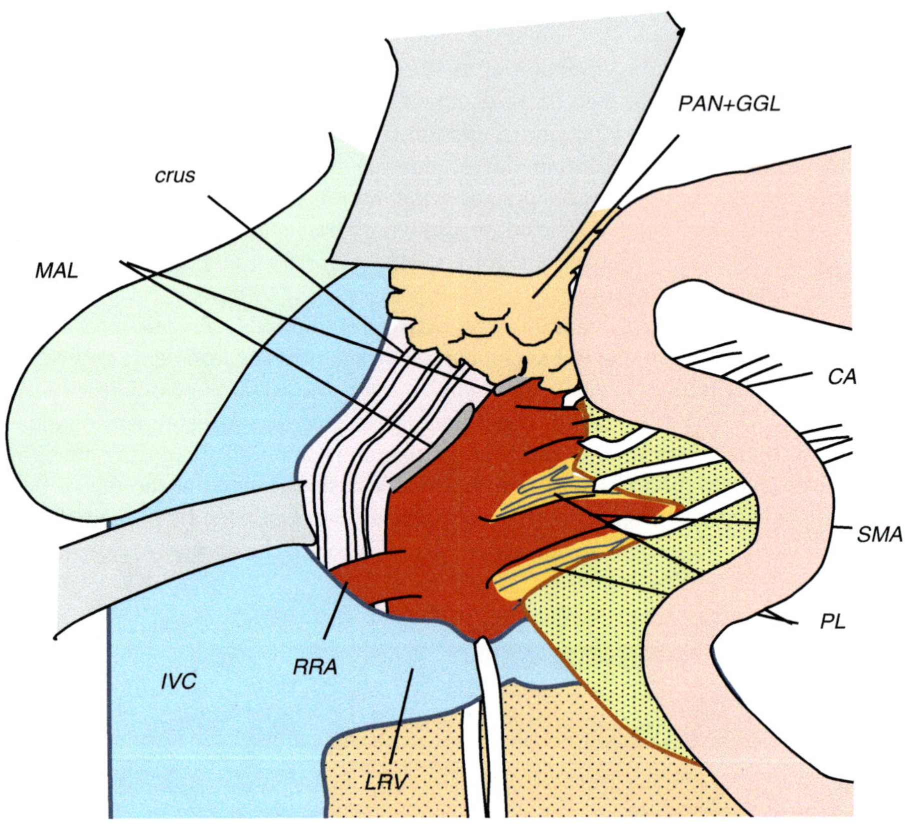

Fig. 13.5 In the right dorsal approach, the plexus of the SMA is first divided in the longitudinal direction following Kocher's maneuver. After eradication of the right celiac ganglion and the right para-aortic nodes by exposing the right crus of the diaphragm, the median arcuate ligament has to be divided to expose just the root of the CA where it should be divided. *CA* celiac axis, *crus* crus of the diaphragm, *IVC* inferior vena cava, *LRV* left renal vein, *MAL* median arcuate ligament, *PAN + GGL* right para-aortic lymph nodes and celiac ganglion, *PL* plexus around the superior mesenteric artery, *RRA* right renal artery, *SMA* superior mesenteric artery

the root of the CA where it should be divided (Fig. 13.5). In the left dorsal approach, en bloc resection of the retroperitoneal fat, together with the upper part of the perirenal fat, including the left adrenal gland cranial to the left renal vessels are performed in exposing the left crus. The left adrenal artery and vein were divided during the procedure. In this approach, the left para-aortic nodes and ganglions are

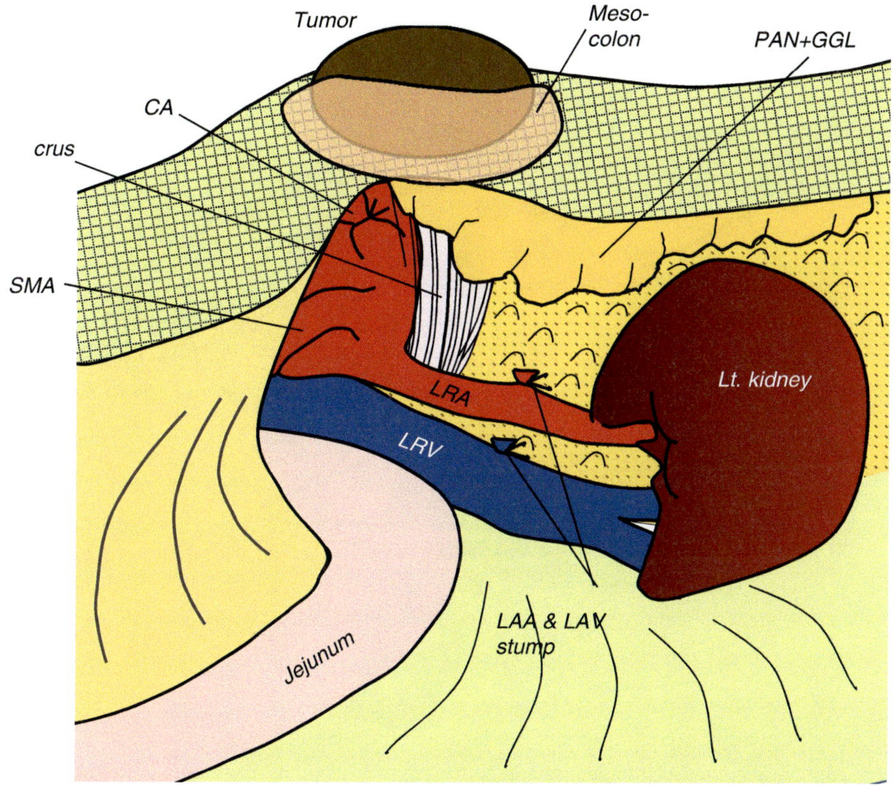

Fig. 13.6 In the left dorsal approach, en bloc resection of the retroperitoneal fat, together with the upper part of the perirenal fat, including the left adrenal gland cranial to the left renal vessels are performed in exposing the left crus. *CA* celiac axis, *crus* crus of the diaphragm, *LAA* left adrenal artery, *LAV* left adrenal vein, *LRA* left renal artery, *LRV* left renal vein, *LSV* left suprarenal vein, *MAL* median arcuate ligament, *PAN + GGL* right para-aortic lymph nodes and celiac ganglion, *RRA* right renal artery, *SMA* superior mesenteric artery

completely dissected. The partial mesocolon covering the tumor was cautiously dissected with the pancreatic parenchyma (Fig. 13.6).

Then, moved ventrally to the pancreas head, transection of the pancreas is performed after dividing the common hepatic artery. When a tumor is located near the GDA, it should be mobilized laterally in order to obtain a cancer-free margin at the site of division of the pancreatic parenchyma. Reconstruction of the portal and/or superior mesenteric vein should be performed in this step, if necessary (Fig. 13.7).

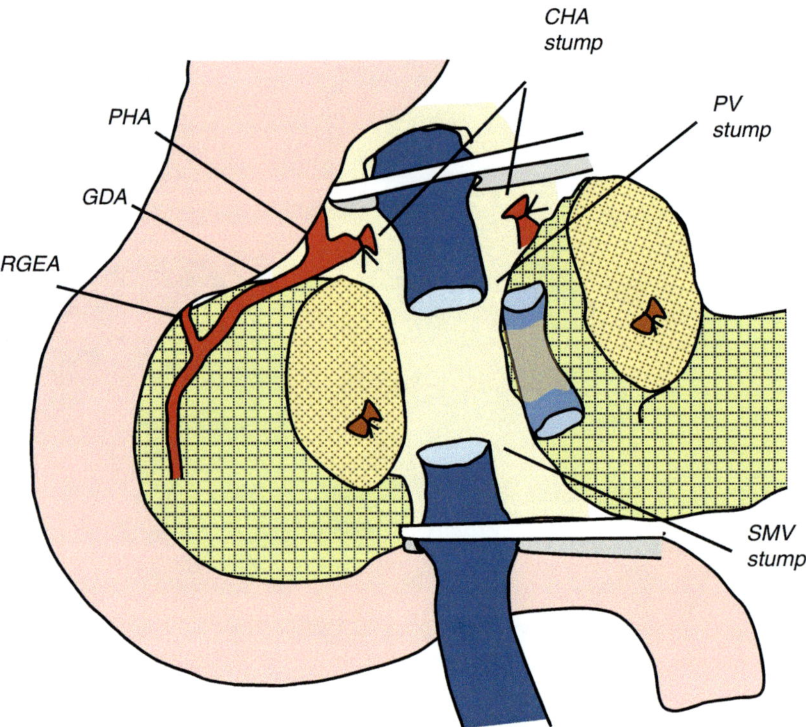

Fig. 13.7 Transection of the pancreas is performed after dividing the common hepatic artery. Reconstruction of the portal and/or superior mesenteric vein should be performed in this step. *CHA* common hepatic artery, *GDA* gastroduodenal artery, *PHA* proper hepatic artery, *PV* portal vein, *RGEA* right gastroepiploic artery, *SMV* superior mesenteric vein

In the next step, division of the SMA plexus in the dorsal side that was performed in the first step is extended longitudinally to just proximal to the inferior pancreaticoduodenal artery (IPDA) to achieve complete resection of the plexus. After the excision of the plexus goes transversally to the right side of the SMA, dissection between the SMA plexus and the uncinate process of the pancreas is performed cranially toward the root of the CA (Fig. 13.8). Then, dividing the tissues between the lesser curvature of the stomach and the distal pancreas with the spleen in dividing the left gastric artery and the short gastric vessels, the specimen can be retrieved.

Accidental injury to the inferior pancreatoduodenal or gastroduodenal artery compromises collateral blood flow and leads to fatal complications, such as gastric necrosis and/or liver infarction. If this occurs, microscopic anastomosis between the proper hepatic artery and middle colic artery (MCA) [8], or the right gastroepiploic artery and MCA [9] could be a possible option for maintaining arterial flow to both the stomach and the liver.

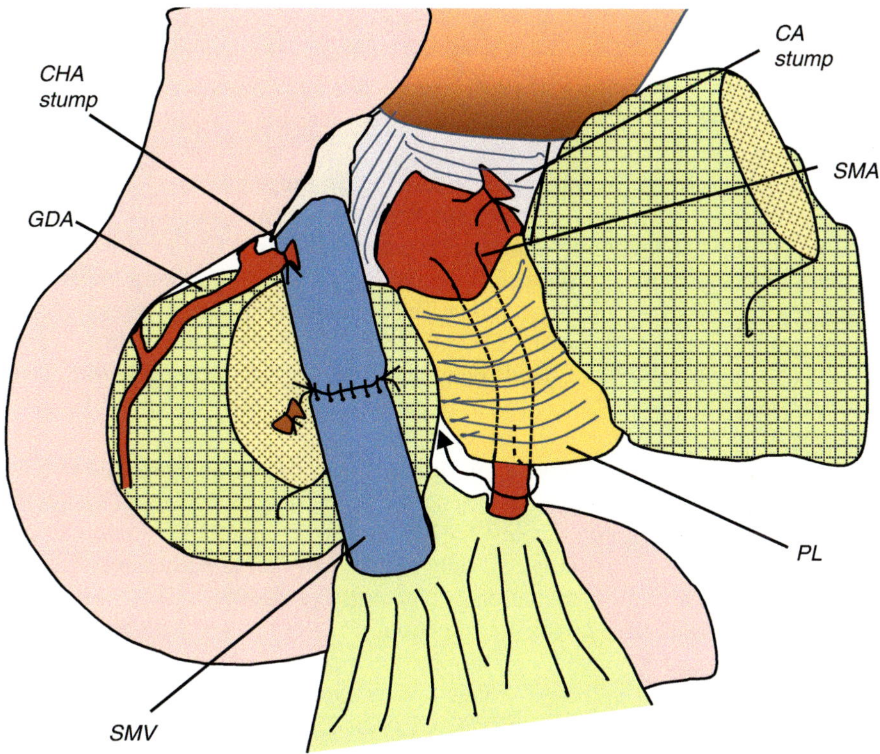

Fig. 13.8 Division of the SMA plexus in the dorsal side is extended longitudinally to just proximal to the inferior pancreaticoduodenal artery (IPDA). The procedure is completed after dissecting between the SMA plexus and the uncinate process of the pancreas (*arrow* shows the direction of the dissection). *CA* celiac axis, *CHA* common hepatic artery, *GDA* gastroduodenal artery, *PL* plexus around the superior mesenteric artery, *RGEA* right gastroepiploic artery, *SMA* superior mesenteric artery, *SMV* superior mesenteric vein

13.5 Short- and Long-Term Outcomes of DP-CAR

The most frequent morbidity after DP-CAR is pancreatic fistula, which occurs relatively easily because the pancreatic parenchyma needs to be divided at the pancreatic head in patients with a tumor extending to the proximal end of the pancreas, beyond the portal vein. In such cases, the cut surface of the pancreas becomes wider than that following usual distal pancreatectomy, in which the pancreatic parenchyma is divided at the neck of the pancreas. It is rather important to insert an indwelling drain at an appropriate position beside the pancreatic stump during surgery, so as to avoid postoperative hemorrhage from a pseudoaneurysm in the stump of the CHA. The second most common morbidity is ischemic gastropathy due to decreased gastric blood flow [10]. According to data from 50 consecutive patients who underwent DP-CAR [11], postoperative morbidity occurred in 27 (54%) patients including those with more than one complication; pancreatic fistula defined by the ISGPF (the International Study Group on Pancreatic Fistula) [12] and ischemic gastropathy occurred in 20 (40%) and 6 (12%) patients, respectively. Two patients out of 50 (4%) died in the hospital of myocardial infarction and multiple organ failure due to anastomotic insufficiency following partial resection of the antrum of the stomach. Postoperative hospital stays ranged from 17 to 208 days, with a median of 39 days [11]. A recent systematic review and meta-analysis [13] of data from 18 articles including more than 6 patients published up to 2014 revealed the morbidity and mortality rates of the were highly variable among the studies; ranged 36–92%, and 0–13%, respectively. The meta-analysis of both rates indicated no significant differences between DP-CAR and distal pancreatectomy. In the paper, pooled incidence of pancreatic fistula defined by ISGPF and gastric ischemic events were 31.31% (95% CI: 23.69–40.12%) and 12.87% (95% CI: 8.30–19.42%), respectively.

One of the other postoperative complications is stubborn diarrhea due to complete dissection of the nerve system around the SMA, CA, and bilateral ganglions. From a published data, approximately half of the patients regularly required antidiarrheal agents, and the remaining half only occasionally required or never used the agents over a median follow-up period of 39 months [14].

Contrary to the adverse effects of resection of nerve tissues, patients enjoy the complete disappearance of pain, even if it has been controlled by opioids just before surgery [5]. The data from the systematic review paper revealed that the proportion of cancer-related pain relief was 89.20% (95% CI: 77.85–95.10%) [13].

In 2007, the long-term outcomes of DP-CAR were first reported in a series of 23 patients with locally advanced pancreatic body cancer who underwent DP-CAR under a policy of "surgery first" [6]. With R0 resectability in 91% of the cases and a median follow-up time of 27.4 months, the estimated 5-year survival rate was 42% and the median survival was 21 months. Seven years after the first report, a second report that included 50 patients was published from the same institute, which indicated estimated disease-specific 1-, 3-, and 5-year survival rates of 80.7%, 32.3%, and 24.3%, respectively, and a median survival time of 24.7 months after a median follow-up period of 45.3 months [11]. Despite the excellent local control with an R0 resection rate of more than 90% in the report, early recurrence (predominantly in the liver) occurred after surgery, which resulted in poor survival time [11].

13.6 Modification of the Indications and Procedure of DP-CAR

Some problems concerning difficulty in achieving R0 resection and patient selection has been reported. Some authors believe that DP-CAR should be reserved for patients without tumor infiltration of either the portal vein or artery because the survival rate of patients with these conditions was poor in their series [15]. A recent article revealed that preoperative factors such as CRP, platelet count, and the level of CA19-9 could assist in the selection of patients who could survive long-term without recurrence following DP-CAR [11]. To reduce the occurrence of postoperative hepatic metastasis while maintaining the complete local control that is achievable by DP-CAR, the strategy of upfront surgery is most likely to change in the current era of advancements in chemo- and chemoradiotherapy. Long-term survival after DP-CAR might be improved by employing neoadjuvant and/or adjuvant chemotherapy.

Another serious problem of DP-CAR to be resolved is ischemic gastropathy. For this, preserving the left gastric artery in limited cases [16] or reconstruction of the artery might be a possible future modification [8, 9].

References

1. Kondo S, Katoh S, Hirano S, Ambo Y, Tanaka E, Okushiba S, Morikawa T, Kanai M, Yano T. Results of radical distal pancreatectomy with en bloc resection of the celiac artery for locally advanced cancer of the pancreatic body. Langenbecks Arch Surg. 2003;388:101–6.
2. Appleby LH. The coeliac axis in the expansion of the operation for gastric carcinoma. Cancer. 1953;6:707.
3. Nimura Y, Hattori T, Miura K, Nakajima N, Hibi M. A case of advanced carcinoma of the body and tail of the pancreas resected by the Appleby operation (in Japanese). Operation. 1976;30:885–9.
4. Hishinuma S, Ogata Y, Matsui J, Ozawa I, Inada T, Shimizu H, Kobu K, Ikeda T, Koyama Y. Two cases of cancer of the pancreatic body undergoing preservation with distal pancreatectomy combined with resection of the celiac axis. Jpn J Gastroenterol Surg. 1991;24:2782–6. In Japanese with English Abstract
5. Kondo S, Katoh H, Omi M, Hirano S, Ambo Y, Tanaka E, Okushiba S, Morikawa T, Kanai M, Yano T. Radical distal pancreatectomy with en bloc resection of the celiac artery, plexus, and ganglions for advanced cancer of the pancreatic body: a preliminary report on perfect pain relief. JOP. 2001;2:93–7.
6. Hirano S, Kondo S, Hara T, Ambo Y, Tanaka E, Shichinohe T, Suzuki O, Hazama K. Distal pancreatectomy with en bloc celiac axis resection for locally advanced pancreatic body cancer: long-term results. Ann Surg. 2007;246:46–51.
7. Abo D, Hasegawa Y, Sakuhara Y, Terae S, Shimizu T, Tha KK, Tanaka E, Hirano S, Kondo S, Shirato H. Feasibility of a dual microcatheter-dual interlocking detachable coil technique in preoperative embolization in preparation for distal pancreatectomy with en bloc celiac axis resection for locally advanced pancreatic body cancer. J Hepatobiliary Pancreat Sci. 2012;19:431–7.
8. Suzuki H, Hosouchi Y, Sasaki S, Araki K, Kubo N, Watanabe A, Kuwano H. Reconstruction of the hepatic artery with the middle colic artery is feasible in distal pancreatectomy with celiac axis resection: a case report. World J Gastrointest Surg. 2013;5:224–8.
9. Kondo S, Ambo Y, Katoh H, Hirano S, Tanaka E, Okushiba S, Morikawa T, Igawa H, Yamamoto Y, Sugihara T. Middle colic artery-gastroepiploic artery bypass for compromised collateral flow in distal pancreatectomy with celiac artery resection. Hepato-Gastroenterology. 2003;50:305–7.
10. Kondo S, Katho H, Hirano S, Ambo Y, Tanaka E, Maeyama Y, Morikawa T, Okushiba S. Ischemic gastropathy after distal pancreatectomy with celiac axis resection. Surg Today. 2004;34:337–40.
11. Miura T, Hirano S, Nakamura T, Tanaka E, Shichinohe T, Tsuchikawa T, Kato K, Matsumoto J, Kondo S. A new preoperative prognostic scoring system to predict prognosis in patients with locally advanced pancreatic body cancer who undergo distal pancreatectomy with en bloc celiac axis resection: a retrospective cohort study. Surgery. 2014;155:457–67.

12. Bassi C, Dervenis C, Butturini G, Fingerhut A, Yeo C, Izbicki J, Neoptolemos J, Sarr M, Traverso W, Buchler M. International Study Group on Pancreatic Fistula Definition. Postoperative pancreatic fistula: an international study group (ISGPF) definition. Surgery. 2005;138:8–13.
13. Gong H, Ma R, Gong J, Cai C, Song Z, Xu B. Distal pancreatectomy with en bloc celiac axis resection for locally advanced pancreatic cancer: a systematic review and meta-analysis. Medicine (Baltimore). 2016;95:e3061. doi:10.1097/MD.0000000000003061.
14. Hirano S, Kondo S, Tanaka E, Shichinohe T, Tsuchikawa T, Kato K, Matsumoto J. Postoperative bowel function and nutritional status following distal pancreatectomy with en-bloc celiac axis resection. Dig Surg. 2010;27:212–6.
15. Okada K, Kawai M, Tani M, Hirono S, Miyazawa M, Shimizu A, Kitahata Y, Yamaue H. Surgical strategy for patients with pancreatic body/tail carcinoma: who should undergo distal pancreatectomy with en-bloc celiac axis resection? Surgery. 2013;153:365–72.
16. Okada K, Kawai M, Tani M, Hirono S, Miyazawa M, Shimizu A, Kitahata Y, Yamaue H. Preservation of the left gastric artery on the basis of anatomical features in patients undergoing distal pancreatectomy with celiac axis en-bloc resection (DP-CAR). World J Surg. 2014;38:2980–5.

14

Ken-ichi Okada and Hiroki Yamaue

14.1 Introduction

14.1.1 The Procedure for Borderline Resectable Pancreatic Body Cancer

The application of distal pancreatectomy with celiac axis en bloc resection (DP-CAR) for borderline resectable pancreatic body/tail carcinoma remains controversial because of the lack of large number of study. One of the advantages of this procedure is its radicality with wide margin behind the tumor through dividing the root of the celiac axis. In addition, the procedure is capable of resolving preoperative cancer pain according to the tumor invasion into the nerve plexuses. R0 resection has also been suggested to be an essential requirement for long survival. In contrast, an R0 resection is not the only consideration for the impact of survival in advanced pancreatic carcinoma [1]. Long-term survivors after DP-CAR have been recently reported [2], with a median survival time of 9.5–12 months in a meta-analysis of 43 patients [3]. In spite of these reports, the indications for DP-CAR remain controversial with regard to its curability and survival benefit. Taken together, one should consider the issue of tumor biology and acknowledge that most pancreatic carcinomas recur systemically, and that tumor involving arterial structures recur rapidly even after an R0 resection. Therefore, we must carefully balance between tumor biology as a systemic disease and the potential benefits of surgery [1]. This procedure can provide clinical benefits for patients with borderline resectable pancreatic body/tail carcinoma after neoadjuvant therapy. In addition, stronger and more precise preoperative therapy for patients with borderline resectable pancreatic body/tail carcinoma will be required to improve their survival.

K.-i. Okada • H. Yamaue (✉)
Second Department of Surgery, Wakayama Medical University,
Kimiidera, Wakayama 641-8510, Japan
e-mail: yamaue-h@wakayama-med.ac.jp

© Springer Science+Business Media Singapore 2017
H. Yamaue (ed.), *Innovation of Diagnosis and Treatment for Pancreatic Cancer*,
DOI 10.1007/978-981-10-2486-3_14

14.1.2 History of DP-CAR for Pancreatic Cancer

In 1973, Fortner introduced the regional resection of pancreatic cancer with major vascular en bloc resection as a new approach [4]. In this literature, 8 of the 15 individuals (53%) who survived the operation lived for periods ranging from 4 to 17 months. Six lived for more than 1 year after regional pancreatectomy. Actual survival estimation was 62% at 1 year, compared with 1-year survival rate of 36% for 17 patients who underwent pancreaticoduodenectomy for less advanced cancer at the same institution from 1959 to 1969 [5]. This approach described regional pancreatectomy to potentially be the most beneficial for patients with small pancreatic cancer, where regional resection would give a wide margin. The Appleby operation was first reported as resection of the celiac axis for complete lymphadenectomy in radical resection of gastric carcinoma in 1953 [6, 7]. Nimura et al. reported the adaptation of the Appleby operation for the resection of pancreatic body/tail carcinoma involving the celiac axis and/or common hepatic artery in 1976 [8]. In 1991, Hishinuma et al. modified this procedure with preservation of the entire stomach, which improved postoperative nutritional status and quality of life (QOL) [9]. In 2000, Konishi et al. reported reconstruction of the hepatic artery when pulsation in the proper hepatic artery was weak after test occlusion of the celiac axis [10]. Since then, several institutions have reported their experience with the modified Appleby operation for advanced pancreatic body/tail carcinoma, i.e., distal pancreatectomy combined with celiac axis en bloc resection, which was named DP-CAR by Kondo et al. [11]. Despite reports of a few long-term survivors, the overall survival benefit and the risks of this challenging operation are unknown because previous reports have only involved a small number of patients [12–15]. However, with the safer modification of the Appleby operation and the emergence of the concept of borderline resectable pancreatic carcinoma [16–25], this procedure once again appeals to pancreatic surgeons as a radical pancreatectomy for borderline resectable pancreatic body/tail carcinoma.

14.2 Anatomical Knowledge of DP-CAR

14.2.1 The Anatomical Features of Celiac Trunk and Its Branches

In 1917, Eaton reported a normal type of celiac axis which gives off the left gastric artery as a collateral branch before it bifurcates into the hepatic and splenic arteries (62.1% of 541 cases), and subsequently trifurcates, which occurs in only 24% of the 541 cases [26]. A recent study described that the celiac trunk gave rise to three main arteries—the left gastric artery, common hepatic artery, and splenic artery. The celiac trunk bifurcates into the splenic and the common hepatic artery, while the left gastric artery had originated between the aortas over the celiac trunk up to a trifurcation. This type of celiac trunk was observed in 72% of 90 cadavers [27]. Malnar et al. described the length of the celiac trunk measured by vernier caliper from its origin to the point where it gives off main branches varied from 1.0 to 3.5 cm. They reported that in the form of trifurcation, its length was 1.9 ± 0.08 cm while in the form of bifurcation, the length was 2.0 ± 0.08 cm. When the diameters of the celiac trunk normal main branches were measured, it was found that the splenic artery had the largest diameter (0.61 ± 0.05 cm) followed by the mean arterial diameter of the common hepatic artery (0.57 ± 0.04 cm) while the left gastric artery had the smallest diameter (0.38 ± 0.03 cm) [27–30].

14.2.2 The Organs and Tissues Resected by DP-CAR

Hirano and Kondo et al. described [1] the en bloc resections of the resected organ and tissues using this procedure that included the celiac, common hepatic, left gastric arteries, celiac plexus and ganglions, nerve plexus around the superior mesenteric artery, a part of the crus of the diaphragm, Gerota fascia, left adrenal gland, retroperitoneal fat tissues bearing lymph nodes above the left renal vein, transverse mesocolon covering the body of the pancreas, and the inferior mesenteric vein. Resections of the portal vein and the middle colic vessels are optional. In general, no reconstruction of the arterial system is required because of early development of the collateral arterial pathways via the pancreaticoduodenal arcades from the superior mesenteric artery. Preoperative coil embolization of the common hepatic artery is routinely used to enlarge the collateral pathways and prevent ischemia-related complications. In addition, with the preservation of the stomach, no reconstruction of the alimentary tract is required. Based on the anatomical features and the relationship between the tumor and artery, the left gastric artery and inferior phrenic arteries can be preserved. Various institutions perform left gastric artery reconstruction in patients who undergo DP-CAR. Table 14.1 shows the list of organs, vessels,

Table 14.1 Reprinted and partially altered from [1]

	Resection	Preservation	Optional resection
Organ	Pancreas (body/tail), left adrenal gland, gallbladder[a], spleen	Stomach, duodenum	
Vessels	Celiac artery, common hepatic artery, splenic artery, dorsal pancreatic artery, short gastric vessels, posterior gastric artery, inferior mesenteric vein	Inferior pancreaticoduodenal artery, gastroduodenal artery (pancreaticoduodenal arcades), proper hepatic artery, the right gastric and right gastroepiploic vessels, gastrocolic trunk	Portal vein, middle colic vessels. Left gastric artery[a] and inferior phrenic arteries can be preserved based on the anatomical features
Other tissues	Part of the crus of the diaphragm, the Gerota fascia, the celiac plexus and ganglions, the nerve plexus around the superior mesenteric artery, the retroperitoneal fat tissues bearing lymph nodes above the left renal vein, the transverse mesocolon covering the body of the pancreas	Right adrenal gland, bilateral kidneys	

[a]Several institutions routinely resect the left gastric artery while others preserve under definite condition or reconstruct it

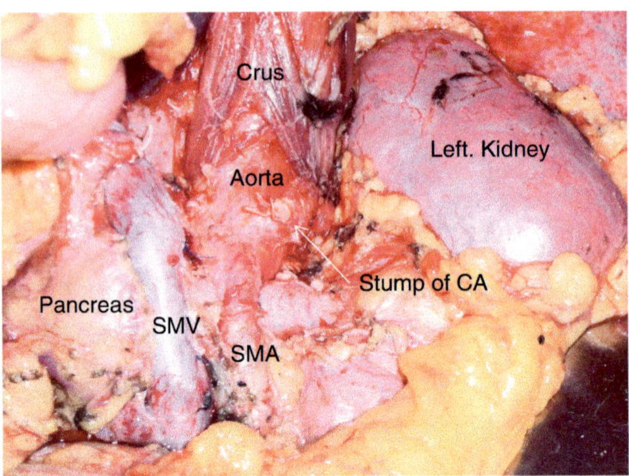

Fig. 14.1 The surgical field after the modified Appleby operation (DP-CAR). *CA* celiac axis, *SMV* superior mesenteric vein, *SMA* superior mesenteric artery (Reprinted from [1])

and other tissues which is resected and preserved in this procedure. Figure 14.1 shows the surgical field after DP-CAR.

14.2.3 Indications of DP-CAR for Patients with Pancreatic Body/tail Carcinoma

Firstly, this procedure should be performed in selected institutions where well-trained and skillful staffs are available. In the early period of the adaptation of DP-CAR, this procedure is indicated for patients with pancreatic body/tail carcinoma involving the celiac axis and/or common hepatic artery (Fig. 14.2). Recent literature reported that this procedure can be suitable for the patients whose pancreatic body/tail tumors involved or touched by at least one of the common hepatic artery, the root of the splenic artery, or the celiac axis [2] (Fig. 14.2), which means a part of the resectable pancreatic body/ tail carcinomas situated near the root of the splenic artery are also indicated for this procedure. Our investigation regarding the relationship between curability and the distance between the edge of the tumor and the splenic artery root in patients who underwent standard DP revealed that the microscopically positive margins were detected more frequently in patients with tumors situated ≤10 mm from the splenic artery than those with a distance of >10 mm from the splenic artery [31]. Therefore, we suggest that DP-CAR should be performed to obtain an R0 resection in those patients with potentially resectable pancreatic body/tail carcinoma who would otherwise receive a standard DP. In addition to that, our study demonstrated the overall survival rate in patients with pathologically negative invasion for portal venous system and artery (double negative invasion) was greater than that of the other patients. With regard to artery invasion, Kanda and colleagues reported that invasion of the splenic artery is a crucial prognostic factor in patients with carcinoma of the body/tail of the pancreas [32].

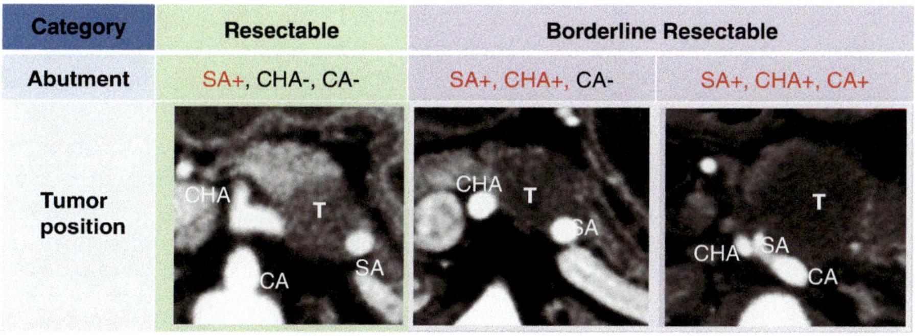

Fig. 14.2 The association between resectability and the tumor abutment to celiac axis and its branches with imaging of computed tomography. *SA* splenic artery, *CHA* common hepatic artery, *CA* celiac axis (Reprinted and partially altered from [1])

Moreover, an extended pancreatectomy with a major arterial resection did not result in any long-term survivors in numerous reports [33–39]. Therefore, patients with a double negative invasion into portal venous system and artery are carefully evaluated using preoperative imaging study for DP-CAR. However, even in the latest modern imaging study modality, the accuracy is not equivalent to that of microscope, and the abutment to the vascular wall itself does not mean pathological invasion. As such, there is room for neoadjuvant intervention to decrease the rate of microscopically positive margins.

14.2.4 The Role of Arterial En Bloc Resection

Recent studies reported arterial en bloc resection in patients undergoing pancreatectomy for pancreatic cancer is associated with poor short- and long-term outcomes. These studies on arterial en bloc resection for pancreatic carcinoma described that it can result in overall survival that is comparable to that obtained with standard resection and better than that after palliative bypass [13, 34, 35]. Nevertheless, arterial resection is associated with significantly higher morbidity and mortality rates, counterbalancing the overall survival and limiting the overall oncological benefit [33]. They concluded that pancreatectomy with artery en bloc resection may be justifiable in selected patients owing to the potential survival benefit compared with patients without resection. These patients should be treated within the boundaries of clinical trials to assess the outcomes after artery en bloc resection given the rise of modern pancreatic surgery and multimodal therapy [33–35]. One of the advantages of the modified Appleby operation is the ability to take surgical margin in pancreatic body/tail carcinoma. In borderline resectable pancreatic head carcinoma abuts to the superior mesenteric artery, the superior mesenteric artery and its plexus itself are the "limit line" of surgical dissection. On the other hand, DP-CAR can take surgical margin by controlling the level of dissection layer behind the tumor as a boundary of aortic surface unless the tumor abuts to the aorta. However, previous study reported high R0 resection rate after this procedure, the surgery first strategy for the tumor adjacent to the aorta often revealed high R1 rates even in patients whose tumor abuts to the celiac axis. As Fortner reported, the greatest potential benefit of DP-CAR may appear to be in patients with small pancreatic cancer where regional resection would give a wide margin. Another advantage of this procedure is its ability to relieve cancer pain by celiac axis en bloc resection combined with the removal of the tumor infiltrating plexuses. Recent studies have reported high resolution rates of 86–100% for cancer pain after this procedure [2, 13, 14] and also improved the QOL after the procedure. The nutritional status and QOL of patients after this surgery was well maintained, and planned adjuvant therapy was completed [40].

14.3 Clinical Preparation

14.3.1 Preoperative Preparation for DP-CAR

The necessity for preoperative coil embolization remains controversial. Several investigators have reported DP-CAR without preoperative coil embolization of the common hepatic artery (CHA) [14]. However, several severe accidents occurred intraoperatively or at the early phase after surgery, it may decrease the risk of critical ischemia-related complications. The safety and efficacy issues are essential to be evaluated in clinical trials. Preoperative coil embolization of the CHA should be performed as collaborative work between the surgeons and interventional radiologists. Surgeons should precisely indicate the planned ligation/division site to the interventional radiologists while the latter ensure that the coil is safely placed in the requested position without causing coil migration into the arteries that are intended to be preserved [41, 42]. The diameter of the inferior pancreaticoduodenectomy usually increases about 1.5–2 times from the procedure.

14.3.2 Preparation of Instruments and Tools for DP-CAR

The surgical instruments used in DP-CAR are basically similar to those of ordinary pancreatic resection. The aortic clamps should be prepared in case of injury or short ligation margin of celiac trunk. Doppler ultrasonography should be routinely prepared for intraoperative evaluation of intrahepatic arterial and portal flow. Where there is a need to suture damaged aortic wall around the root of celiac axis, 6-0 prolene® with nonabsorbable pad made of polytetrafluoroethylene called pledget® (Covidien, USA) are helpful to decompress the damage from arterial suture.

14.4 Procedure and Perioperative Management

14.4.1 The Procedure and Pitfalls of DP-CAR

The specific procedure for DP-CAR is as follows: firstly, the right gastroepiploic artery/vein and right gastric artery/vein are encircled by vessel tape for preservation purpose. Before the transection of the neck of the pancreas, the bifurcation of the gastroduodenal artery (GDA) and the common hepatic artery (CHA) are first to be exposed, followed by the exposure of the origin of the proper hepatic artery (PHA). At this point, it is necessary to harvest the periarterial nerve plexus around the bifurcation to confirm negative cancer cell infiltration. This is to evaluate the resectability in patients whose tumor is adjacent this region. Kocher's maneuver should be performed in case of accidental bleeding from the portal venous system. The gastrocolic trunk is preserved for venous returning from the stomach. Transection of the pancreas is performed with wide surgical margin from the tumor to confirm negative cancer cell infiltration. In patients whose tumor involves the portal vein, the resection and reconstruction of the portal vein are performed antecedently. After the pancreatic transaction, the dissection of the retroperioteum must be performed from the right side to the left side in the manner of a radical antegrade modular pancreatosplenectomy procedure. This is because the surgical field for this procedure is better and safer for surgeon and assistant in case of accidental bleeding [43]. By en bloc dissecting the lymph nodes around the CHA, the right celiac ganglion and celiac nerve plexus (the origin of the celiac axis) is exposed. Then, palpation is performed to confirm blood flow through the PHA, the right gastric artery, and the right gastroepiploic artery. Intrahepatic arterial flow is also checked by intraoperative Doppler ultrasonography after clamping the end of the CHA in patients who had undergone preoperative embolization of the CHA. The CHA is divided just proximal to the origin of the GDA (Fig. 14.3). In cases with dog-leg branching of PHA and GDA, both arteries are preserved by carefully avoiding the ligation of bifurcation site (Figs. 14.4 and 14.5). Lifting the cut end of the distal pancreas and the CHA into the left caudal side, the superior mesenteric artery (SMA) is dissected from the surrounding lymph node and nerve plexus toward its origin. The inferior pancreaticoduodenal artery (IPDA) arising from the SMA or the first jejunal artery is

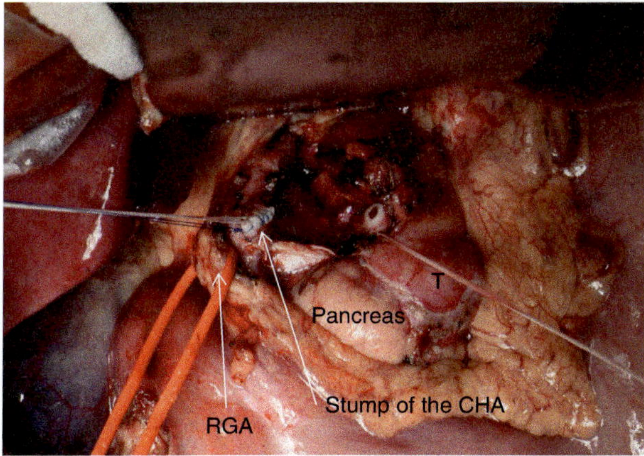

Fig. 14.3 The common hepatic artery was divided just proximal to the origin of the gastroduodenal artery. *T* pancreatic adenocarcinoma, *CHA* common hepatic artery, *RGA* right gastric artery (Reprinted from [1])

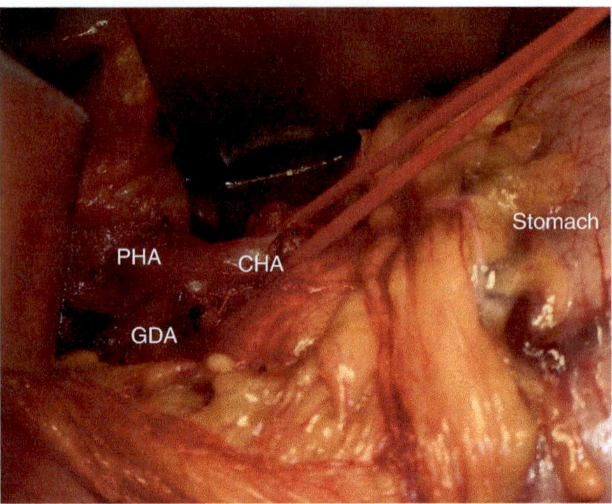

Fig. 14.4 In the cases with dog-leg branching of proper hepatic artery and gastroduodenal artery, both arteries were carefully preserved by avoiding the ligation of bifurcation site. *CHA* common hepatic artery, *PHA* proper hepatic artery, *GDA* gastroduodenal artery (Reprinted from [1])

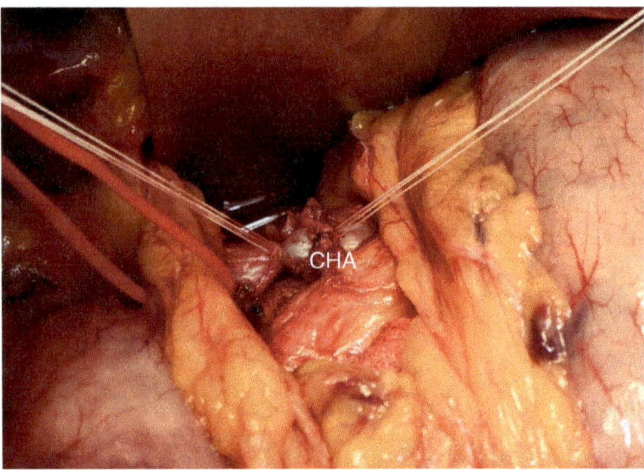

Fig. 14.5 The common hepatic artery was ligated in the distal side. Pulsations of proper hepatic artery and gastroduodenal artery were reconfirmed after ligation. *CHA* common hepatic artery (Reprinted from [1])

carefully preserved. The dissecting layer around the SMA is connected to that of the celiac axis (CA) from the caudal side to dorsal side. The origin of the celiac axis is identified circumferentially just above the aorta and as divided. It is important to note the origin and the direction of inferior phrenic arteries when dissecting around the CA in front of the aorta (Fig. 14.6).

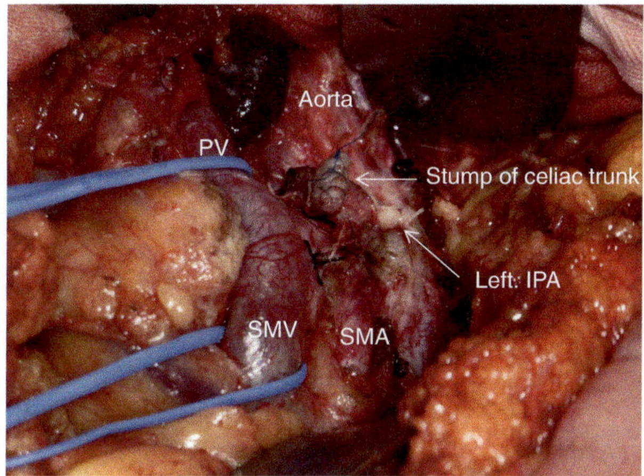

Fig. 14.6 The origin and direction of the inferior phrenic arteries should be noted when dissecting around the celiac axis in front of the aorta. *PV* portal vein, *SMV* superior mesenteric artery, *SMA* superior mesenteric artery, *IPA* inferior phrenic artery (Reprinted from [1])

Table 14.2 Reprinted from [1]

Author (Reference)	Reported year	Number of cases (n)	MST[a] (month)	1-year survival rate (%)[a]	Ischemia-related complication (%)[b]	Morbidity (%)	Mortality (n)
Hishinuma et al. [11]	2007	7	19	30	0	29	0
Hirano et al. [1]	2007	23	21	42	13[c]	48	0
Wu et al. [12]	2010	11	14	9	0[c]	36	1
Takahashi et al. [13]	2011	16	10	35	0[c]	56	1
Yamamoto et al. [14]	2012	13	21	25	38[c]	92	0
Okada et al. [30]	2013	16	25	42	6	44	0

[a]Data included estimated survival time/rates
[b]Ischemia-related complications in the stomach, duodenum, and liver
[c]Preventive combined resection of the total stomach was performed

14.4.2 Postoperative Complications After DP-CAR

The rate of morbidity after this procedure is not low as shown in Table 14.2. The presence of postoperative hemorrhage from the resected stump of the common hepatic artery due to a pancreatic fistula after DP-CAR is difficult to rescue using interventional radiology (IVR) techniques because of the common hepatic artery resection. To that end, a novel procedure to reduce the risk of pancreatic fistula formation is urgently

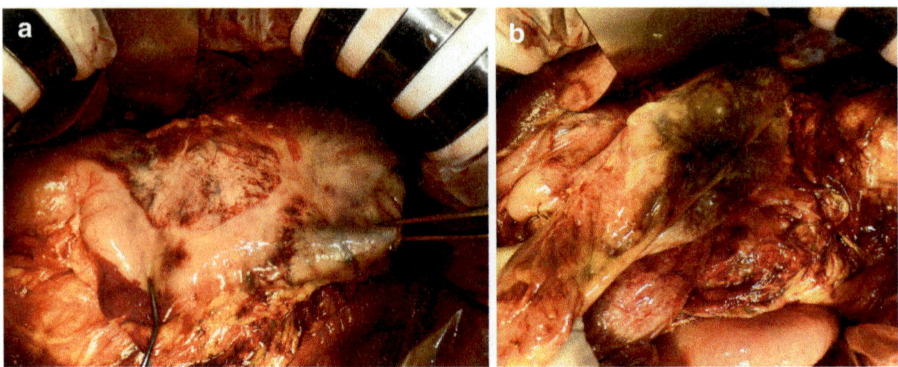

Fig. 14.7 Intraoperative finding of gastric ischemia after DP-CAR. (**a**) a region of lesser curvature of the stomach to which blood supply from the left gastric artery presented necrotic change; (**b**) the fundic area of the stomach to which blood supply from the left gastric and left inferior phrenic arteries presented completely necrotic change

needed for DP-CAR. This is especially the case for patients with thick pancreatic parenchyma, in which the pancreatic transection with a large cross-section surface is usually located on the right side of the portal vein [44, 45]. In addition, DP-CAR is associated with significant morbidities such as severe gastropathy or hepatic ischemia. Total gastrectomy is performed if severe ischemia of the stomach is observed during operation and if surgeons could not exclude the possibility of future necrosis of the remnant stomach in several institutions. Unplanned arterial reconstruction is required in patients with accidental injury [2]. The possible ischemic gastropathy includes irregular, shallow, and wide ulcerations usually in the cardia of the stomach thought to be ischemic in the origin and delayed gastric emptying after surgery. We experienced ischemia of the stomach which required total gastrectomy in a patient who underwent DP-CAR on the postoperative day 2 (Fig. 14.7a, b). Particular care should be taken for simultaneous division of the left gastric and left inferior phrenic arteries for the progress of stomach ischemia intra/postoperatively. The issue would directly affect the postoperative recovery and the schedule for adjuvant chemotherapy. On hepatic ischemia, recent studies reported low incidence of clinically relevant hepatic infarction requiring drainage of abscess, and that abnormal liver function are usually observed to recover within several days. However, there is no evidence of decreased risk of these ischemia-related complications from preoperative embolization of the common hepatic artery. Preoperative angiography should be carried out and variations of the inferior pancreaticoduodenal artery (IPDA) should be examined to ensure safety of the procedure. Postoperative necrotic cholecystitis occurrence is also reported potentially due to the spasm of the gastroduodenal artery and/or proper hepatic artery reported from various institutions (Fig. 14.8). One main concern is the onset of diarrhea after the removal of the plexus around the celiac axis and the superior mesenteric artery. This is because diarrhea would influence the nutritional status and quality of life after surgery. In many studies, diarrhea after this procedure is reported to be within a controllable degree to maintain QOL and nutritional status by medication, usually with loperamide hydrochloride, and occasionally with a tincture of opium [2].

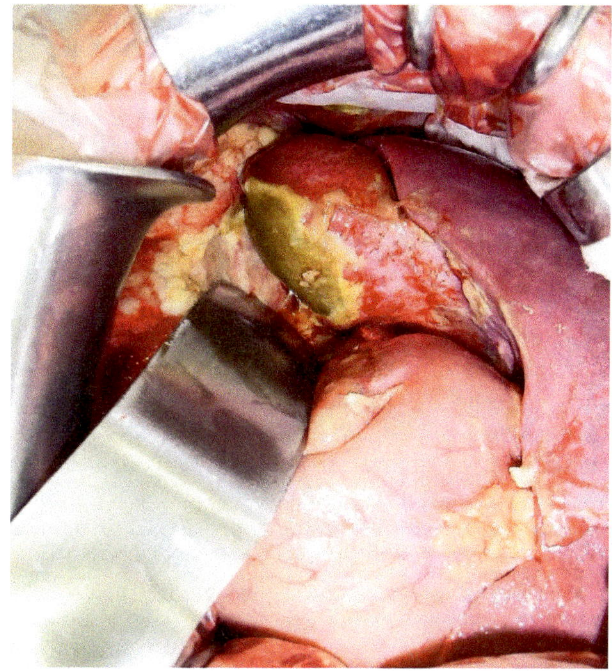

Fig. 14.8 Intraoperative findings of ischemic cholecystitis after DP-CAR

14.4.3 Feasibility and Safety Compared with the Standard Distal Pancreatectomy

While the mean operative time is significantly longer due to the extended and radical dissections, there is no difference in the mean estimated blood loss and mean postoperative hospital stay. In terms of postoperative complications, previous studies reported the incidence of postoperative pancreatic fistula based on the International Study Group of Pancreatic Fistula (ISGPF) [46] revealed no significant differences between the modified Appleby operation and standard distal pancreatectomy, but delayed gastric emptying (DGE) was more common in the modified Appleby operation. Otherwise, the mortality for the procedure was reportedly low in recent literatures [47] (Table 14.2).

14.5 Modified DP-CAR

14.5.1 Preservation of the Left Gastric Artery on the Basis of Anatomical Features

Despite recent favorable surgical outcomes, delayed gastric emptying (DGE) or ischemic gastropathy after the modified Appleby operation (DP-CAR) is a continuous challenging complication. DGE induced by ischemic gastropathy, with an incidence rate varying from 13.0% to 30.8% [2, 15], is not a life-threatening complication, but results in a prolonged hospital stay and leads to a decreased QOL, poorer nutritional status, and delayed administration of postoperative adjuvant chemotherapy. In a recent study, several patients underwent combined total gastrectomy to prevent gastric ischemic complications during the modified Appleby operation (DP-CAR) [2, 15]. The left gastric artery (LGA) develops as the first branch of the celiac trunk embryologically, and it was reported to branch antecedently in 68–72% of cases as a first branch of trifurcation described above [26, 27]. However, the procedures used for the modified Appleby operation (DP-CAR) routinely included en bloc resection of the LGA [2] although pancreas body cancer requiring DP-CAR does not always involve the LGA or the nerve plexus surrounding the LGA. We prospectively attempted to preserve the LGA with enough margins in patients whose LGA branched antecedently and in whom the distance between the LGA and carcinoma was more than 10 mm to clarify whether LGA preservation in DP-CAR (modified DP-CAR) could reduce the incidence of DGE and other postoperative complications [48]. Medical records of 37 consecutive patients who underwent DP-CAR were evaluated. The incidence of DGE occurred in 23 patients (62%) with left gastric artery (LGA)-resecting DP-CAR (conventional DP-CAR) compared with 14 patients (38%) who underwent distal pancreatectomy with resection of the common hepatic artery and splenic artery, with preservation of the LGA (modified DP-CAR) for pancreatic carcinoma. The patients with tumors situated more than 10 mm away from the antecedent branching LGA underwent modified DP-CAR (Fig. 14.9a–c). The antecedent branching of the LGA was found in 19 patients (51%) in this study. In the conventional DP-CAR group, the LGA was involved in 20 patients (87.0%). Clinically relevant DGE according to the ISGPS grades were: 30% in the conventional DP-CAR group and 0% in the modified DP-CAR group ($p = 0.035$). The R0 rate was higher in the modified DP-CAR group (79%) compared with the conventional DP-CAR group (43%) ($p = 0.048$). Univariate and multivariate analyses demonstrated that resection of the LGA was an independent risk factor for increased incidence of DGE (Table 14.3). Therefore, modified DP-CAR significantly reduced the incidence of DGE in comparison with conventional DP-CAR [48]. In this series, distal stomach blood/nerve supply including right gastric, right gastroepiploic arteries, and antral nerve branch were preserved, but proximal stomach blood supply including the left gastroepiploic and short gastric arteries were resected in all cases. A recent study reported resection of LGA-induced ischemia of the proximal remnant stomach during distal pancreatectomy, demonstrating the only circulation of blood from the esophagogastric junction through the intramural capillary network by intraoperative indocyanine green (ICG) fluorescence angiography [49]. In addition, we experienced slow development of the right gastric and right gastroepiploic arteries as whole stomach blood supply following DP-CAR by CT or angiography in several cases. Regarding major venous drainage, the right gastric and right gastroepiploic veins were preserved, while the left gastric and short gastric veins were resected in all cases. Therefore, the venous flow of the stomach following DP-CAR were similar between the two groups in this study. In particular, the development of gastric/duodenal ischemia apparently leads to DGE after DP-CAR. Therefore, the LGA should be preserved if it is anatomically and oncologically feasible. The LGA preservation can

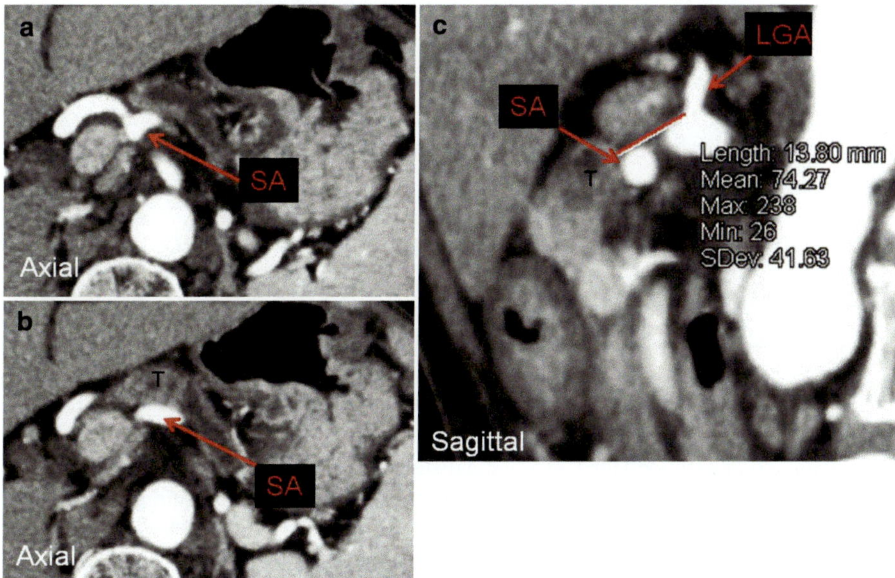

Fig. 14.9 Patients with tumors situated more than 10 mm away from the antecedent branching left gastric artery underwent distal pancreatectomy with resection of the common hepatic artery and splenic artery, with preservation of the left gastric artery (modified DP-CAR); (**a**) an axial image shows the root of the splenic artery; (**b**) an axial image revealed the tumor abuts to the splenic artery; (**c**) a sagittal image demonstrated the distance between the tumor and the left gastric artery was 13.8 mm. *SA* splenic artery; *LGA* left gastric artery (Reprinted from [1])

Table 14.3 Reprinted from [48]

Factor	Univariate analysis			Multivariate analysis		
	DGE(−) (n = 23)	DGE(+) (n = 14)	*p*-Value	OR	95% CI	*P*-Value
Tumor size >4 cm	9	8	0.328			
NAC(R)T	8	7	0.493			
LGA resection	10	13	0.004	10.071	1.035–98.011	0.047
Portal vein resection	3	5	0.215			
Operative time > 360 min	8	9	0.101			
EBL >700 ml	8	9	0.101			
Residual tumor (R1)	6	10	0.015	3.702	0.666–20.579	0.135
Pancreatic fistula (Grade B, C)	2	6	0.035	3.975	0.456	0.211
Ischemic gastroduodenal complication	0	2	0.137			

DGE delayed gastric emptying, *OR* odds ratio, *NAC(R)T* neoadjuvant chemo (radiation) therapy, *LGA* left gastric artery, *EBL* estimated blood loss

reduce the ischemic gastropathy after DP-CAR, and this approach (preservation of the LGA when feasible) provides another option for surgeons in performing DP-CAR. Furthermore, patients whose collateral flow had been injured or proved to be insufficient during the surgery, arterial reconstruction by saphenous vein or middle colic artery-gastroepiploic artery bypass would compromise the collateral flow [50].

14.5.2 Surgical Technique Preserving Left Gastric Artery

Apart from the intention to preserve the left gastric artery preoperatively, the right gastroepiploic and right gastric arteries/veins are also encircled by vessel tape for preservation. We rule out cancer cell infiltration into the periarterial nerve plexuses around GDA or CHA as soon as possible to evaluate resectability. We check the pulsation of GDA and PHA before clamping. After clamping the CHA, we reconfirm the pulsation, and subsequently ligated and divided the CHA at the distal part described earlier. We encircled the left gastric artery by vessel tape for preservation in the early phase of surgery as a destination of dissection. Lifting the distal pancreas and the CHA by en bloc dissecting of lymph nodes with arteries around the CHA, the origin of the celiac axis is exposed, and the celiac axis is encircled (Fig. 14.10). After confirming that the patients have negative cancer cell infiltration into the nerve plexus surrounding the LGA by an intraoperative histopathological diagnosis of several frozen sections (Fig. 14.11), the celiac artery was divided just after the branching of the LGA (Fig. 14.12). The resection and reconstruction of the portal vein is performed antecedently before the radical antegrade modular pancreatosplenectomy procedure. The depth of dissecting layer of retroperitoneum was controlled with wide margin according to the tumor position. Figure 14.13 shows the surgical field after modified DP-CAR.

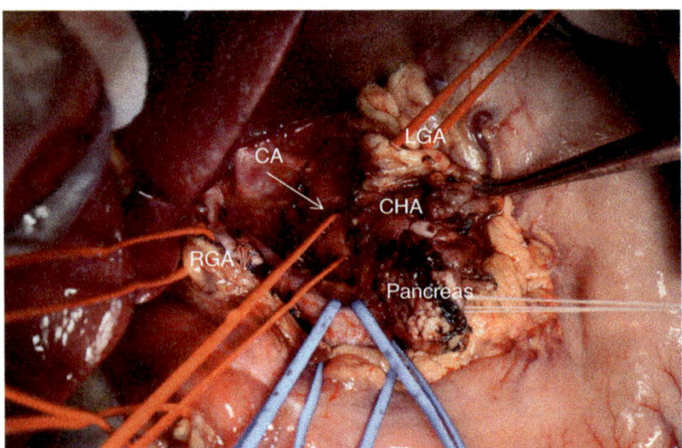

Fig. 14.10 Lifting up the distal pancreas and the common hepatic artery by en bloc dissecting of lymph nodes with arteries, the origin of the celiac axis was exposed, and encircled. *CA* celiac axis, *RGA* right gastric artery, *CHA* common hepatic artery, *LGA* left gastric artery (Reprinted from [1])

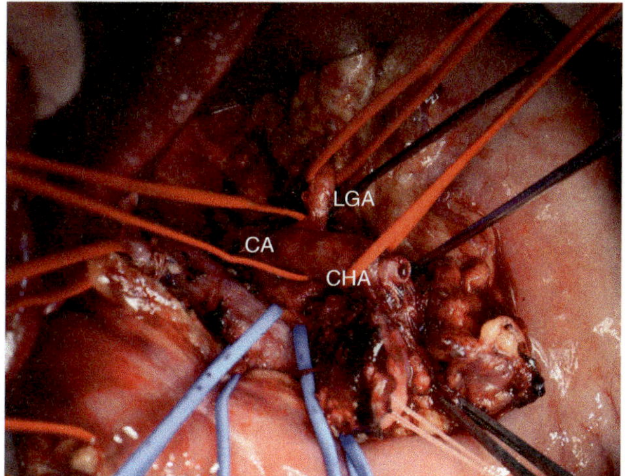

Fig. 14.11 Several frozen sections were harvested to confirm that the patients were negative for cancer cell infiltration into the nerve plexus surrounding the left gastric artery by an intraoperative histopathological examination. *CA* celiac axis, *CHA* common hepatic artery, *LGA* left gastric artery (Reprinted from [1])

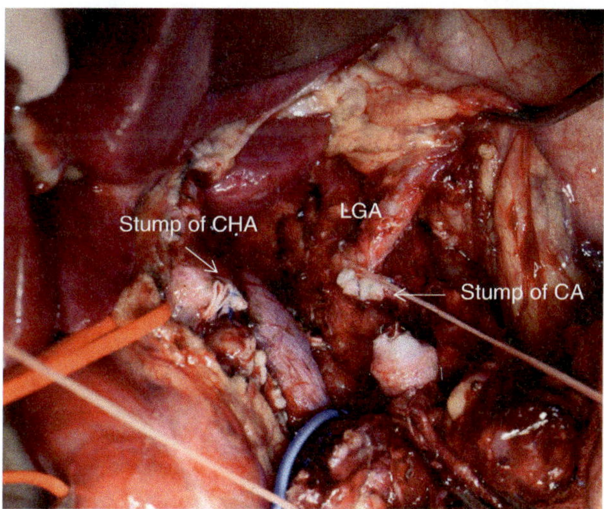

Fig. 14.12 The celiac artery was divided just after the branching of the left gastric artery. *CA* celiac axis, *RGA* right gastric artery, *CHA* common hepatic artery, *LGA* left gastric artery (Reprinted from [1])

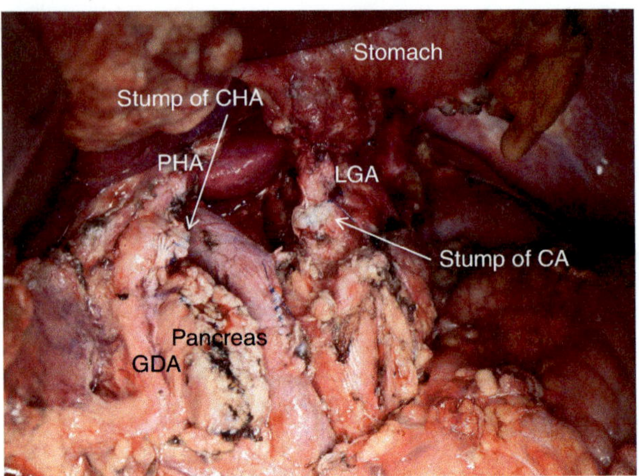

Fig. 14.13 The surgical field after modified DP-CAR. *CA* celiac axis, *RGA* right gastric artery, *CHA* common hepatic artery, *LGA* left gastric artery, *PHA* proper hepatic artery, *GDA* gastroduodenal artery (Reprinted from [1])

14.6 Postoperative Issues

14.6.1 Survivals After DP-CAR

A few long-term survivors were reported in previous small-number studies. Table 14.2 also shows the survivals after this procedure reported in recent literatures. The (estimated) median survival time was 9–42 months after the procedure. Several investigators have reported better survival in patients who underwent DP-CAR compared to those with R2/M1 resection or those who underwent surgery. The value of modified Appleby operation in pancreatic body/tail carcinoma is now convincing, especially in the first and second years after surgery. In our series, there were no differences in survival between patients who underwent standard DP and DP-CAR between 2005 and 2010. Fifty-two consecutive patients underwent distal pancreatectomy with D2 node dissection, including 36 standard DP and 16 DP-CAR, for pancreatic body/tail carcinoma [31]. Neoadjuvant chemotherapy based on the metastatic pancreatic carcinoma and early recovery to the adjuvant surgery after this procedure are indicators to improve the survival time.

14.6.2 DP-CAR as an Adjuvant Surgery

Adjuvant surgery for patients with initially unresectable pancreatic cancer has a major role to play with the improvement of chemotherapy [51]. Chemotherapy may occasionally reduce the size of a pancreatic body/tail carcinoma (that initially abuts to celiac axis and aorta) enough to be resected by surgery. Satoi et al. reported ten cases (17%) of DP-CAR as adjuvant surgery in 58 initially unresectable pancreatic cancer patients including 41 locally advanced and 17 metastatic who underwent adjuvant surgery with a favorable response to non-surgical anti-cancer treatments over 6 months. They concluded that adjuvant surgery for initially unresectable pancreatic cancer patients including DP-CAR can be a safe and effective treatment. Recent advancement of chemotherapy will be all the more effective in allowing more patients to be downstaged and develop a surgical opportunity in patients with initially unresectable pancreatic cancer [52–54].

14.7 Specimen

14.7.1 Specimen of DP-CAR

In our study, the histopathologic examination revealed positive margins for tumor infiltration in ten patients (63%) [31]. Microscopically positive margins were frequently identified in two dissected sites. The surface in front of the aorta at the root of the celiac axis in the periarterial nerve plexuses was found in four patients. The retropancreatic tissue around the periarterial nerve plexuses of the celiac artery was found in six patients. These positive margins were situated at the posterior surface of the resected specimens (Fig. 14.14) [55]. These areas should be carefully noted for in the histopathological examination. They could also be the potential targets to focus on for non-surgical anti-cancer treatment for locally advanced/borderline resectable pancreatic cancer. The arterial wall invasion is also investigated precisely. The findings around major arteries which were

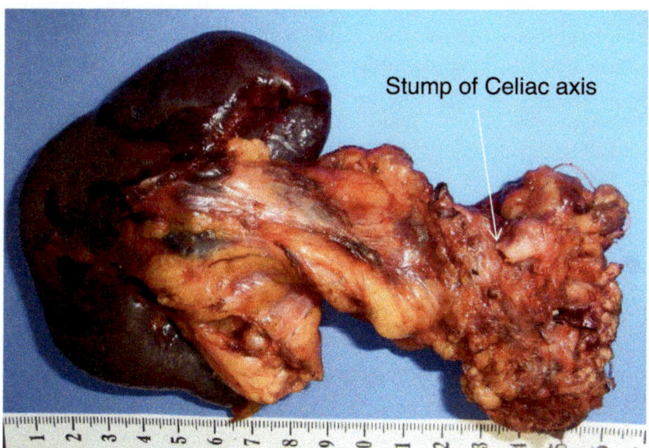

Fig. 14.14 The posterior side of resected specimen of modified DP-CAR. The bifurcations of the splenic artery and common hepatic artery were not exposed at the dissection surface (Reprinted from [1])

diagnosed as abutment or encasement in preoperative imaging studies should be supported by histopathological examination in regard to the presence of cancer cells or other desmoplastic reaction to improve the preoperative strategy for pancreatic carcinoma.

Conclusion

In 2015, the description of pancreatic body/tail carcinoma was added to the borderline resectable category in the National Comprehensive Cancer Network Guidelines. Because most pancreatic carcinomas recur systemically, and tumor involving arterial structures recur rapidly even after the complete resection [31]. One should consider whether the presence of just an R0 resection should be the primary issue of cure in borderline resectable pancreatic carcinoma. The modified Appleby operation (DP-CAR) is feasible and safe compared with standard DP if it is performed in the selected institutions where well-trained and skillful staff are available. This procedure with artery en bloc resection may be justifiable in selected patients owing to the potential survival benefit compared with patients without resection, and these patients should be treated in multimodal therapy. Recent additional modification of DP-CAR can lead the procedure to be a significantly safer modality [1].

References

1. Okada K, Yamaue H. The role of the appleby operation and arterial resection in the multimodality management of borderline resectable pancreatic cancer. In: Katz MH, Ahmad SA, editors. Multimodality management of borderline resectable pancreatic cancer. Springer US; 2016. p. 247–264.
2. Hirano S, Kondo S, Hara T, et al. Distal pancreatectomy with en bloc celiac axis resection for locally advanced pancreatic body cancer: long-term results. Ann Surg. 2007;246:46–51.
3. Wu YL, Yan HC, Chen LR, et al. Extended Appleby's operation for pancreatic cancer involving celiac axis. J Surg Oncol. 2007;96:442–6.
4. Fortner JG. Regional resection of cancer of the pancreas: a new surgical approach. Surgery. 1973;73:307–20.
5. Fortner JG, Kim DK, Cubilla A, et al. Regional pancreatectomy: en bloc pancreatic, portal vein and lymph node resection. Ann Surg. 1977;186:42–50.
6. Appleby LH. The coeliac axis in the expansion of the operation for gastric carcinoma. Cancer. 1953;6:704–7.
7. Appleby LH. Removal of the celiac axis in gastrectomy for carcinoma of the stomach in selected cases: a ten-year assessment. J Int Coll Surg. 1960;34:143–7.
8. Nimura Y, Hattori T, Miura K, et al. Experience of Appleby's operation for advanced carcinoma of the pancreatic body and tail (in Japanese). Shujutsu. 1976;30:885–9.
9. Hishinuma S, Ogata Y, Matsui J, et al. Two cases of cancer of the pancreatic body undergoing gastric preservation with distal pancreatectomy combined with resection of the celiac axis. Jpn J Gastroenterol Surg. 1991;24:2782–6. (in Japanese with English abstract)
10. Konishi M, Kinoshita T, Nakagori T, et al. Distal pancreatectomy with resection of the celiac axis and reconstruction of the hepatic artery for carcinoma of the body and tail of the pancreas. J Hepato-Biliary-Pancreat Surg. 2000;7:183–7.

11. Kondo S, Katoh H, Hirano S, et al. Results of radical distal pancreatectomy with en bloc resection of the celiac artery for locally advanced cancer of the pancreatic body. Langenbeck's Arch Surg. 2003;388:101–6.

12. Hishinuma S, Ogata Y, Tomikawa M, et al. Stomach-preserving distal pancreatectomy with combined resection of the celiac artery: radical procedure for locally advanced cancer of the pancreatic body. J Gastrointest Surg. 2007;11:743–9.

13. Wu X, Tao R, Lei R, et al. Distal pancreatectomy combined with celiac axis resection in treatment of carcinoma of the body/tail of the pancreas: a single-center experience. Ann Surg Oncol. 2010;17:1359–66.

14. Takahashi Y, Kaneoka Y, Maeda A, et al. Distal pancreatectomy with celiac axis resection for carcinoma of the body and tail of the pancreas. World J Surg. 2011;35:2535–42.

15. Yamamoto Y, Sakamoto Y, Ban D, et al. Is celiac axis resection justified for T4 pancreatic body cancer? Surgery. 2012;151:61–9.

16. Evans DB, Rich TA, Byrd DR, et al. Preoperative chemoradiation and pancreaticoduodenectomy for adenocarcinoma of the pancreas. Arch Surg. 1992;127:1335–9.

17. Varadhachary GR, Tamm EP, Abbruzzese JL, et al. Borderline resectable pancreatic cancer: definitions, management, and role of preoperative therapy. Ann Surg Oncol. 2006;13:1035–46.

18. Katz MH, Pisters PW, Evans DB, et al. Borderline resectable pancreatic cancer: the importance of this emerging stage of disease. J Am Coll Surg. 2008;206:833–46.

19. Callery MP, Chang KJ, Fishman EK, et al. Pretreatment assessment of resectable and borderline resectable pancreatic cancer: expert consensus statement. Ann Surg Oncol. 2009;16:1727–33.

20. Katz MH, Wang H, Fleming JB, et al. Long-term survival after multidisciplinary management of resected pancreatic adenocarcinoma. Ann Surg Oncol. 2009;16:836–47.

21. Evans DB, Farnell MB, Lillemoe KD, et al. Surgical treatment of resectable and borderline resectable pancreas cancer: expert consensus statement. Ann Surg Oncol. 2009;16:1736–44.

22. Evans DB, Erickson BA, Ritch P. Borderline resectable pancreatic cancer: definitions and the importance of multimodality therapy. Ann Surg Oncol. 2010;17:2803–5.

23. Walters DM, Lapar DJ, de Lange EE, et al. Pancreas-protocol imaging at a high-volume center leads to improved preoperative staging of pancreatic ductal adenocarcinoma. Ann Surg Oncol. 2011;18:2764–71.

24. Schwarz L, Lupinacci RM, Svrcek M, et al. Para-aortic lymph node sampling in pancreatic head adenocarcinoma. Br J Surg. 2014;101:530–8.

25. Tol JA, Gouma DJ, Bassi C, et al. Definition of a standard lymphadenectomy in surgery for pancreatic ductal adenocarcinoma: a consensus statement by the international study group on pancreatic surgery (ISGPS). Surgery. 2014;156:591–600.

26. Eaton PB. The coeliac axis. Anat Rec. 1917;13:369–74.

27. Malnar D, Klasan GS, Miletić D, et al. Properties of the celiac trunk—anatomical study. Coll Anthropol. 2010;34:917–21.

28. Vandamme JP, Bonte J. The branches of the celiac trunk. Acta Anat. 1985;122:110–4.

29. Cavdar S, Gürbüz J, Zeybek A, et al. A variation of coeliac trunk. Kaibogaku Zasshi. 1998;73:505–8.

30. Hiatt JR, Gabbay J, Busuttil RW. Surgical anatomy of the hepatic arteries in 1000 cases. Ann Surg. 1994;220:50–2.

31. Okada K, Kawai M, Tani M, et al. Surgical strategy for patients with pancreatic body/tail carcinoma: who should undergo distal pancreatectomy with en-bloc celiac axis resection? Surgery. 2013;153:365–72.

32. Kanda M, Fujii T, Sahin TT, et al. Invasion of the splenic artery is a crucial prognostic factor in carcinoma of the body and tail of the pancreas. Ann Surg. 2010;251:483–7.

33. Mollberg N, Rahbari NN, Koch M, et al. Arterial resection during pancreatectomy for pancreatic cancer: a systematic review and meta-analysis. Ann Surg. 2011;254:882–93.

34. Stitzenberg KB, Watson JC, Roberts A, et al. Survival after pancreatectomy with major arterial resection and reconstruction. Ann Surg Oncol. 2008;15:1399–406.

35. Bockhorn M, Burdelski C, Bogoevski D, et al. Arterial en bloc resection for pancreatic carcinoma. Br J Surg. 2011;98:86–92.

36. Christians KK, Pilgrim CH, Tsai S, et al. Arterial resection at the time of pancreatectomy for cancer. Surgery. 2014;155:919–26.

37. Ozaki H, Kinoshita T, Kosuge T, et al. An aggressive therapeutic approach to carcinoma of the body and tail of the pancreas. Cancer. 1996;77:2240–5.

38. Mayumi T, Nimura Y, Kamiya J, et al. Distal pancreatectomy with en bloc resection of the celiac artery for carcinoma of the body and tail of the pancreas. Int J Pancreatol. 1997;22:15–21.

39. Bachellier P, Rosso E, Lucescu I, et al. Is the need for an arterial resection a contraindication to pancreatic resection for locally advanced pancreatic adenocarcinoma? A case-matched controlled study. J Surg Oncol. 2011;103:75–84.

40. Hirano S, Kondo S, Tanaka E, et al. Postoperative bowel function and nutritional status following distal pancreatectomy with en-bloc celiac axis resection. Dig Surg. 2010;27:212–6.

41. Kondo S, Katoh H, Shimizu T, et al. Preoperative embolization of the common hepatic artery in preparation for radical pancreatectomy for pancreas body cancer. Hepatogastroenterology. 2000;47:1447–9.

42. Abo D, Hasegawa Y, Sakuhara Y, et al. Feasibility of a dual microcatheter-dual interlocking detachable coil technique in preoperative embolization in preparation for distal pancreatectomy with en bloc celiac axis resection for locally advanced pancreatic body cancer. J Hepatobiliary Pancreat Sci. 2012;19:431–7.

43. Strasberg SM, Linehan DC, Hawkins WG. Radical antegrade modular pancreatosplenectomy procedure for adenocarcinoma of the body and tail of the pancreas: ability to obtain negative tangential margins. J Am Coll Surg. 2007;204:244–9.

44. Okada K, Kawai M, Tani M, et al. Isolated Roux-en-Y anastomosis of the pancreatic stump in a duct-to-mucosa fashion in patients with distal pancreatectomy with en-bloc celiac axis resection. J Hepatobiliary Pancreat Sci. 2014;21:193–8.

45. Kawai M, Tani M, Okada K, et al. Stump closure of a thick pancreas using stapler closure increases pancreatic fistula after distal pancreatectomy. Am J Surg. 2013;206:352–9.

46. Bassi C, Dervenis C, Butturini G, et al. International study group on pancreatic fistula definition. Postoperative pancreatic fistula: an international study group (ISGPF) definition. Surgery. 2005;138:8–13.

47. Wente MN, Bassi C, Dervenis C, et al. Delayed gastric emptying (DGE) after pancreatic surgery: a suggested definition by the international study group of pancreatic surgery (ISGPS). Surgery. 2007;142:761–8.

48. Okada K, Kawai M, Tani M, et al. Preservation of the left gastric artery on the basis of anatomical features in patients undergoing distal pancreatectomy with celiac axis en-bloc resection (DP-CAR). World J Surg. 2014;38:2980–5.

49. Takahashi H, Nara S, Ohigashi H, et al. Is preservation of the remnant stomach safe during distal pancreatectomy in patients who have undergone distal gastrectomy? World J Surg. 2013;37:430–6.

50. Kondo S, Ambo Y, Katoh H, et al. Middle colic artery-gastroepiploic artery bypass for compromised collateral flow in distal pancreatectomy with celiac artery resection. Hepato-Gastroenterology. 2003;50:305–7.

51. Satoi S, Yamaue H, Kato K, et al. Role of adjuvant surgery for patients with initially unresectable pancreatic cancer with a long-term favorable response to non-surgical anti-cancer treatments: results of a project study for pancreatic surgery by the Japanese society of hepato-biliary-pancreatic surgery. J Hepatobiliary Pancreat Sci. 2013;20:590–600.

52. Conroy T, Desseigne F, Ychou M, et al. FOLFIRINOX versus gemcitabine for metastatic pancreatic cancer. N Engl J Med. 2011;364:1817–25.

53. Von Hoff DD, Ervin T, Arena FP, et al. Increased survival in pancreatic cancer with nab-paclitaxel plus gemcitabine. N Engl J Med. 2013;369:1691–703.
54. Boone BA, Steve J, Krasinskas AM, et al. Outcomes with FOLFIRINOX for borderline resectable and locally unresectable pancreatic cancer. J Surg Oncol. 2013;108:236–41.
55. Konstantinidis IT, Warshaw AL, Allen JN, et al. Pancreatic ductal adenocarcinoma: is there a survival difference for R1 resections versus locally advanced unresectable tumors? What is a "true" R0 resection? Ann Surg. 2013;257:731–6.

Laparoscopic Distal Pancreatectomy for Pancreatic Cancer

15

Chang Moo Kang

15.1 Rationale of Laparoscopic Distal Pancreatectomy for Pancreatic Cancer

With the advance in laparoscopic techniques, laparoscopic distal pancreatectomy (LDP) has proven to be safe and effective through multiple clinical trials. Now, LDP is regarded as a standard approach in treating benign and low-grade, malignant, pancreatic lesions. Unlike other fields of gastrointestinal surgery, clinical efforts to use laparoscopic approaches to treat pancreatic cancer have only recently begun, and it still remains controversial. However, there is a great deal of evidence showing that radical LDP is feasible and oncologically safe.

First, many studies reporting the perioperative outcomes of LDP suggest that LDP is safe and effective for treating pathologic conditions arising from the left-sided pancreas [1]. The evidence supporting this statement provides fundamental concepts that can be applied to LDP in treating pancreatic cancer. Second, after dissecting the pancreatic neck at the confluence of the superior mesenteric, splenic, and portal veins, the pancreas can be divided at the pancreatic neck [2, 3]. An extended or subtotal distal pancreatectomy is the maximum extent of resection for this procedure. Therefore, to ensure adequate resection margins, techniques for laparoscopic division of the pancreatic neck are necessary. Third, it has already been proven that laparoscopic perigastric lymph node dissection is feasible and safe in gastric cancer surgery [4, 5]. Therefore, laparoscopic radical gastrectomy has become one of the standard options for

C.M. Kang, M.D., Ph.D.
Division of Hepatobiliary and Pancreatic Surgery, Department of Surgery, Yonsei University College of Medicine, Seoul, South Korea

Pancreatobiliary Cancer Clinic, Yonsei Cancer Center, Severance Hospital, Seoul, South Korea
e-mail: cmkang@yuhs.ac

© Springer Science+Business Media Singapore 2017
H. Yamaue (ed.), *Innovation of Diagnosis and Treatment for Pancreatic Cancer*,
DOI 10.1007/978-981-10-2486-3_15

treating early gastric cancer. The topographical extent of regional lymph node dissection in pancreatic cancer may be similar to that of gastric cancer. The common practice of this technique in gastric cancer surgery can indirectly support the rationale for radical LDP. Fourth, until now, as a monotherapy, surgical resection with clear resection margins was thought to be the most effective treatment; however, postoperative chemotherapy is actively considered because early recurrence, especially to the liver, is very common in pancreatic cancer. Minimally invasive surgery can enhance postoperative recovery and reduce surgical stress [6, 7]. Theoretically, LDP can allow for earlier administration of postoperative chemotherapy, and it enhances the likelihood of completing the course of chemotherapy by reducing physical and immunological impairment in the perioperative period. Fifth, with the advances in axial imaging technology, increasing concerns about personal health care, a greater number of routine medical check-ups, the incidence of localized pancreatic cancer may increase. This form of pancreatic cancer would be more appropriately treated with minimally invasive pancreatectomy.

Based on these rationales, LDP can be an option for treating left-sided pancreatic cancer in well-selected patients. Due to the controversy surrounding LDP, we need to evaluate the technical feasibility and the clinical outcomes of this procedure in treating left-sided pancreatic cancer.

15.2 Oncologic Concept of Laparoscopic Distal Pancreatectomy for Pancreatic Cancer

Local control should be a priority in radical surgery. Resection margins and lymph node clearance are important aspects that surgeons need to consider when performing radical surgery to treat cancers. These two surgical components are possibly influenced by the surgeon's techniques. In addition, the long-term oncologic outcomes of radical surgery are significantly associated with these two factors [8–11].

The oncologic concept of radical LDP in treating pancreatic cancer should be the same as open surgery. The pancreas is a retroperitoneal organ, and therefore, there are two resection margins to be considered in radical distal pancreatectomy. One is based on the "horizontal" concept, which states that the pancreatic resection margin should have enough normal pancreatic parenchyma bordering the pancreatic cancer. Another is based on the "vertical" concept, which has been newly developed as a result of surgical detachment of the pancreas from the retroperitoneum (posterior margin, or tangential margin).

In theory, during distal pancreatectomy, if surgeons mobilize or grasp the tumor before controlling the surrounding splenic artery and vein, this may increase the risk of squeezing and shedding the cancer cells into the splenic vein and peritoneal cavity [12, 13]. The "no touch isolation technique" was originally proposed as a strategy to protect against cancer cell spreading related to handling malignant tumors during both colon and eye cancer surgery [14, 15].

When performing a conventional distal pancreatectomy (left-to-right dissection), it is hard to adhere to the no touch isolation technique because isolation and division of the splenic artery and vein is performed at the last stage of the procedure. In addition, due to a lack of anatomic landmarks, it might be difficult to secure posterior (tangential) margin clearance. Therefore, radical antegrade modular distal pancreatosplenectomy (RAMPS) was developed as an oncologically sound approach for treating left-sided pancreatic cancer [16, 17]. All involved regional lymph nodes are supposed to be included in surgical specimens because the surgical procedure is based on en bloc resection of the left-sided pancreas and surrounding peripancreatic soft tissue. There are no randomized control studies investigating which surgical approach is better for treating left-sided pancreatic cancer. Some literature suggests that RAMPS is superior to the conventional technique. On the other hand, several reports showed similar survival outcomes between the conventional technique and RAMPS [18, 19].

15.3 Indications and Surgical Technique

As long as there is no clinical evidence suggesting distant metastasis, peritoneal seeding, or major vascular involvement, for example, invasion to superior mesenteric artery, and celiac axis, LDP can be considered for radical surgery in treating resectable left-sided pancreatic cancer. However, in order to increase oncological safety and technical feasibility of margin-negative, bloodless resection [20], our group previously suggested that radical LDP should be limited to anterior RAMPS (Fig. 15.1). The Yonsei Criteria [21], which are determined by preoperative CT scan, have been developed to select eligible patients for radical LDP. The criteria include the following tumor conditions: (1) Tumor confined to the pancreas, (2) Intact fascial layer between the distal pancreas and the left adrenal gland and kidney, (3) Tumor located at least 1–2 cm away from the celiac axis. According to recent literature [22], minimally invasive radical distal pancreatectomy performed in patients who met the Yonsei Criteria showed quite favorable survival outcomes. This study revealed an overall disease-specific 5-year survival rate of 55.6%. In particular, patients without lymph node metastasis had an excellent 5-year survival rate of 77.8%, suggesting that this group may be categorized as having "practical" early pancreatic cancer. With the advance of surgical techniques, indications for radical LDP will extended based on surgeons' laparoscopic skills and patient tumor conditions.

In brief [23, 24], radical LDP is performed according to the following surgical process. Patients are placed in the supine position with their head [25] and left side elevated. After dividing the gastrocolic and gastrosplenic ligaments, the

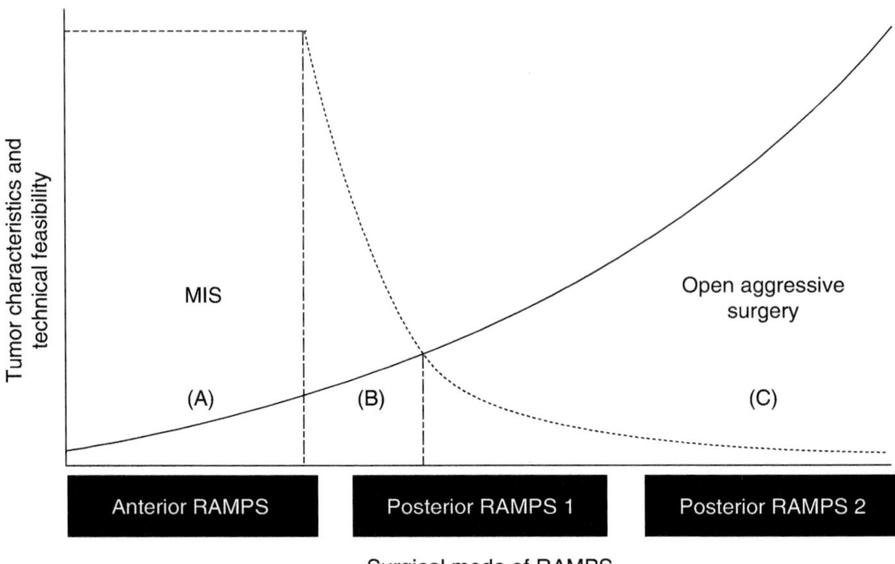

Fig. 15.1 Determining the extent of minimally invasive radical antegrade modular pancreato-splenectomy (RAMPS). The *dotted line* shows the technical feasibility of bloodless and margin-negative radical antegrade modular pancreatosplenectomy (RAMPS) using a minimally invasive approach. The *solid line* represents the biological aggressiveness of tumors according to the appropriate mode of RAMPS for margin-negative resection. Presently, minimally invasive anterior RAMPS is thought to be a generally accepted surgical method for bloodless and margin-negative resections. Oncologically safe posterior RAMPS 1 and 2 may be difficult to perform using a minimally invasive approach. Note the marginal zone of (B). Only a few expert laparoscopic surgeons can be fully responsible for this region. Future directions include widening the area of (B) by means of technical improvements (shifting the *dotted line* to the *left*) and by improving early tumor detection (attenuating the slope of the *solid line*). *MIS* minimally invasive surgery. Figure 15.1 is from Kang CM, minimally invasive radical pancreatectomy for left-sided pancreatic cancer: current status and future perspectives. World J Gastroenterol. Mar 7, 2014; 20(9): 2343–51 [21]

pancreas is exposed in its entirety. After careful dissection of the pancreatic neck, a complete window can be made via the avascular plane between the pancreatic neck and the superior mesenteric vein-portal vein-splenic vein (SMV-PV-SV) confluence. Using the endo-GIA, division of the pancreas at the level of the pancreatic neck is performed. The coronary vein is ligated and divided with the soft tissue around the left gastric artery. Dissection of the soft tissue around the common hepatic artery and the celiac trunk is then performed. The splenic artery is dissected and ligated at the origin of the celiac trunk, and the splenic vein is isolated and divided at the junction of the SV and SMV. Dissection of the pancreas is subsequently performed in a right-to-left fashion including the soft tissue around the celiac trunk and the splenic vessels (Fig. 15.2). After en bloc resection of the tissue, an endo-pouch is used for safe retrieval of the specimen through a small vertical umbilical wound.

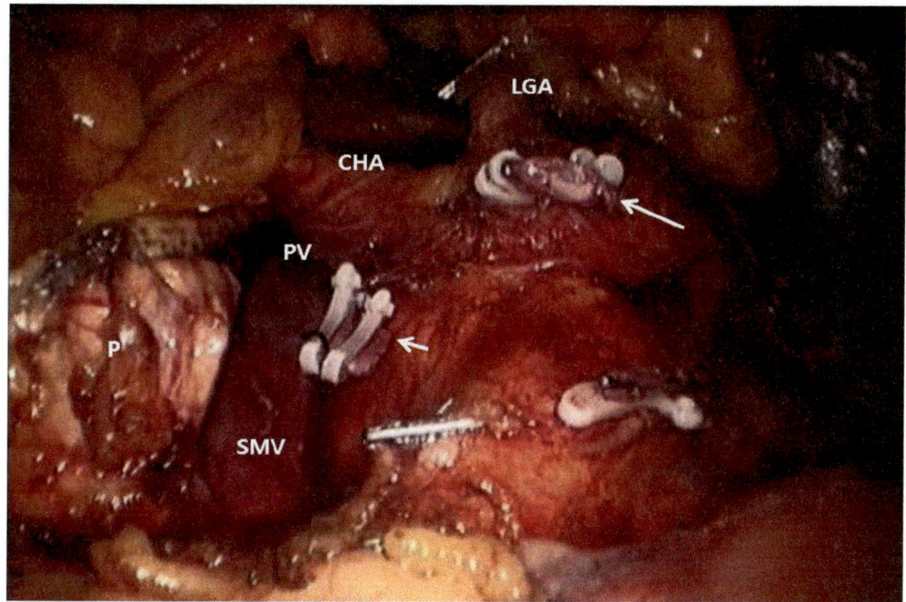

Fig. 15.2 Operation field after radical laparoscopic distal pancreatosplenectomy. Radical laparoscopic DPS is performed in patients meeting the Yonsei criteria. These tumors do not typically invade posteriorly (note that one of the tumor conditions is an intact fascial layer between the left adrenal gland, kidney, and left-sided pancreas). Retroperitoneal tissue is not always peeled off. *P* pancreas, *SMV* superior mesenteric vein, *PV* portal vein, *CHA* common hepatic artery, *LGA* left gastric artery, *short arrow* splenic vein control, *long arrow* splenic artery control [23].

15.4 Current Advanced Evidence

In the past, only a few case series reported the laparoscopic approach for treating left-sided pancreatic cancer. Most reported cases of pancreatic cancer (ductal adenocarcinoma) treated by LDP were incidentally included in those case series. As a result, it is difficult to fully assess the surgical quality of these procedures based on relevant oncologic concepts [25–31]. In addition, important perioperative oncologic short-term and long-term outcomes, such as pT stage, pN stage, number of retrieved lymph nodes, margin status, and survival outcomes were not documented, making it difficult to determine the feasibility of the laparoscopic approach for left-sided pancreatic cancer.

Based on the growing literature reporting short-term and long-term oncologic outcomes, there are several meta-analyses and review articles that show the feasibility of minimally invasive left-sided pancreatic cancer. Table 15.1 summarizes recent publications with perioperative short-term and long-term outcomes of laparoscopically resected left-sided pancreatic cancer. Some observational reports [33] assessing nationwide observational analyses are limited in detailing short-term oncologic outcomes. Although no randomized control study comparing open and laparoscopic radical DP is currently available, these data are enough to suggest that radical LDP is feasible and safe with acceptable long-term survival in well-selected patients.

Table 15.1 Recent publications reporting short-term and long-term oncologic outcomes of radical laparoscopic distal pancreatosplenectomy

Authors	N	Operation time, min	EBL, Ml	Retrieved LNs	R0, %	Mortality, %	Oncologic outcome
Sahakyan [32][a]	191	220 (66)	250 (0–3040)	10 (0–48)	83.8	0	31.3 months 30%
Sulpice [33][b]	347	NA	NA	NA	NA	1.2 2.6	62.5 months 50.6%
Rooij [34][c]	141	194 (150–270)	800 (495–1618)	9 (4–14)	50	3 6	17 months 22%
Kawaguchi [35]	23	203 (54)	208 (264)	19.8 (9.3)	100	0	10 months 33%
Shin [36]	70	NA	NA	12 (1–34)	75.7	0	33.4 months 32.5%
Lee [22]	12	324.3 (154.2)	445.8 (346.1)	10.5 (7.1)	100	0	39 months 55.9%
Rehman [37]	8	376 (300–534)	306 (250–535)	14 (0–26)	88	1.2	33 months
Mitchem [38]	37	243.6 (93.5)	744.3 (570.4)	18.0 (11.7)	81	0	25.9 months 30.4%

Continuous values were described as the mean (standard deviation) or median (range). Mortality includes 30-day mortality and 90-day mortality. Oncologic outcome includes median survival time in months and 5-year survival %
[a]International multicenter trial
[b]French national observation study
[c]Dutch national observation study

15.5 Special Considerations

15.5.1 Spleen Preservation

When pancreatic cancer directly invades the spleen or spleen hilum, a concomitant splenectomy should be performed for a margin-negative resection. This allows for the potential clearance of regional lymph node metastasis around splenic hilar area when the cancer is located near the body of the pancreas [16, 17]. Then, the following questions become relevant: What do we know about the incidence of splenic hilar lymph node metastasis in left-sided pancreatic cancer? What is the oncologic impact of splenic hilar lymph node metastasis?

It is quite interesting to note that these questions were not seriously studied in the past. Only a few reports evaluated lymph node metastasis in resected left-sided pancreatic cancer. According to previously published literature [39, 40], splenic hilar lymph node metastasis was reported in 0–3.3% of resected left-sided pancreatic cancers, and there is little concern about the oncologic impact of splenic hilar lymph node metastasis in resected left-sided pancreatic cancer. Recently, a joint

Korean and Japanese multicenter trial [41] evaluated the incidence of splenic hilar lymph node metastasis in resected left-sided pancreatic cancer, which was found to be 4.4%. It was also found that a small tumor size (<3 cm), proximal (neck/body) location, and no combined organ resection are predictive of no splenic hilar lymph node metastasis.

So far, there are two distal pancreatectomy techniques that allow for the spleen to be preserved. One is a splenic vessels-conserving technique [42], and another one is a splenic vessels-sacrificing approach, or the Warshaw's procedure [43]. From the oncologic point of view, the splenic vessel-conserving technique is not appropriate for treating left-sided pancreatic cancer because lymph nodes surrounding the splenic vessels (No. 11) are the most frequent sites for lymph node metastasis, and pancreatic cancer frequently shows direct invasion to these vessels. Therefore, considering that the risk of splenic hilar lymph node metastasis is very low in left-side pancreatic cancer, modification of the splenic vessel-sacrificing technique for spleen-preserving LDP can lead to performing a radical pancreatectomy. This procedure involves removing the cancer and splenic hilar lymph node group using RAMPS while leaving the spleen intact.

In addition, the minimally invasive extended Warshaw procedure has been reported to be technically feasible [2, 3]. In fact, recent literature [44] demonstrated the oncologic reliability of spleen-preserving radical distal pancreatectomy for pancreatic cancer. They applied the Warshaw technique for radical pancreatectomy and reported 17 cases of spleen-preserving LDP. The average tumor size was 32±12 mm, and the average number of retrieved lymph nodes was 19.8±9.3. All resectional margin were found to be negative. Survival rates of the patients after 1, 3, and 5 years were 64.7, 52.9, and 41.2%, respectively, with similar outcomes observed in spleen-resecting LDP and open distal pancreatectomy (ODP) surgeries. No splenic hilar lymph node metastasis was reported. The role of spleen preservation as a postoperative adjuvant strategy for resected left-sided pancreatic cancer remains to be investigated [45–50].

15.5.2 Combined Vascular Resection

In the case of pancreatic cancer invading the celiac axis and superior mesenteric vein-splenic vein-portal vein confluence, radical DPS combined with celiac axis excision and venous vascular resection can result in favorable outcomes in select patient groups [51–53]. It is also reported that the laparoscopic approach is also feasible in this kind of aggressive surgery, but only a few studies are currently available [54, 55]. Although the minimally invasive approach is technically feasible, the surgical technique is quite demanding. Only a few expert surgeons are able to execute this approach. Aggressive tumor biology and technical difficulty beg the question of oncologic efficacy and practical feasibility of minimally invasive surgery in this specific case (Fig. 15.1). Minimally invasive combined arterial or venous vascular resection in treating left-sided pancreatic cancer may not be generalized.

15.5.3 Prospective Randomized Controlled Trial

In order to lay the foundation for an evidence-based surgical approach, a randomized controlled trial (RCT) should be performed to test the reliability of laparoscopic radical DPS for treating left-sided pancreatic cancer. However, it is very difficult to organize a successful trial. There are not many surgeons capable of performing laparoscopic radical DPS, and the incidence of resectable pancreatic cancer that is potentially manageable by both laparoscopy and open radical DPS will be very low [38]. Considering that margin-negative resection is critical in treating pancreatic cancer, it may not be possible to randomize all resectable left-sided pancreatic cancers because some cases should be treated with open surgery due to the technical difficulty of obtaining a margin-negative resection. Therefore, in order to have a successful RCT for treating left-sided pancreatic cancer, a multicenter collaboration allow for a greater number of patients to be enrolled. In addition, among the patients with resectable pancreatic cancer, clinical subgroup needs to be defined in whom both laparoscopic and open radical DPS can easily produce margin-negative resection. Randomization should be done in those specific patients group. Surgical technique and postoperative management should also be standardized to minimize bias.

Alternatively, propensity score matching (PSM) is a statistical matching technique that minimizes selection bias and mimics randomization [56, 57]. Radical LDP remains controversial, and its clinical application to left-sided pancreatic cancer should be carefully considered based on the surgeons' technique and oncologic philosophy, as margin-negative resection is critical for patient outcomes. As shown in Table 15.1, the number of the cases of radical LDP used to treating left-sided pancreatic cancer is increasing. To avoid ethical and scientific problems related to RCT in treating left-sided pancreatic cancer, a multicenter retrospective case collection with PSM analysis will be currently available potential strategies to validate the oncologic role of radical LDP [58–61].

References

1. Postlewait LM, Kooby DA. Laparoscopic distal pancreatectomy for adenocarcinoma: safe and reasonable? J Gastrointest Oncol. 2015;6(4):406–17. doi:10.3978/j.issn.2078-6891.2015.034.
2. Choi SH, Kang CM, Kim JY, Hwang HK, Lee WJ. Laparoscopic extended (subtotal) distal pancreatectomy with resection of both splenic artery and vein. Surg Endosc. 2013;27(4):1412–3. doi:10.1007/s00464-012-2605-9.
3. Kang CM, Choi SH, Hwang HK, Kim DH, Yoon CI, Lee WJ. Laparoscopic distal pancreatectomy with division of the pancreatic neck for benign and borderline malignant tumor in the proximal body of the pancreas. J Laparoendosc Adv Surg Tech A. 2010;20(7):581–6. doi:10.1089/lap.2009.0348.
4. Hayashi H, Ochiai T, Shimada H, Gunji Y. Prospective randomized study of open versus laparoscopy-assisted distal gastrectomy with extraperigastric lymph node dissection for early gastric cancer. Surg Endosc. 2005;19(9):1172–6. doi:10.1007/s00464-004-8207-4.
5. Cai J, Wei D, Gao CF, Zhang CS, Zhang H, Zhao T. A prospective randomized study comparing open versus laparoscopy-assisted D2 radical gastrectomy in advanced gastric cancer. Dig Surg. 2011;28(5-6):331–7. doi:10.1159/000330782.

6. Okholm C, Goetze JP, Svendsen LB, Achiam MP. Inflammatory response in laparoscopic vs. open surgery for gastric cancer. Scand J Gastroenterol. 2014;49(9):1027–34. doi:10.3109/003 65521.2014.917698.

7. Carter JJ, Whelan RL. The immunologic consequences of laparoscopy in oncology. Surg Oncol Clin N Am. 2001;10(3):655–77.

8. Leng KM, Wang ZD, Zhao JB, Cui YF, Zhong XY. Impact of pancreatic margin status and lymph node metastases on recurrence after resection for invasive and noninvasive intraductal papillary mucinous neoplasms of the pancreas: a meta-analysis. Dig Surg. 2012;29(3):213–25. doi:10.1159/000339334.

9. Tol JA, Eshuis WJ, Besselink MG, van Gulik TM, Busch OR, Gouma DJ. Non-radical resection versus bypass procedure for pancreatic cancer—a consecutive series and systematic review. Eur J Surg Oncol. 2015;41(2):220–7. doi:10.1016/j.ejso.2014.11.041.

10. Liu L, Katz MH, Lee SM, Fischer LK, Prakash L, Parker N, et al. Superior mesenteric artery margin of posttherapy pancreaticoduodenectomy and prognosis in patients with pancreatic ductal adenocarcinoma. Am J Surg Pathol. 2015;39(10):1395–403. doi:10.1097/pas.0000000000000491.

11. La Torre M, Nigri G, Petrucciani N, Cavallini M, Aurello P, Cosenza G, et al. Prognostic assessment of different lymph node staging methods for pancreatic cancer with R0 resection: pN staging, lymph node ratio, log odds of positive lymph nodes. Pancreatology. 2014;14(4):289–94. doi:10.1016/j.pan.2014.05.794.

12. Kuroki T, Eguchi S. No-touch isolation techniques for pancreatic cancer. Surg Today. 2017;47(1):8–13. doi:10.1007/s00595-016-1317-5.

13. Hirota M, Shimada S, Yamamoto K, Tanaka E, Sugita H, Egami H, et al. Pancreatectomy using the no-touch isolation technique followed by extensive intraoperative peritoneal lavage to prevent cancer cell dissemination: a pilot study. JOP. 2005;6(2):143–51.

14. Barnes JP. Physiologic resection of the right colon. Surg Gynecol Obstet. 1952;94(6):722–6.

15. Turnbull Jr RB, Kyle K, Watson FR, Spratt J. Cancer of the colon: the influence of the no-touch isolation technic on survival rates. Ann Surg. 1967;166(3):420–7.

16. Strasberg SM, Drebin JA, Linehan D. Radical antegrade modular pancreatosplenectomy. Surgery. 2003;133(5):521–7. doi:10.1067/msy.2003.146.

17. Strasberg SM, Linehan DC, Hawkins WG. Radical antegrade modular pancreatosplenectomy procedure for adenocarcinoma of the body and tail of the pancreas: ability to obtain negative tangential margins. J Am Coll Surg. 2007;204(2):244–9. doi:10.1016/j.jamcollsurg.2006.11.002.

18. Park HJ, You DD, Choi DW, Heo JS, Choi SH. Role of radical antegrade modular pancreatosplenectomy for adenocarcinoma of the body and tail of the pancreas. World J Surg. 2014;38(1):186–93. doi:10.1007/s00268-013-2254-8.

19. Marangos IP, Buanes T, Rosok BI, Kazaryan AM, Rosseland AR, Grzyb K, et al. Laparoscopic resection of exocrine carcinoma in central and distal pancreas results in a high rate of radical resections and long postoperative survival. Surgery. 2012;151(5):717–23. doi:10.1016/j. surg.2011.12.016.

20. Kang CM, Kim DH, Lee WJ. Ten years of experience with resection of left-sided pancreatic ductal adenocarcinoma: evolution and initial experience to a laparoscopic approach. Surg Endosc. 2010;24(7):1533–41. doi:10.1007/s00464-009-0806-7.

21. Kang CM, Lee SH, Lee WJ. Minimally invasive radical pancreatectomy for left-sided pancreatic cancer: current status and future perspectives. World J Gastroenterol. 2014;20(9):2343–51. doi:10.3748/wjg.v20.i9.2343.

22. Lee SH, Kang CM, Hwang HK, Choi SH, Lee WJ, Chi HS. Minimally invasive RAMPS in well-selected left-sided pancreatic cancer within Yonsei criteria: long-term (>median 3 years) oncologic outcomes. Surg Endosc. 2014;28(10):2848–55. doi:10.1007/s00464-014-3537-3.

23. Choi SH, Kang CM, Lee WJ, Chi HS. Laparoscopic modified anterior RAMPS in well-selected left-sided pancreatic cancer: technical feasibility and interim results. Surg Endosc. 2011;25(7):2360–1. doi:10.1007/s00464-010-1556-2.

24. Choi SH, Kang CM, Hwang HK, Lee WJ, Chi HS. Robotic anterior RAMPS in well-selected left-sided pancreatic cancer. J Gastrointest Surg. 2012;16(4):868–9. doi:10.1007/s11605-012-1825-6.

25. Laxa BU, Carbonell 2nd AM, Cobb WS, Rosen MJ, Hardacre JM, Mekeel KL, et al. Laparoscopic and hand-assisted distal pancreatectomy. Am Surg. 2008;74(6):481–6. discussion 486–7

26. Lebedyev A, Zmora O, Kuriansky J, Rosin D, Khaikin M, Shabtai M, et al. Laparoscopic distal pancreatectomy. Surg Endosc. 2004;18(10):1427–30. doi:10.1007/s00464-003-8221-y.

27. Melotti G, Butturini G, Piccoli M, Casetti L, Bassi C, Mullineris B, et al. Laparoscopic distal pancreatectomy: results on a consecutive series of 58 patients. Ann Surg. 2007;246(1):77–82. doi:10.1097/01.sla.0000258607.17194.2b.

28. Taylor C, O'Rourke N, Nathanson L, Martin I, Hopkins G, Layani L, et al. Laparoscopic distal pancreatectomy: the Brisbane experience of forty-six cases. HPB (Oxford). 2008;10(1):38–42. doi:10.1080/13651820701802312.

29. Eom BW, Jang JY, Lee SE, Han HS, Yoon YS, Kim SW. Clinical outcomes compared between laparoscopic and open distal pancreatectomy. Surg Endosc. 2008;22(5):1334–8. doi:10.1007/s00464-007-9660-7.

30. Jayaraman S, Gonen M, Brennan MF, D'Angelica MI, DeMatteo RP, Fong Y, et al. Laparoscopic distal pancreatectomy: evolution of a technique at a single institution. J Am Coll Surg. 2010;211(4):503–9. doi:10.1016/j.jamcollsurg.2010.06.010.

31. Borja-Cacho D, Al-Refaie WB, Vickers SM, Tuttle TM, Jensen EH. Laparoscopic distal pancreatectomy. J Am Coll Surg. 2009;209(6):758–65. quiz 800 doi:10.1016/j.jamcollsurg.2009.08.021.

32. Sahakyan MA, Kazaryan AM, Rawashdeh M, Fuks D, Shmavonyan M, Haugvik SP, et al. Laparoscopic distal pancreatectomy for pancreatic ductal adenocarcinoma: results of a multicenter cohort study on 196 patients. Surg Endosc. 2016;30(8):3409–18. doi:10.1007/s00464-015-4623-x.

33. Sulpice L, Farges O, Goutte N, Bendersky N, Dokmak S, Sauvanet A, et al. Laparoscopic distal pancreatectomy for pancreatic ductal adenocarcinoma: time for a randomized controlled trial? Results of an all-inclusive national observational study. Ann Surg. 2015;262(5):868–73. discussion 73–4 doi:10.1097/SLA.0000000000001479.

34. de Rooij T, Tol JA, van Eijck CH, Boerma D, Bonsing BA, Bosscha K, et al. Outcomes of distal pancreatectomy for pancreatic ductal adenocarcinoma in the Netherlands: a nationwide retrospective analysis. Ann Surg Oncol. 2016;23(2):585–91. doi:10.1245/s10434-015-4930-4.

35. Kawaguchi Y, Fuks D, Nomi T, Levard H, Gayet B. Laparoscopic distal pancreatectomy employing radical en bloc procedure for adenocarcinoma: technical details and outcomes. Surgery. 2015;157(6):1106–12. doi:10.1016/j.surg.2014.12.015.

36. Shin SH, Kim SC, Song KB, Hwang DW, Lee JH, Lee D, et al. A comparative study of laparoscopic vs. open distal pancreatectomy for left-sided ductal adenocarcinoma: a propensity score-matched analysis. J Am Coll Surg. 2015;220(2):177–85. doi:10.1016/j.jamcollsurg.2014.10.014.

37. Rehman S, John SK, Lochan R, Jaques BC, Manas DM, Charnley RM, et al. Oncological feasibility of laparoscopic distal pancreatectomy for adenocarcinoma: a single-institution comparative study. World J Surg. 2014;38(2):476–83. doi:10.1007/s00268-013-2268-2.

38. Mitchem JB, Hamilton N, Gao F, Hawkins WG, Linehan DC, Strasberg SM. Long-term results of resection of adenocarcinoma of the body and tail of the pancreas using radical antegrade modular pancreatosplenectomy procedure. J Am Coll Surg. 2012;214(1):46–52. doi:10.1016/j.jamcollsurg.2011.10.008.

39. Fujita T, Nakagohri T, Gotohda N, Takahashi S, Konishi M, Kojima M, et al. Evaluation of the prognostic factors and significance of lymph node status in invasive ductal carcinoma of the body or tail of the pancreas. Pancreas. 2010;39(1):e48–54. doi:10.1097/MPA.0b013e3181bd5cfa.

40. Nakao A, Harada A, Nonami T, Kaneko T, Nomoto S, Koyama H, et al. Lymph node metastasis in carcinoma of the body and tail of the pancreas. Br J Surg. 1997;84(8):1090–2.

41. Kim SH, Kang CM, Satoi S, Sho M, Nakamura Y, Lee WJ. Proposal for splenectomy-omitting radical distal pancreatectomy in well-selected left-sided pancreatic cancer: multicenter survey study. J Hepatobiliary Pancreat Sci. 2013;20(3):375–81. doi:10.1007/s00534-012-0549-z.

42. Kimura W, Yano M, Sugawara S, Okazaki S, Sato T, Moriya T, et al. Spleen-preserving distal pancreatectomy with conservation of the splenic artery and vein: techniques and its significance. J Hepatobiliary Pancreat Sci. 2010;17(6):813–23. doi:10.1007/s00534-009-0250-z.

43. Warshaw AL. Distal pancreatectomy with preservation of the spleen. J Hepatobiliary Pancreat Sci. 2010;17(6):808–12. doi:10.1007/s00534-009-0226-z.

44. Sun Z, Zhu Y, Zhang N. The detail of the en bloc technique and prognosis of spleen-preserving laparoscopic distal pancreatectomy for pancreatic cancer. World J Surg Oncol. 2015;13:322. doi:10.1186/s12957-015-0735-y.

45. Higashijima J, Shimada M, Chikakiyo M, Miyatani T, Yoshikawa K, Nishioka M, et al. Effect of splenectomy on antitumor immune system in mice. Anticancer Res. 2009;29(1):385–93.

46. Imai S, Nio Y, Shiraishi T, Tsubono M, Morimoto H, Tseng CC, et al. Effects of splenectomy on pulmonary metastasis and growth of SC42 carcinoma transplanted into mouse liver. J Surg Oncol. 1991;47(3):178–87.

47. Shiratori Y, Kawase T, Nakata R, Tanaka M, Hikiba Y, Okano K, et al. Effect of splenectomy on hepatic metastasis of colon carcinoma and natural killer activity in the liver. Dig Dis Sci. 1995;40(11):2398–406.

48. Miwa H, Kojima K, Ono F, Kobayashi T, Tsurumi T, Hatosaki A, et al. Effect of splenectomy and immunotherapy on advanced gastric cancer associated with total gastrectomy. Jpn J Surg. 1983;13(1):20–4.

49. Okinaga K, Iinuma H, Kitamura Y, Yokohata T, Inaba T, Fukushima R. Effect of immunotherapy and spleen preservation on immunological function in patients with gastric cancer. J Exp Clin Cancer Res. 2006;25(3):339–49.

50. Miwa H, Kojima K, Kobayashi T, Inoue T, Nakamura K, Moriyama M, et al. The tumor—immunological significance of splenectomy for cancer therapy. Nihon Geka Gakkai Zasshi. 1983;84(9):970–3.

51. Miura T, Hirano S, Nakamura T, Tanaka E, Shichinohe T, Tsuchikawa T, et al. A new preoperative prognostic scoring system to predict prognosis in patients with locally advanced pancreatic body cancer who undergo distal pancreatectomy with en bloc celiac axis resection: a retrospective cohort study. Surgery. 2014;155(3):457–67. doi:10.1016/j.surg.2013.10.024.

52. Okada K, Kawai M, Tani M, Hirono S, Miyazawa M, Shimizu A, et al. Surgical strategy for patients with pancreatic body/tail carcinoma: who should undergo distal pancreatectomy with en-bloc celiac axis resection? Surgery. 2013;153(3):365–72. doi:10.1016/j.surg.2012.07.036.

53. Hirano S, Kondo S, Hara T, Ambo Y, Tanaka E, Shichinohe T, et al. Distal pancreatectomy with en bloc celiac axis resection for locally advanced pancreatic body cancer: long-term results. Ann Surg. 2007;246(1):46–51. doi:10.1097/01.sla.0000258608.52615.5a.

54. Cho A, Yamamoto H, Kainuma O, Ota T, Park S, Ikeda A, et al. Pure laparoscopic distal pancreatectomy with en bloc celiac axis resection. J Laparoendosc Adv Surg Tech A. 2011;21(10):957–9. doi:10.1089/lap.2011.0300.

55. Giulianotti PC, Addeo P, Buchs NC, Ayloo SM, Bianco FM. Robotic extended pancreatectomy with vascular resection for locally advanced pancreatic tumors. Pancreas. 2011;40(8):1264–70. doi:10.1097/MPA.0b013e318220e3a4.

56. Kang CM. Should we randomize our patients in the name of the "scientific evidence"? Surgery. 2015;158(6):1742–3. doi:10.1016/j.surg.2015.02.010.

57. Kooby DA, Vollmer CM. Laparoscopic versus open distal pancreatectomy: is a randomized trial necessary? J Hepatobiliary Pancreat Sci. 2015;22(10):737–9. doi:10.1002/jhbp.279.

58. Shiomi A, Ito M, Maeda K, Kinugasa Y, Ota M, Yamaue H, et al. Effects of a diverting stoma on symptomatic anastomotic leakage after low anterior resection for rectal cancer: a propensity score matching analysis of 1,014 consecutive patients. J Am Coll Surg. 2015;220(2):186–94. doi:10.1016/j.jamcollsurg.2014.10.017.

59. Katsuno H, Shiomi A, Ito M, Koide Y, Maeda K, Yatsuoka T, et al. Comparison of symptomatic anastomotic leakage following laparoscopic and open low anterior resection for rectal cancer: a propensity score matching analysis of 1014 consecutive patients. Surg Endosc. 2015; doi:10.1007/s00464-015-4566-2.

60. Nishikawa H, Osaki Y, Endo M, Takeda H, Tsuchiya K, Joko K, et al. Comparison of standard-dose and halfdose sorafenib therapy on clinical outcome in patients with unresectable hepatocellular carcinoma in field practice: a propensity score matching analysis. Int J Oncol. 2014;45(6):2295–302. doi:10.3892/ijo.2014.2654.
61. Uccella S, Bonzini M, Palomba S, Fanfani F, Ceccaroni M, Seracchioli R, et al. Impact of obesity on surgical treatment for endometrial cancer: a multicenter study comparing laparoscopy vs open surgery, with propensity-matched analysis. J Minim Invasive Gynecol. 2016;23(1):53–61. doi:10.1016/j.jmig.2015.08.007.

Part IV

Immunotherapy and Gene Therapy for Pancreatic Cancer

Development of Cancer Vaccine and Targeted Immune Checkpoint Therapies

Yuwen Zhu, Alessandro Paniccia, Barish H. Edil, and Richard D. Schulick

16.1 Introduction

The immune system's natural capacity to detect and destroy abnormal cells may prevent the development of many cancers [1, 2]. However, cancer cells are capable of evading detection and destruction by the immune system. They create a heterogeneous environment to favor or facilitate their progression, the so-called tumor microenvironment (TME) [3–5]. Besides tumor cells, the TME comprises many different stromal cells. These include vascular or lymphatic endothelial cells, supporting pericytes, fibroblasts, and infiltrating immune cells. These nonimmune stromal cells provide support to tumor cells, with growth factors and cytokines, and promote angiogenesis, tissue invasion, and metastasis [6]. In addition, the stroma provides a chemoresistant barrier to the tumor, preventing chemotherapeutics from reaching their targets [7].

The major immune cells at TME include myeloid-derived suppressor cells (MDSCs), tumor-associated macrophages (TAMs), dendritic cells (DCs), natural killer (NK) cells, and T and B lymphocytes [8, 9]. Generally, immune cells can exert both tumor suppressive and promoting effects [10]. T lymphocytes have a paramount role in tumor-specific cellular adaptive immunity. The main components of this population are CD8+ cytotoxic T lymphocytes (CTLs), CD4+ helper T cells, and regulatory T cells (T_{reg}). CD8+ CTLs are the major cell type that can directly kill cancer cells, and their presence is associated with prolonged survival. However, most CD8+ T cells at tumor sites exhibit dysfunctional or exhausted phenotypes and are reluctant to proliferate [11]. The presence of Th1 and Th2 lymphocytes in the tumor microenvironment appears to have opposite prognostic significance in the setting of tumor progression [12]. DCs are important for

Y. Zhu • A. Paniccia • B.H. Edil • R.D. Schulick (✉)
Department of Surgery, University of Colorado Anschutz Medical Campus, Aurora, CO 80045, USA
e-mail: richard.schulick@ucdenver.edu

© Springer Science+Business Media Singapore 2017
H. Yamaue (ed.), *Innovation of Diagnosis and Treatment for Pancreatic Cancer*,
DOI 10.1007/978-981-10-2486-3_16

antigen presentation and T cell activation during antitumor immunity. However, the immunosuppressive TME always turns DCs into a suppressive or regulatory DC phenotype [13]. T_{reg} cells, which are positive for CD4+, CD25+, and Foxp3, are enriched in the tumor microenvironment [14]. T_{reg} cells effectively suppress the adaptive immune response, and their presence in the tumor microenvironment leads to decreased anticancer immunity and often correlates with poor prognosis [14]. TAMs are polarized macrophages with a protumoral phenotype; they suppress antitumor T cell responses, and promote tumor angiogenesis and metastasis [15]. MDSCs are mobilized during tumorigenesis, and infiltrate developing tumors where they promote tumor vascularization and disrupt major mechanisms of immunosurveillance by T cells, DCs, and NK cells [16, 17]. Neutrophils can play both tumor-promoting and tumoricidal functions, depending on their differentiation status and the presence of TGF-β [18]. The role of B cells in tumor immunity remains unclear: some reports showed that B cell depletion promotes antitumor immune responses while some studies found that activated B cells increase T cell activation and suppress tumor growth [19].

16.2   A Unique Immunosuppressive Microenvironment of Pancreatic Cancer

Pancreatic cancers present an enormous challenge, as they are insensitive to traditional therapies. One prime contributing factor is the uniquely abundant tumor stromal content present in the microenvironment of pancreatic cancer [20–22]. The epithelial and stromal compartments interact and communicate to enhance the aggressive nature of this disease, ultimately culminating in an extremely effective immunosuppressive network [23]. Pancreatic cancer cells release various factors that stimulate the formation of stroma. Stromal cells, in turn, release mutagenic substances that stimulate tumor growth, invasion, and resistance to therapy. Structurally, the presence of an enormous number of stromal cells forms a physical shield, preventing immune cells from reaching and attacking cancer cells [24, 25]. Furthermore, pancreatic cancer cells utilize multiple pathways to create an immunosuppressive microenvironment and evade immune cell attack. Several cytokines appear to be dysregulated and contribute to cancer progression in pancreatic ductal adenocarcinoma (PDAC). In particular, higher levels of circulating interleukin-6 (IL-6) are identified in patients with PDAC and appear to promote cancer progression through enhancement of pro-tumorigenic Stat3 signaling [26, 27]. Furthermore, members of the IL-1 family (e.g., IL-α, IL-ß, and IL-1 receptor antagonist (IL-1ra)) seem to play a role in PDAC development [28, 29]. Immunosuppressive cytokine IL-10 is upregulated in PDAC, which leads to a reduction in effector cell function in the PDAC microenvironment and indicates a worse prognosis [30]. Finally, pancreatic cancer is a non-immunogenic cancer type with low frequency of mutations [31]. As a result, the frequency of tumor-specific T cells at cancer sites is relatively low, and intraepithelial CD8$^+$ T cells infiltration is very rare in PDAC [23]. This poses a great challenge to active immunotherapies, such as cancer vaccines and immune checkpoint inhibitors, which would rely on the existing anticancer immunity in cancer patients. Therefore, a better understanding of the complex interactions between the cancer cells and their associated stromal cells could be key to the development of new therapeutic options for patients [32].

16.3   Principles for Cancer Immunotherapy

The immune system is capable of detecting carcinogenesis though the extent and efficiency of anticancer effect are generally not strong enough to eradicate established cancer [1]. Therefore, the strategies of cancer immunotherapy are to launch a strong anticancer response by mobilizing endogenous anticancer immunity or by infusing immune effector cells to combat cancer. Based on the reliance of the existing immune system, the approaches of immunotherapy can be classified into two types: passive and active (Table 16.1) [51]. Passive immunotherapy comprises antibodies and immune cells that are made outside of the body and are subsequently

Table 16.1 Major immunotherapeutic approaches in pancreatic cancer

Type of immunotherapy		Passive or active	Example	Advantages	Disadvantage	References
Adaptive cellular therapy	TIL	Passive	N/A	Limited TILs for *in vitro* expansion	A personalized approach and costly	N/A
	CAR-T	Passive	Mesothelin	Can be produced in large scale	*A costly personalized approach *Tumor-specific targets yet to be found *Target limited tumor antigens	[33]
Cancer vaccine	Peptide	Active	MUC-1, survivin, telomerase, Ras mutant, VEGFR2	Low cost, high specificity	*Derived from weak antigen (TAA) *Neoantigen yet to be identified * Target limited tumor epitopes	[34]
	DC-based			A good inducer of tumor-specific T cells		[35–38]
	Whole Cell		GVAX, Algenpantucel-L	*Easy to manufacture *Multiple and unknown tumor antigens targeted.	Trigger weak anticancer immunity	[39–48]
Checkpoint inhibitor		Active	CTLA-4, PD-1	*Target a broad spectrum of tumor antigens *Does not need the knowledge of antigen identity	The anticancer effect relies on the immunogenicity of cancer	[49, 50]

inoculated into cancer patients, in an attempt to target and destroy cancer cells. It includes but it is not limited to antibody and adaptive cellular therapy (ACT) [52]. On the other end of the spectrum, active immunotherapy interventions aim to trigger or amplify anticancer immunity by mobilizing the host immune system and include at least cancer vaccines and immune checkpoint inhibitors.

The following sections will summarize current major immunotherapy development in research and clinical trials, and their progresses in pancreatic cancer therapy.

16.3.1 Adaptive Cellular Therapy

Adaptive cellular therapy (ACT) is a procedure that aims to first expand T cells in vitro and then re-infuse the expanded T cell pool back into patients for cancer treatment [53]. Compared to peripheral blood of cancer patients, tumor infiltrated lymphocytes (TILs) are enriched in tumor-specific T cells and can be easily expanded in vitro by tumor cells with the presence of growth factors like interleukin-2 [54, 55]. This practice can generate tumor-reactive T cells with a broad range of tumor reactivity, without the knowledge of tumor antigen identities. With the improvement of culturing technology, the degree of expansion and quality control has been greatly enhanced. Isolating and expanding TILs for ACT is a very efficacious treatment strategy in melanoma [56]. However, the number of TILs that can be successfully recovered from the vast majority of solid tumors is very limited, especially for those cancers with few TILs. In addition, the majority of TILs display exhausted or dysfunctional phenotypes, which might cause the poor persistence of expansion tumor-specific T cell clones upon intravenous infusion [57, 58]. Therefore, the current approach of expanding TILs for ACT is mainly practiced in melanoma patients.

Genetically, engineering of lymphocytes is a new approach that aims to eliminate the obstacle posed by many tumors with a limited number of tumor-reactive T cells for ACT [52, 59, 60]. This strategy involves transducing immune cells with genes that redirect T cells to recognize cancer cells. The specificity of T cells can be redirected by the incorporation of genes encoding either conventional alpha-beta TCRs or chimeric antigen receptors (CARs) [61]. In this case, T cells from patient blood can be directly used as a source for ACT. CARs are constructed by linking the variable regions of the antibody heavy and light chains to intracellular signaling chains, such as CD3-zeta. The new generation of CARs is also composed of costimulatory domains of CD28 and/or CD137 to promote T cell expansion [62]. Because CARs are derived from antibodies, recognition of tumor-associated antigens (TAAs) by CARs is strong and is not restricted by major histocompatibility complex (MHC) [62].

However, a major hurdle for CAR-T therapy in human cancer is the identification requirement of appropriate tumor antigens that are exclusively expressed on the cancer cells, but not normal self-tissues. Most of the currently identified tumor-specific antigens are self-antigens that are normally expressed in early fetal development and that are aberrantly expressed during malignancy [63]. Examples include

NY-ESO1 and the MAGE family antigens. The phenomenon known as "off-tumor, on-target," where CAR-T cells recognize non-cancer cells expressing the tumor antigen, is responsible for severe immune-mediated toxicities that have limited the applicability of this treatment strategy [64, 65]. Therefore, careful monitoring and screening of targets for CAR-T therapy is extremely important. As a result, current successes of CAR-T therapy in clinic are mainly limited to certain types of lymphoma/leukemia [66]. Testing the feasibility of this approach can only be carried out in clinical trials, as preclinical models have proven to be insufficiently predictive of both efficacy and toxicity in humans. Whole-genome sequencing of cancer cells is generating abundant information about specific mutations in tumor cells, which may lead to the identification of tumor-specific antigens, also called neoantigens [67]. Innovative ways of generating antigen receptors that recognize these, including CARs that directly recognize intracellular molecules presented by MHC, may generate T cells with even greater specificities for tumor cells. It is worth noting that another potential obstacle for ACT is that the majority of the inoculated T cells die before reaching the cancer site, which can be a challenging obstacle for patients with solid cancers [68]. Therefore, selection of T cell subsets with better capacity for survival and proliferation is a critical step in ACT, and methods to selectively enrich central memory and stem cell memory T cell subsets from human lymphocytes may enable more effective anticancer responses in humans, similar to those observed in mouse models [68–70]. Although the range of CARs currently available is sufficient to cover most types of malignancy, tumor cells can lose the expression of TAAs to evade immune attack during ACT [60]. Therefore, using several CAR genes that target multiple TAAs simultaneously may be needed for future ACT to better accommodate the heterogeneity in human cancers.

Animal models of pancreatic cancer have shown encouraging results with the use of ACT [71, 72], and clinical trials using CAR engineered T cells for pancreatic cancer are currently ongoing in many cancer centers (NCT01897415, NCT02465983) [33]. The recently completed PDAC genomic analysis by Bailey et al. led to a deeper understanding of the molecular evolution of PDAC and to the identification of a specific immunogenic PDAC subtype [73]. This new and long awaited information may open the way to new and more accurate therapeutic targets for ACT.

16.3.2 Cancer Vaccines

Vaccine is an active therapeutic approach aiming to mobilize the immune system to generate or amplify tumor-specific immune response to combat cancer [74]. The primary mechanism for therapeutic cancer vaccines is to increase the presentation of tumor-associated antigens (TAAs) to the immune system, so as to mount a potent immune response against tumors. Cancer vaccines attempt to copy the achievements made in vaccinations against pathogens though more work is necessary to bring it to fruition. Based on the formats utilized, cancer vaccine can be classified into three major categories: protein/peptide vaccines, whole cell vaccines, and DNA vaccines [51].

16.3.2.1 Peptide Vaccines

Protein/peptide vaccines attempt to immunize patients with a peptide or a protein derived from cancer antigens in the formation of adjuvant or cellular vehicles. This strategy requires the identification of tumor-specific antigens or TAAs that are only expressed on cancer cells or overexpressed on cancer cells.

Peptide vaccine therapy for PDAC has been conducted in clinic for many years [34]. The most commonly used antigens in trials include telomerase, Wilms tumor gene, KIP20A, survivin, mutated Ras protein, mucin MUC1 protein, and vascular endothelial growth factor receptor 2 (VEGFR2). Though overall cancer vaccine is well tolerated, the outcomes of these vaccine trials have been disappointing with many lessons learned [34]. First, the presence of suppressive mechanisms at the cancer sites must be conquered. Immunoconditioning can eliminate some of these immunosuppressive mechanisms, but at the same time it also dampens endogenous anticancer immunity that is needed for cancer vaccines. Examples of cells responsible for this suppressive mechanism include T_{reg} cells, MDSCs, as well as the signal generated through the interaction between PD1 and PD-L1 at the cancer site [75, 76]. Second, the antigen/peptides used in trials are mainly tumor-associated antigens (TAAs), which may be well tolerated and thus incapable of triggering anticancer immunity strong enough to destroy PDAC [77]. Emerging data in clinical immunotherapy suggest that the recognition and response to neoantigens, which arise as a consequence of tumor-specific mutation, is the major player, and neoantigen loads correlate with overall response rates to therapy [67]. Recent technological advancements have made it possible to dissect the immune response to patient-specific neoantigens [78]. It remains to be seen whether a neoantigen-based vaccine is capable of triggering potent anticancer immunity for cancer therapy.

16.3.2.2 Whole Cell-based Vaccines

Whole cell vaccines are conceptually easy to understand as this strategy, as the name indicates, proposes to utilize the whole tumor cell to elicit a specific anticancer immune response [79]. The tumor cell can be either autologous (i.e., patient-specific tumor cell) or allogenic (i.e., established human tumor cell line). The rationale for this approach is that cancer cells express the entire spectrum of tumor antigens (i.e., for that specific tumor in that specific patient) as well as specific epitopes for CD8+ and CD4+ T cells that can be presented to the patient's immune system [80]. This approach is considered polyvalent (as it presents a wide range of tumor antigens to the immune system) and therefore, at least in theory, it is less susceptible to tumor immune evasion as seen in peptide-based vaccine (i.e., where mutation of TAAs under selective pressure leads to loss of the immune target). In addition, this approach is applicable to cancers even without the knowledge of antigen identity [80]. In the autologous approach, tumor cells are required to be isolated from the patient, irradiated, combined with an immunostimulating agent and ultimately infused back into the patient [79]. Therefore, this technique is limited by the availability of sufficient tumor sample that at times can be difficult to obtain, especially in certain cancer types. In this case, allogenic cell lines offer a valid alternative, as they are readily available and can be produced on a large scale [81].

GVAX is an allogenic irradiated whole cell vaccine composed of two irradiated cancer cell lines (PANC 6.03 and PANC 10.05) engineered to express granulocyte macrophage-colony stimulating factor (GM-CSF) [39, 40]. GM-CSF is a potent cytokine that functions to promote the growth of granulocytes and monocytes and also to attract dendritic cells for better antigen presentation. GVAX alone or in combination with other therapies has been investigated in multiple phase I and II studies [41–43]. A phase I trial of GVAX in 14 patients with resectable pancreatic cancer showed a mean disease-free survival (DFS) of 13 months, with three patients disease-free from 25 to 30 months [44]. Though a following phase II trial of GVAX in combination with cyclophosphamide (CY) in patients with metastatic pancreatic cancer failed to show improvement of overall survival (OS), a higher rate of induced mesothelin-specific T cell responses could correlate with longer progression-free survival (PFS) and OS [41]. Similarly, a phase II study of patients with resected PDAC using GVAX plus chemoradiation displayed median DFS of 17.3 and median survival of 24.8 months. This demonstrated an association between mesothelin-specific T cell induction and improved overall survival [42]. GVAX also has been tested in combination with *Live-Attenuated Listeria monocytogenes (CRS-207),* in an attempt to use the ability of *Listeria* to stimulate both innate and adaptive immunity to ultimately boost the overall response to the cancer vaccine [45, 46]. In a recent phase II trial, the authors showed a 2-month improvement in overall survival in patients treated with GVAX–cyclophosphamide and CRS-207, compared with GVAX–cyclophosphamide (median 6 months vs. 4 months; HR 0.60; $P = 0.02$) [46]. Based on that, it is anticipated that a larger study of the GVAX/CRS-207 combination on patient survival will launch soon.

Algenpantucel-L is another major whole cell cancer vaccine being developed for PDAC [47]. It is composed of two human pancreatic cancer cells expressing the enzyme alpha-1, 3-galactosyl transferase (αGT) [48]. Humans lack a functional αGT gene and are not tolerant to αGT; therefore, αGT-labeled tumor cells could lead to enhanced antitumor response, as has been demonstrated in mouse tumor models [82, 83, 84]. In an open labeled, phase II trial of algenpantucel-L with gemcitabine and 5-fluorouracil (FU) for patients with resected PDAC, 12-month DFS of 62% and OS of 86% were achieved as compared to historical controls (45% and 65%, respectively) [48]. Another positive sign was that patients with algenpantucel-L therapy experienced minimal side effects, mainly consisting of injection site pain and induration. Based upon these encouraging results, a phase III study in patients with surgically resected PDAC was launched in 2010 [NCT01072981]. Another ongoing phase III trial (ClinicalTrials.gov: NCT01836432) involving Algenpantucel-L in PDAC is to combine with FOLFIRINOX or gemcitabine/nab-paclitaxel, and results of the trial are expected to be released in June 2017.

16.3.2.3 DC and DNA Vaccine

Similar to peptide vaccine, DC and DNA vaccines require the knowledge of TAAs or neoantigens. Genetic vaccine consists of a DNA-based vaccine that aims to introduce genetic material into a live host [85]. This allows the chosen gene products to be expressed and ultimately triggers a specific immune reaction to the gene-derived antigen. The advantage of a genetic vaccine is that it allows the expression of antigens that resemble native viral epitopes more closely than live-attenuated or killed vaccines that often alter the protein structure and antigenicity [85]. DCs are one of the most effective APCs which function to process and present antigens on MHC molecules to trigger T cell responses [86]. DC vaccines use DCs as a vehicle for peptide/DNA vaccine, and this strategy has the potential of bridging the gap between innate and adaptive immunity [87]. This approach requires isolation of patient's DC that are eventually pulsed with peptides, and finally injected back to the patient. A successful example of peptide vaccines is Sipuleucel-T, the first FDA-approved drug for the treatment of hormone refractory prostate cancer, which is capable of extending the overall survival of cancer patients [88].

Early clinical trials of PDAC patients demonstrated that DC vaccine is well tolerated and capable of inducing detectable antigen-specific immune response in patient blood though no clear clinical benefit is observed [35]. In a phase I/II study, Lepisto and colleagues evaluated the use of an MUC1 peptide pulsed autologous DC vaccine as adjuvant therapy in patients with resectable pancreatic and biliary tumor [36]. In this study, patients were followed for over 4 years and 4 out of the 12 enrolled patients (10 had pancreatic cancer) were alive and without any evidence of recurrence. Other TAAs, such as CEA and hTERT, were used for early clinical trials of DC vaccine, with only minor objective clinical responses reported [37, 38]. Because neoantigens are more immunogenic and trigger a more potent immune response in cancer patients, the future development of DC vaccine for PDAC will likely utilize neoantigen-based DC vaccine.

16.3.3 Immune Checkpoint Inhibitors

T cell response is largely controlled by an array of cellular surface signaling molecules, also known as cosignaling molecules [89]. Modulating these cosignaling pathways increases anticancer immunity, either through the amplification of costimulatory pathways or blockade of negative signals, also known as immune checkpoints [90]. The major immune checkpoints under clinical investigation include at least CTLA-4, PD-1, TIM-3, LAG3, and TIGIT [91, 92]. Many of the ligands for immune checkpoints are upregulated at cancer sites and contribute to the induction of tumor-specific T cell exhaustion/dysfunction at cancer sites [91, 93]. Using monoclonal antibodies or fusion proteins are the main strategy to block or amplify cosignaling pathways. The immunomodulation strategy strives to promote or liberate internal anticancer immunity in a patient with an established cancer [94]. One of the advantages of this therapeutic strategy is that immunomodulation does not require the knowledge of specific cancer antigens but rather focuses on the manipulation of known leukocyte receptors. These provide several potential therapeutic targets that are characterized by a broad spectrum of antigen diversity that could ultimately avoid the mechanism of cancer immune evasion, caused by mutation of cancer-specific antigens [95].

Targeting immune checkpoints has been a major breakthrough in cancer treatment in recent years [96]. CTLA-4 is transiently expressed on the T cell surface upon activation and attenuates ongoing T cell response by competing ligands B7-1 (CD80) and B7-2 (CD86) with the costimulatory receptor CD28 [97, 98]. In addition, CTLA-4 also transduces a suppressive signal to T cell via the recruitment of phosphatases SHP-2 and PP2A [90]. Ipilimumab, an anti-CTLA-4 mAb, is the first FDA-approved immunotherapy drug to treat patients with late-stage melanoma [99, 100]. Administration of ipilimumab activates T cells systemically, leading to extensive antitumor immunity and therefore a survival benefit in 10–15% of patients with advanced metastatic melanoma. Furthermore, this antitumor response significantly increases overall patient survival in advanced melanoma cases [99]. However, antitumor activity is frequently accompanied by significant immune-related adverse events. PD-1 is another inducible immune checkpoint on T cells that suppresses T cell response upon interaction with its two ligands, PD-L1 (B7-H1) and PD-L2 (B7-DC) [36, 101]. The PD-1 pathway is heavily involved in the immunosuppressive cancer microenvironment: PD-1 is highly expressed in TILs while the ligand PD-L1 is found on tumor cells, tumor-associated DCs, macrophages, and fibroblasts [94, 102]. Targeting the PD-1 pathway has elicited durable antitumor responses and long-term remissions in patients with a broad spectrum of cancers. The objective response rates varies in different cancer types, with bladder cancer, melanoma, mismatch repair-deficient colorectal cancer and certain hematopoietic malignancies among the most responsive cancer types [102]. Compared to CTLA-4 blockade, the antitumor efficacy of PD-1 blockade is higher, and the side effect is significantly milder and manageable [49, 103–105]. Currently, PD-1/PD-L1 mAbs have been approved by FDA to treat late-stage melanoma, non-small cell lung cancer, and kidney cancer [102]. It is anticipated that PD-1 mAb will be approved for treating more cancer types and become the frontline therapy for future cancer treatment.

Ipilimumab alone, or in combination with peptide vaccine, did not have any clinical benefit in treating PDAC patients. In a phase II trial of 27 patients with advanced PDAC, single-agent ipilimumab failed to detect any responder by response evaluation criteria in solid tumors [50]. However, a significant delayed response in one subject of this trial suggests that this immunotherapeutic approach to PDAC deserves further exploration [50]. With tremendous success in many cancer types, early trials of anti-PD-1 mAb alone showed no effect in treating patients with advanced PDAC, though the number of patients in the study was small [49]. PD-1 mAb alone is ineffective in treating cancers with few neoantigen loads [49]. PDAC happens to be a low immunogenic cancer [31]. It is not surprising that targeting immune checkpoints alone is incapable of launching an effective anticancer immunity in PDAC patients. Therefore, additional procedures are needed to increase the number of TILs surrounding PDAC cancers, so as to prime PDAC for immune checkpoint therapy [106].

16.3.4 Combined Therapy

The low immunogenicity and unique stromal structure of PDAC cancer poses a great challenge for immunotherapy [22]. The disappointing outcomes in clinical trials using single-agent immunotherapy propel the launch of combinatory approaches. Combination therapy targets more than one aspect and can be classified as the combination of two different arms of immunotherapeutic approaches, or the combination of immunotherapy with traditional therapy (chemotherapy or radiotherapy).

Examples of combinatory approaches that combine two different arms of immunotherapy could include the combination of cancer vaccine with immune checkpoint blockade or the simultaneous use of both active and passive immune therapy. Immune checkpoint inhibitors alone are not effective in the treatment of PDAC, much due to the lack of tumor-infiltrating T cells at tumor sites [23]. Cancer vaccine is known to be a very efficient method of expanding tumor-reactive T cells, while blockade of immune checkpoints will further promote antitumor immune responses at tumor sites. In fact, several preclinical studies exist that demonstrate the synergistic role of cancer vaccine therapy, which is responsible for stimulation of the immune system, and the use of immune checkpoint blockade, which allows for the unopposed effector function of cytotoxic T cells [107–109]. Consistently, clinical examination of resected PDAC tumors demonstrated that vaccine therapy can alter the immunosuppressive cancer microenvironment [106]. The majority of PDAC patients receiving GVAX vaccine had vaccine-induced intratumoral tertiary lymphoid aggregates in resected tumors, accompanied with increased intratumoral T_{eff}/T_{reg} ratios [106]. As such, a phase Ib, open-label randomized study demonstrated the feasibility and safety of an approach based on the combination of Ipilimumab with GVAX in patients with previously treated PDAC [47]. One of the most interesting aspects of this study was the difference in 12-month OS: 27% vs. 7% and the median OS: 5.7 vs. 3.6 months (HR = 0.51; P = 0.072), respectively, for combination therapy vs. monotherapy (i.e., Ipilimumab alone).

Given that PD-1/PD-L1 blockade is safer and more effective than CTLA-4 blockade in the treatment of many cancers, it is interesting to see how the combination of GVAX with PD-1/PD-L1 blockade performs in the treatment of PDAC [104]. Interestingly, PD-L1 expression was observed in all these lymphoid aggregates in GVAX-treated PDAC patients [106]. Currently, a phase I/II study with GVAX and anti-PD-1 mAb (nivolumab) has started to recruit patients with PDAC (NCT02451982). Similarly, a randomized phase II trial of GVAX and CRS-207 with or without nivolumab has also launched (NCT02243371).

Combinational therapy involving PD-1/PD-L1 blockade has also been investigated with chemotherapy or radiotherapy in PDAC [110]. These approaches are based on the observation that chemotherapy or radiotherapy can kill cancer cells to increase the supply of tumor antigens for presentation, so as to promote tumor-reactive immune responses [111–113]. In addition, many conventional cancer treatments in chemotherapy and radiotherapy have immune potentiating mechanisms of action, such as the elimination of immunosuppressive cells, including T_{reg} and MDSC (Zitvogel L, JCI 2008). A phase I trial (NCT02303990) of pembrolizumab (anti-PD-1 mAb) with the combination of hypofractionated radiotherapy has started to treat patients with metastatic pancreatic cancer. In another phase I study of PDAC (NCT02546531), PD-1 blockade (pembrolizumab) is proposed to be combined with gemcitabine and defactinib, an inhibitor of focal adhesion kinase (FAK), which promotes stromal fibrosis. Because immune effector cells are also sensitive to chemotherapy and radiotherapy, early phase clinical investigations into optimizing dose and schedule in patients are necessary.

16.4 Perspective

Despite recent advancements in PDAC treatment modalities, modest success has been achieved and the curative goal remains unmet. Surgical resection remains to be the only potential cure for early-stage PDAC. Immunotherapy emerges as a promising treatment for metastatic PDAC, with the potential of targeting disseminated disease as well as preventing cancer recurrence. With the technological advancement in genome sequencing, neoantigens in PDAC will be identified as better targets for vaccine therapy or ACT. Together with further interrogation of the PDAC microenvironment, it is promising that more PDAC immunosuppressive mechanisms, by which PDAC evades immune attack, will be revealed for future immune interventions.

Early clinical trials in immunotherapy also demonstrated that the complexity of the PDAC microenvironment and the formidable immunosuppressive nature of this cancer might require a combination of different therapeutic strategies [110]. These therapies need to be able to simultaneously target the stroma-cell population, where the tumor cells locate, as well as the cytotoxic T lymphocytes (manipulating different immune checkpoint inhibitors) or directly the tumor cells (traditional chemotherapeutic, vaccination, ACT). For instance, besides cancer vaccine, other therapeutic approaches, including chemotherapy, radiotherapy, and ACT may prime PDAC to become susceptible for immune checkpoint inhibitor therapy. Moving forward, the focus of modern clinical immunotherapy will be to identify the most efficacious, synergistic therapy that is able to obtain the maximum antitumor activity with the least systemic toxicity. Finally, it is imperative to identify reliable biomarkers to predict tumor susceptibility to immunotherapy in clinic, to identify those patients that are more likely to benefit from this unique therapeutic approach.

References

1. Finn OJ. Immuno-oncology: understanding the function and dysfunction of the immune system in cancer. Ann Oncol. 2012;23(Suppl 8):viii6–9. PubMed PMID: 22918931. Pubmed Central PMCID: 4085883
2. Disis ML. Immune regulation of cancer. J Clin Oncol. 2010;28(29):4531–8. PubMed PMID: 20516428. Pubmed Central PMCID: 3041789
3. Quail DF, Joyce JA. Microenvironmental regulation of tumor progression and metastasis. Nat Med. 2013;19(11):1423–37. PubMed PMID: 24202395. Pubmed Central PMCID: 3954707
4. Hanahan D, Weinberg RA. Hallmarks of cancer: the next generation. Cell. 2011;144(5):646–74. PubMed PMID: 21376230
5. Turley SJ, Cremasco V, Astarita JL. Immunological hallmarks of stromal cells in the tumour microenvironment. Nat Rev Immunol. 2015;15(11):669–82. PubMed PMID: 26471778
6. Pietras K, Ostman A. Hallmarks of cancer: interactions with the tumor stroma. Exp Cell Res. 2010;316(8):1324–31. PubMed PMID: 20211171

7. Cairns R, Papandreou I, Denko N. Overcoming physiologic barriers to cancer treatment by molecularly targeting the tumor microenvironment. Mol Cancer Res. 2006;4(2):61–70. PubMed PMID: 16513837

8. Gajewski TF, Schreiber H, Fu YX. Innate and adaptive immune cells in the tumor microenvironment. Nat Immunol. 2013;14(10):1014–22. PubMed PMID: 24048123. Pubmed Central PMCID: 4118725

9. Shiao SL, Ganesan AP, Rugo HS, Coussens LM. Immune microenvironments in solid tumors: new targets for therapy. Genes Dev. 2011;25(24):2559–72. PubMed PMID: 22190457. Pubmed Central PMCID: 3248678

10. Chew V, Toh HC, Abastado JP. Immune microenvironment in tumor progression: characteristics and challenges for therapy. J Oncol. 2012;2012:608406. PubMed PMID: 22927846. Pubmed Central PMCID: 3423944

11. Joyce JA, Fearon DT. T cell exclusion, immune privilege, and the tumor microenvironment. Science. 2015;348(6230):74–80. PubMed PMID: 25838376

12. Tatsumi T, Kierstead LS, Ranieri E, Gesualdo L, Schena FP, Finke JH, et al. Disease-associated bias in T helper type 1 (Th1)/Th2 CD4(+) T cell responses against MAGE-6 in HLA-DRB10401(+) patients with renal cell carcinoma or melanoma. J Exp Med. 2002;196(5):619–28. PubMed PMID: 12208877. Pubmed Central PMCID: 2193999

13. Tran Janco JM, Lamichhane P, Karyampudi L, Knutson KL. Tumor-infiltrating dendritic cells in cancer pathogenesis. J Immunol. 2015;194(7):2985–91. PubMed PMID: 25795789. Pubmed Central PMCID: 4369768

14. Zou W. Regulatory T cells, tumour immunity and immunotherapy. Nat Rev Immunol. 2006;6(4):295–307. PubMed PMID: 16557261

15. Noy R, Pollard JW. Tumor-associated macrophages: from mechanisms to therapy. Immunity. 2014;41(1):49–61. PubMed PMID: 25035953. Pubmed Central PMCID: 4137410

16. Gabrilovich DI, Nagaraj S. Myeloid-derived suppressor cells as regulators of the immune system. Nat Rev Immunol. 2009;9(3):162–74. PubMed PMID: 19197294. Pubmed Central PMCID: 2828349

17. Li H, Han Y, Guo Q, Zhang M, Cao X. Cancer-expanded myeloid-derived suppressor cells induce anergy of NK cells through membrane-bound TGF-beta 1. J Immunol. 2009;182(1):240–9. PubMed PMID: 19109155

18. Fridlender ZG, Sun J, Kim S, Kapoor V, Cheng G, Ling L, et al. Polarization of tumor-associated neutrophil phenotype by TGF-beta: "N1" versus "N2" TAN. Cancer Cell. 2009;16(3):183–94. PubMed PMID: 19732719. Pubmed Central PMCID: 2754404

19. He Y, Qian H, Liu Y, Duan L, Li Y, Shi G. The roles of regulatory B cells in cancer. J Immunology Res. 2014;2014:215471. PubMed PMID: 24991577. Pubmed Central PMCID: 4060293

20. Tjomsland V, Niklasson L, Sandstrom P, Borch K, Druid H, Bratthall C, et al. The desmoplastic stroma plays an essential role in the accumulation and modulation of infiltrated immune cells in pancreatic adenocarcinoma. Clin Dev Immunol. 2011;2011:212810. PubMed PMID: 22190968. Pubmed Central PMCID: 3235447

21. Zischek C, Niess H, Ischenko I, Conrad C, Huss R, Jauch KW, et al. Targeting tumor stroma using engineered mesenchymal stem cells reduces the growth of pancreatic carcinoma. Ann Surg. 2009;250(5):747–53. PubMed PMID: 19826249

22. Feig C, Gopinathan A, Neesse A, Chan DS, Cook N, Tuveson DA. The pancreas cancer microenvironment. Clin Cancer Res. 2012;18(16):4266–76. PubMed PMID: 22896693. Pubmed Central PMCID: 3442232

23. von Bernstorff W, Voss M, Freichel S, Schmid A, Vogel I, Johnk C, et al. Systemic and local immunosuppression in pancreatic cancer patients. Clin Cancer Res. 2001;7(3 Suppl):925s–32s. PubMed PMID: 11300493

24. Merika EE, Syrigos KN, Saif MW. Desmoplasia in pancreatic cancer. Can we fight it? Gastroenterol Res Pract. 2012;2012:781765. PubMed PMID: 23125850. Pubmed Central PMCID: 3485537

25. Whatcott CJ, Posner RG, Von Hoff DD, Han H. Desmoplasia and chemoresistance in pancreatic cancer. In: Grippo PJ, Munshi HG, editors. Pancreatic cancer and tumor microenvironment. Trivandrum (India); 2012

26. Lesina M, Kurkowski MU, Ludes K, Rose-John S, Treiber M, Kloppel G, et al. Stat3/Socs3 activation by IL-6 transsignaling promotes progression of pancreatic intraepithelial neoplasia and development of pancreatic cancer. Cancer Cell. 2011;19(4):456–69. PubMed PMID: 21481788

27. Okada S, Okusaka T, Ishii H, Kyogoku A, Yoshimori M, Kajimura N, et al. Elevated serum interleukin-6 levels in patients with pancreatic cancer. Jpn J Clin Oncol. 1998;28(1):12–5. PubMed PMID: 9491135

28. Ling J, Kang Y, Zhao R, Xia Q, Lee DF, Chang Z, et al. KrasG12D-induced IKK2/beta/NF-kappaB activation by IL-1alpha and p62 feedforward loops is required for development of pancreatic ductal adenocarcinoma. Cancer Cell. 2012;21(1):105–20. PubMed PMID: 22264792. Pubmed Central PMCID: 3360958

29. Muerkoster S, Wegehenkel K, Arlt A, Witt M, Sipos B, Kruse ML, et al. Tumor stroma interactions induce chemoresistance in pancreatic ductal carcinoma cells involving increased secretion and paracrine effects of nitric oxide and interleukin-1beta. Cancer Res. 2004;64(4):1331–7. PubMed PMID: 14973050

30. Poch B, Lotspeich E, Ramadani M, Gansauge S, Beger HG, Gansauge F. Systemic immune dysfunction in pancreatic cancer patients. Langenbeck Arch Surg. 2007;392(3):353–8. PubMed PMID: 17235586

31. Alexandrov LB, Nik-Zainal S, Wedge DC, Aparicio SA, Behjati S, Biankin AV, et al. Signatures of mutational processes in human cancer. Nature. 2013;500(7463):415–21. PubMed PMID: 23945592. Pubmed Central PMCID: 3776390

32. Swartz MA, Iida N, Roberts EW, Sangaletti S, Wong MH, Yull FE, et al. Tumor microenvironment complexity: emerging roles in cancer therapy. Cancer Res. 2012;72(10):2473–80. PubMed PMID: 22414581. Pubmed Central PMCID: 3653596

33. Beatty GL, Haas AR, Maus MV, Torigian DA, Soulen MC, Plesa G, et al. Mesothelin-specific chimeric antigen receptor mRNA-engineered T cells induce anti-tumor activity in solid malignancies. Canc Immunol Res. 2014;2(2):112–20. PubMed PMID: 24579088. Pubmed Central PMCID: 3932715

34. Gaudernack G. Prospects for vaccine therapy for pancreatic cancer. Best Pract Res Clin Gastroenterol. 2006;20(2):299–314. PubMed PMID: 16549329

35. Mule JJ. Dendritic cell-based vaccines for pancreatic cancer and melanoma. Ann N Y Acad Sci. 2009;1174:33–40. PubMed PMID: 19769734

36. Lepisto AJ, Moser AJ, Zeh H, Lee K, Bartlett D, McKolanis JR, et al. A phase I/II study of a MUC1 peptide pulsed autologous dendritic cell vaccine as adjuvant therapy in patients with resected pancreatic and biliary tumors. Canc Ther. 2008;6(B):955–64. PubMed PMID: 19129927. Pubmed Central PMCID: 2614325

37. Kimura Y, Tsukada J, Tomoda T, Takahashi H, Imai K, Shimamura K, et al. Clinical and immunologic evaluation of dendritic cell-based immunotherapy in combination with gemcitabine and/or S-1 in patients with advanced pancreatic carcinoma. Pancreas. 2012;41(2):195–205. PubMed PMID: 21792083

38. Suso EM, Dueland S, Rasmussen AM, Vetrhus T, Aamdal S, Kvalheim G, et al. hTERT mRNA dendritic cell vaccination: complete response in a pancreatic cancer patient associated with response against several hTERT epitopes. Canc Immunol Immunother. 2011;60(6):809–18. PubMed PMID: 21365467. Pubmed Central PMCID: 3098983

39. Jaffee EM, Thomas MC, Huang AY, Hauda KM, Levitsky HI, Pardoll DM. Enhanced immune priming with spatial distribution of paracrine cytokine vaccines. J Immunother Emp Tumor Immunol. 1996;19(3):176–83. PubMed PMID: 8811492

40. Dranoff G, Jaffee E, Lazenby A, Golumbek P, Levitsky H, Brose K, et al. Vaccination with irradiated tumor cells engineered to secrete murine granulocyte-macrophage colony stimulating factor stimulates potent, specific, and long-lasting anti-tumor immunity. Proc

Natl Acad Sci U S A. 1993;90(8):3539–43. PubMed PMID: 8097319. Pubmed Central PMCID: 46336

41. Laheru D, Lutz E, Burke J, Biedrzycki B, Solt S, Onners B, et al. Allogeneic granulocyte macrophage colony-stimulating factor-secreting tumor immunotherapy alone or in sequence with cyclophosphamide for metastatic pancreatic cancer: a pilot study of safety, feasibility, and immune activation. Clin Canc Res. 2008;14(5):1455–63. PubMed PMID: 18316569. Pubmed Central PMCID: 2879140

42. Lutz E, Yeo CJ, Lillemoe KD, Biedrzycki B, Kobrin B, Herman J, et al. A lethally irradiated allogeneic granulocyte-macrophage colony stimulating factor-secreting tumor vaccine for pancreatic adenocarcinoma. A Phase II trial of safety, efficacy, and immune activation. Ann Surg. 2011;253(2):328–35. PubMed PMID: 21217520. Pubmed Central PMCID: 3085934

43. Chawla S, Henshaw R, Seeger L, Choy E, Blay JY, Ferrari S, et al. Safety and efficacy of denosumab for adults and skeletally mature adolescents with giant cell tumour of bone: interim analysis of an open-label, parallel-group, phase 2 study. Lancet Oncol. 2013;14(9):901–8. PubMed PMID: 23867211

44. Jaffee EM, Hruban RH, Biedrzycki B, Laheru D, Schepers K, Sauter PR, et al. Novel allogeneic granulocyte-macrophage colony-stimulating factor-secreting tumor vaccine for pancreatic cancer: a phase I trial of safety and immune activation. J Clin Oncol Off J Am Soc Clin Oncol. 2001;19(1):145–56. PubMed PMID: 11134207

45. Le DT, Brockstedt DG, Nir-Paz R, Hampl J, Mathur S, Nemunaitis J, et al. A live-attenuated Listeria vaccine (ANZ-100) and a live-attenuated Listeria vaccine expressing mesothelin (CRS-207) for advanced cancers: phase I studies of safety and immune induction. Clin Canc Res. 2012;18(3):858–68. PubMed PMID: 22147941. Pubmed Central PMCID: 3289408

46. Le DT, Wang-Gillam A, Picozzi V, Greten TF, Crocenzi T, Springett G, et al. Safety and survival with GVAX pancreas prime and *Listeria Monocytogenes*-expressing mesothelin (CRS-207) boost vaccines for metastatic pancreatic cancer. J Clin Oncol Off J Am Soc Clin Oncol. 2015;33(12):1325–33. PubMed PMID: 25584002. Pubmed Central PMCID: 4397277

47. Coveler AL, Rossi GR, Vahanian NN, Link C, Chiorean EG. Algenpantucel-L immunotherapy in pancreatic adenocarcinoma. Immunotherapy. 2016;8(2):117–25. PubMed PMID: 26787078

48. Hardacre JM, Mulcahy M, Small W, Talamonti M, Obel J, Krishnamurthi S, et al. Addition of algenpantucel-L immunotherapy to standard adjuvant therapy for pancreatic cancer: a phase 2 study. J Gastrointest Sur. 2013;17(1):94–100. discussion p -1. PubMed PMID: 23229886

49. Topalian SL, Hodi FS, Brahmer JR, Gettinger SN, Smith DC, McDermott DF, et al. Safety, activity, and immune correlates of anti-PD-1 antibody in cancer. N Engl J Med. 2012;366(26):2443–54. PubMed PMID: 22658127. Pubmed Central PMCID: 3544539

50. Royal RE, Levy C, Turner K, Mathur A, Hughes M, Kammula US, et al. Phase 2 trial of single agent Ipilimumab (anti-CTLA-4) for locally advanced or metastatic pancreatic adenocarcinoma. J Immunother. 2010;33(8):828–33. PubMed PMID: 20842054

51. Paniccia A, Merkow J, Edil BH, Zhu Y. Immunotherapy for pancreatic ductal adenocarcinoma: an overview of clinical trials. Chinese J Can Res. 2015;27(4):376–91. PubMed PMID: 26361407. Pubmed Central PMCID: 4560736

52. Hinrichs CS, Rosenberg SA. Exploiting the curative potential of adoptive T-cell therapy for cancer. Immunol Rev. 2014;257(1):56–71. PubMed PMID: 24329789. Pubmed Central PMCID: 3920180

53. Rosenberg SA, Restifo NP, Yang JC, Morgan RA, Dudley ME. Adoptive cell transfer: a clinical path to effective cancer immunotherapy. Nat Rev Cancer. 2008;8(4):299–308. PubMed PMID: 18354418. Pubmed Central PMCID: 2553205

54. Restifo NP, Dudley ME, Rosenberg SA. Adoptive immunotherapy for cancer: harnessing the T cell response. Nat Rev Immunol. 2012;12(4):269–81. PubMed PMID: 22437939

55. Besser MJ, Shapira-Frommer R, Treves AJ, Zippel D, Itzhaki O, Hershkovitz L, et al. Clinical responses in a phase II study using adoptive transfer of short-term cultured tumor infiltration lymphocytes in metastatic melanoma patients. Clin Cancer Res. 2010;16(9):2646–55. PubMed PMID: 20406835

56. Besser MJ. Is there a future for adoptive cell transfer in melanoma patients? Oncoimmunology. 2013;2(10):e26098. PubMed PMID: 24353909. Pubmed Central PMCID: 3862631

57. Robbins PF, Dudley ME, Wunderlich J, El-Gamil M, Li YF, Zhou J, et al. Cutting edge: persistence of transferred lymphocyte clonotypes correlates with cancer regression in patients receiving cell transfer therapy. J Immunol. 2004;173(12):7125–30. PubMed PMID: 15585832. Pubmed Central PMCID: 2175171

58. Hinrichs CS, Borman ZA, Gattinoni L, Yu Z, Burns WR, Huang J, et al. Human effector CD8+ T cells derived from naive rather than memory subsets possess superior traits for adoptive immunotherapy. Blood. 2011;117(3):808–14. PubMed PMID: 20971955. Pubmed Central PMCID: 3035075

59. Wang M, Yin B, Wang HY, Wang RF. Current advances in T-cell-based cancer immunotherapy. Immunotherapy. 2014;6(12):1265–78. PubMed PMID: 25524383. Pubmed Central PMCID: 4372895

60. Kershaw MH, Westwood JA, Darcy PK. Gene-engineered T cells for cancer therapy. Nat Rev Cancer. 2013;13(8):525–41. PubMed PMID: 23880905

61. Barrett DM, Singh N, Porter DL, Grupp SA, June CH. Chimeric antigen receptor therapy for cancer. Annu Rev Med. 2014;65:333–47. PubMed PMID: 24274181. Pubmed Central PMCID: 4120077

62. Jena B, Dotti G, Cooper LJ. Redirecting T-cell specificity by introducing a tumor-specific chimeric antigen receptor. Blood. 2010;116(7):1035–44. PubMed PMID: 20439624. Pubmed Central PMCID: 2938125

63. Blankenstein T, Coulie PG, Gilboa E, Jaffee EM. The determinants of tumour immunogenicity. Nat Rev Cancer. 2012;12(4):307–13. PubMed PMID: 22378190. Pubmed Central PMCID: 3552609

64. Morgan RA, Yang JC, Kitano M, Dudley ME, Laurencot CM, Rosenberg SA. Case report of a serious adverse event following the administration of T cells transduced with a chimeric antigen receptor recognizing ERBB2. Mol Ther 2010;18(4):843–851. PubMed PMID: 20179677. Pubmed Central PMCID: 2862534

65. Curran KJ, Brentjens RJ. Chimeric antigen receptor T cells for cancer immunotherapy. J Clin Oncol Off J Am Soc Clin Oncol. 2015;33(15):1703–6. PubMed PMID: 25897155

66. Kakarla S, Gottschalk S. CAR T cells for solid tumors: armed and ready to go? Cancer J. 2014;20(2):151–5. PubMed PMID: 24667962. Pubmed Central PMCID: 4050065

67. Schumacher TN, Schreiber RD. Neoantigens in cancer immunotherapy. Science. 2015;348(6230):69–74. PubMed PMID: 25838375

68. Fousek K, Ahmed N. The evolution of T-cell therapies for solid malignancies. Clin Canc Res. 2015;21(15):3384–92. PubMed PMID: 26240290. Pubmed Central PMCID: 4526112

69. Casati A, Varghaei-Nahvi A, Feldman SA, Assenmacher M, Rosenberg SA, Dudley ME, et al. Clinical-scale selection and viral transduction of human naive and central memory CD8+ T cells for adoptive cell therapy of cancer patients. Canc Immunol Immunother. 2013;62(10):1563–73. PubMed PMID: 23903715

70. Gattinoni L, Klebanoff CA, Restifo NP. Paths to stemness: building the ultimate antitumour T cell. Nat Rev Cancer. 2012;12(10):671–84. PubMed PMID: 22996603

71. Chmielewski M, Hahn O, Rappl G, Nowak M, Schmidt-Wolf IH, Hombach AA, et al. T cells that target carcinoembryonic antigen eradicate orthotopic pancreatic carcinomas without inducing autoimmune colitis in mice. Gastroenterology. 2012;143(4):1095–107. e2. PubMed PMID: 22750462

72. Stromnes IM, Schmitt TM, Hulbert A, Brockenbrough JS, Nguyen HN, Cuevas C, et al. T cells engineered against a native antigen can surmount immunologic and physical barriers to treat pancreatic ductal adenocarcinoma. Cancer Cell. 2015;28(5):638–52. PubMed PMID: 26525103. Pubmed Central PMCID: 4724422

73. Bailey P, Chang DK, Nones K, Johns AL, Patch AM, Gingras MC, et al. Genomic analyses identify molecular subtypes of pancreatic cancer. Nature. 2016;531(7592):47–52. PubMed PMID: 26909576

74. Lollini PL, Cavallo F, Nanni P, Forni G. Vaccines for tumour prevention. Nat Rev Cancer. 2006;6(3):204–16. PubMed PMID: 16498443

75. Laheru D, Jaffee EM. Immunotherapy for pancreatic cancer—science driving clinical progress. Nat Rev Cancer. 2005;5(6):459–67. PubMed PMID: 15905855

76. Wachsmann MB, Pop LM, Vitetta ES. Pancreatic ductal adenocarcinoma: a review of immunologic aspects. J Investig Med. 2012;60(4):643–63. PubMed PMID: 22406516. Pubmed Central PMCID: 3319488

77. Melief CJ, van Hall T, Arens R, Ossendorp F, van der Burg SH. Therapeutic cancer vaccines. J Clin Invest. 2015;125(9):3401–12. PubMed PMID: 26214521. Pubmed Central PMCID: 4588240

78. Rajasagi M, Shukla SA, Fritsch EF, Keskin DB, DeLuca D, Carmona E, et al. Systematic identification of personal tumor-specific neoantigens in chronic lymphocytic leukemia. Blood. 2014;124(3):453–62. PubMed PMID: 24891321. Pubmed Central PMCID: 4102716

79. de Gruijl TD, van den Eertwegh AJ, Pinedo HM, Scheper RJ. Whole-cell cancer vaccination: from autologous to allogeneic tumor- and dendritic cell-based vaccines. Cancer Immunol Immunother. 2008;57(10):1569–77. PubMed PMID: 18523771. Pubmed Central PMCID: 2491427

80. Keenan BP, Jaffee EM. Whole cell vaccines—past progress and future strategies. Semin Oncol. 2012;39(3):276–86. PubMed PMID: 22595050. Pubmed Central PMCID: 3356993

81. Srivatsan S, Patel JM, Bozeman EN, Imasuen IE, He S, Daniels D, et al. Allogeneic tumor cell vaccines: the promise and limitations in clinical trials. Human Vaccin Immunother. 2014;10(1):52–63. PubMed PMID: 24064957. Pubmed Central PMCID: 4181031

82. Galili U. Anti-Gal: an abundant human natural antibody of multiple pathogeneses and clinical benefits. Immunology. 2013;140(1):1–11. PubMed PMID: 23578170. Pubmed Central PMCID: 3809700

83. Rossi GR, Mautino MR, Unfer RC, et al. Effective treatment of preexisting melanoma with whole cell vaccines expressing α(1,3)-galactosyl epitopes. Cancer Res. 2005;65:10555–61

84. Rossi GR, et al. Allogeneic melanoma vaccine expressing alphaGal epitopes induces antitumor immunity to autologous antigens in mice without signs of toxicity. Journal of Immunotherapy. 2008;31(6):545–54

85. Rice J, Ottensmeier CH, Stevenson FK. DNA vaccines: precision tools for activating effective immunity against cancer. Nat Rev Cancer. 2008;8(2):108–20. PubMed PMID: 18219306

86. Banchereau J, Steinman RM. Dendritic cells and the control of immunity. Nature. 1998;392(6673):245–52. PubMed PMID: 9521319

87. Palucka K, Banchereau J. Cancer immunotherapy via dendritic cells. Nat Rev Cancer. 2012;12(4):265–77. PubMed PMID: 22437871. Pubmed Central PMCID: 3433802

88. Kantoff PW, Higano CS, Shore ND, Berger ER, Small EJ, Penson DF, et al. Sipuleucel-T immunotherapy for castration-resistant prostate cancer. N Engl J Med. 2010;363(5):411–22. PubMed PMID: 20818862

89. Zhu Y, Yao S, Chen L. Cell surface signaling molecules in the control of immune responses: a tide model. Immunity. 2011;34(4):466–78. PubMed PMID: 21511182. Pubmed Central PMCID: 3176719

90. Chen L. Co-inhibitory molecules of the B7-CD28 family in the control of T-cell immunity. Nat Rev Immunol. 2004;4(5):336–47. PubMed PMID: 15122199

91. Zou W, Chen L. Inhibitory B7-family molecules in the tumour microenvironment. Nat Rev Immunol. 2008;8(6):467–77. PubMed PMID: 18500231

92. Jiang Y, Li Y, Zhu B. T-cell exhaustion in the tumor microenvironment. Cell Death Dis. 2015;6:e1792. PubMed PMID: 26086965. Pubmed Central PMCID: 4669840

93. Wherry EJ. T cell exhaustion. Nat Immunol. 2011;12(6):492–9. PubMed PMID: 21739672

94. Pardoll DM. The blockade of immune checkpoints in cancer immunotherapy. Nat Rev Cancer 2012;12(4):252–264. PubMed PMID: 22437870

95. Naidoo J, Page DB, Wolchok JD. Immune modulation for cancer therapy. Br J Cancer. 2014;111(12):2214–9. PubMed PMID: 25211661. Pubmed Central PMCID: 4264429

96. Couzin-Frankel J. Breakthrough of the year 2013. Canc Immunother Sci. 2013;342(6165):1432–3. PubMed PMID: 24357284

97. Greenwald RJ, Freeman GJ, Sharpe AH. The B7 family revisited. Annu Rev Immunol. 2005;23:515–48. PubMed PMID: 15771580

98. Lenschow DJ, Walunas TL, Bluestone JA. CD28/B7 system of T cell costimulation. Annu Rev Immunol. 1996;14:233–58. PubMed PMID: WOS:A1996UH42900011. English

99. Hodi FS, O'Day SJ, McDermott DF, Weber RW, Sosman JA, Haanen JB, et al. Improved survival with ipilimumab in patients with metastatic melanoma. N Engl J Med. 2010;363(8):711–23. PubMed PMID: 20525992. Pubmed Central PMCID: 3549297

100. Robert C, Thomas L, Bondarenko I, O'Day S, Weber J, Garbe C, et al. Ipilimumab plus dacarbazine for previously untreated metastatic melanoma. N Engl J Med. 2011;364(26):2517–26. PubMed PMID: 21639810

101. Chen L, Han X. Anti-PD-1/PD-L1 therapy of human cancer: past, present, and future. J Clin Invest. 2015;125(9):3384–91. PubMed PMID: 26325035. Pubmed Central PMCID: 4588282

102. Zou W, Wolchok JD, Chen L. PD-L1 (B7-H1) and PD-1 pathway blockade for cancer therapy: mechanisms, response biomarkers, and combinations. Sci Trans Med. 2016;8(328):328rv4. PubMed PMID: 26936508

103. Hamid O, Robert C, Daud A, Hodi FS, Hwu WJ, Kefford R, et al. Safety and tumor responses with lambrolizumab (anti-PD-1) in melanoma. N Engl J Med. 2013;369(2):134–44. PubMed PMID: 23724846. Pubmed Central PMCID: 4126516

104. Robert C, Schachter J, Long GV, Arance A, Grob JJ, Mortier L, et al. Pembrolizumab versus Ipilimumab in Advanced Melanoma. N Engl J Med. 2015;372(26):2521–32. PubMed PMID: 25891173

105. Brahmer JR, Tykodi SS, Chow LQ, Hwu WJ, Topalian SL, Hwu P, et al. Safety and activity of anti-PD-L1 antibody in patients with advanced cancer. N Engl J Med. 2012;366(26):2455–65. PubMed PMID: 22658128. Pubmed Central PMCID: 3563263

106. Lutz ER, Kinkead H, Jaffee EM, Zheng L. Priming the pancreatic cancer tumor microenvironment for checkpoint-inhibitor immunotherapy. Oncoimmunology. 2014;3(11):e962401. PubMed PMID: 25941589. Pubmed Central PMCID: 4292514

107. Soares KC, Rucki AA, Wu AA, Olino K, Xiao Q, Chai Y, et al. PD-1/PD-L1 blockade together with vaccine therapy facilitates effector T-cell infiltration into pancreatic tumors. J Immunother. 2015;38(1):1–11. PubMed PMID: 25415283. Pubmed Central PMCID: 4258151

108. Duraiswamy J, Kaluza KM, Freeman GJ, Coukos G. Dual blockade of PD-1 and CTLA-4 combined with tumor vaccine effectively restores T-cell rejection function in tumors. Cancer Res. 2013;73(12):3591–603. PubMed PMID: 23633484. Pubmed Central PMCID: 3686913

109. Zamarin D, Holmgaard RB, Subudhi SK, Park JS, Mansour M, Palese P, et al. Localized oncolytic virotherapy overcomes systemic tumor resistance to immune checkpoint blockade immunotherapy. Sci Trans Med. 2014;6(226):226ra32. PubMed PMID: 24598590. Pubmed Central PMCID: 4106918

110. Arslan C, Yalcin S. Current and future systemic treatment options in metastatic pancreatic cancer. J Gastrointest Oncol. 2014;5(4):280–95. PubMed PMID: 25083302. Pubmed Central PMCID: 4110498

111. Bernstein MB, Krishnan S, Hodge JW, Chang JY. Immunotherapy and stereotactic ablative radiotherapy (ISABR): a curative approach? Nat Rev Clin Oncol. 2016;13:516–24. PubMed PMID: 26951040

112. Formenti SC, Demaria S. Combining radiotherapy and cancer immunotherapy: a paradigm shift. J Natl Cancer Inst. 2013;105(4):256–65. PubMed PMID: 23291374. Pubmed Central PMCID: 3576324

113. Lake RA, Robinson BW. Immunotherapy and chemotherapy—a practical partnership. Nat Rev Cancer. 2005;5(5):397–405. PubMed PMID: 15864281

Development of Hypoxia: Activated Cytotoxic Prodrug

Takuya Tsunoda

17.1 Tumor Microenvironment and Hypoxia

Hypoxia is defined as a level of oxygen below the physiologic level; physiologic range is different in different organs, due to differences in the blood vessel network [1]. There is specific circumstance in tumor, that of hypoxia, which is established by abnormal expansion of tumor cells and stromal microenvironment. Such tumor tissue is lower in oxygen compared with the normal tissue, and constitutes an oxygen-limited environment. Generally, the level of oxygen in the tissue is determined by the blood flow in that tissue. In tumor, many kinds of factors affect the tissue, the surrounding tumor and stromal cells, collectively referred to as the tumor microenvironment. Hypoxic conditions are developed during progression of cancer and stromal cells, due to rapidly proliferating tumor cells that reduce oxygen diffusion as well as impaired perfusion for the abnormal blood vessels in the tumor. The oxygen level in hypoxic tumor tissues is found to be less than 1.3% O_2, far below the physiologic oxygenation level (5–10% O_2) [2].

In molecular mechanism of hypoxia based on literature review, "prolyl hydroxylase domain (PHD) and factor-inhibiting hypoxia-inducible factor (HIF) 1 (FIH-1) enzymes regulate protein stabilization of HIF subunits (HIF1a, HIF2a, and HIF3a)". In normal cells, "subunits of HIFa might be hydroxylated by both PHD and FIH-1, poly-ubiquitinated and degraded by its proteasome" [3]. On the other hand, in hypoxia, "the PHD enzymes lose their activity and the degradation of the HIF is terminated. The stabilized, non-hydroxylated HIFa are believed to translocate to the nucleus, where constitutively they dimerize the expressed HIFb subunit, and fix to DNA to initiate gene transcription of the adaptive pathways" [4, 5].

T. Tsunoda
Department of Clinical Immuno Oncology, Clinical Research Institute for Clinical Pharmacology and Therapeutics, Showa University,
6-11-11, Kitakarasuyama, Setagaya-ku, Tokyo 157-8577, Japan
e-mail: ttsunoda@med.showa-u.ac.jp

© Springer Science+Business Media Singapore 2017
H. Yamaue (ed.), *Innovation of Diagnosis and Treatment for Pancreatic Cancer*,
DOI 10.1007/978-981-10-2486-3_17

The HIF family is reported to represent the main mediator of the hypoxic response and is upregulated in cancers abundantly. It has been demonstrated that the oxygen-regulated HIF isforms HIF-1α, and in some way HIF-2α, are related to the clinical efficacy of chemotherapy, and association with HIF function contains great promise to improve the efficacy of anticancer therapy. Another molecular mechanism in regard to hypoxia is the HIF-independent pathway, demonstrated by mammalian target of rapamycin kinase, in response to "endoplasmic reticulum stress, p38 MAPK, cyclooxygenase-2, inducible nitric oxide synthase, NF-kB, and alarmins". Hypoxia is clinically associated with "aggressive, invasive, and metastatic phenotypes that involve multiple mechanisms, including the promotion of genetic and epigenetic alternation, decrease of apoptosis, an exchange to glycolytic metabolism, up-regulation of survival factors, stimulation of angiogenic signals, induction of epithelial to mesenchymal transition, and preferential location of cancer stem cells to hypoxic regions" [6–10].

17.2 Pancreatic Cancer and Hypoxia

Pancreatic cancer is one of the worst prognosis of cancer, in which the 5-year survival rate is less than 5% in advanced stages and the median survival is only near 6 months in metastatic disease [11]. For anatomical reasons, pancreatic cancer is very difficult to diagnose at the early stage, and a typical specific symptomatic sign of pancreatic cancer is derived only from the advanced tumor. Only curative surgical resection of pancreatic cancer has cured some patients. Regarding advanced pancreatic cancer, chemotherapy is the main modality for patients. Radiotherapy is not as effective as chemotherapy as a monotherapy. Gemcitabine demonstrated an improvement in clinical benefit, antitumor response, and overall survival (OS). Combination chemotherapies with gemcitabine and erlotinib showed modest incremental improvements in OS compared with gemcitabine alone (6.24 v 5.91 months, respectively) [12]. The combination regimen of fluorouracil, leucovorin, oxaliplatin, and irinotecan (FOLFIRINOX) has been reported a notable advancement in the treatment of pancreatic cancer, demonstrating significant improvements in clinical outcome compared with gemcitabine alone (median progression-free survival [PFS], 6.4 v 3.3 months; and median OS, 11.1 v 6.8 months, respectively) [13]. Although pivotal clinical studies have not been performed yet and not many patients have been enrolled, this was the first phase III study to demonstrate an increase in OS of more than 2 months. However, FOLFIRINOX showed significantly higher hematologic and non-hematologic toxicities, including gastrointestinal toxicity and neuropathy, which strongly limits its applicability to patients. Recently, a phase III pivotal clinical trial comparing nanoparticle albumin-bound (nab)-paclitaxel plus gemcitabine with gemcitabine alone demonstrated significant improvement in survival (median PFS, 5.5 v 3.7 months; median OS, 8.5 v 6.7 months, respectively), positioning this combination as a current standard of care for gemcitabine-based chemotherapy against advanced pancreatic cancer [14]. The most common severe adverse events related with the combination were

Table 17.1 Hypoxia of various types of cancer

Tumor type	Tumor tissue median pO_2 mm Hg (patients)	Normal tissue median pO_2 mm Hg
Pancreas	2 (8 pts)	57
Brain	13 (104 pts)	26
Head and Neck	10 (592 pts)	n/a
Lung	16 (26 pts)	n/a
Breast	10 (212 pts)	52
Cervix	9 (730 pts)	42
Liver	6 (4 pts)	30
Sarcoma	14 (283 pts)	51
Melanoma	12 (18 pts)	41

Ref. [15]

neutropenia, fatigue, and neuropathy. In Japan, nanoparticle albumin-bound (nab)-paclitaxel plus gemcitabine is one of the most common regimens against advanced pancreatic cancer as a first-line chemotherapy. However, there are still only very limited modalities against advanced pancreatic cancer, and the clinical outcome remains far from satisfactory.

Tumor hypoxia is a routinely and generally observed phenotype derived from chemoresistance, causing major therapeutic difficulties. One of the common features of the microenvironment of many solid tumors is tumor hypoxia, or a low-oxygen condition [15]. In pancreatic cancer, the oxygen partial pressure (pO_2) of tumor tissue is 2 mmHg, compared with normal pancreas tissue with pO_2 of 57 mmHg. In sarcoma, tumor tissue pO_2 is 14 mmHg, compared with normal tissue pO_2 of 51 mmHg. In breast cancer, tumor tissue pO_2 is 10 mmHg, compared with normal breast tissue pO_2 of 52 mmHg (Table 17.1). Pancreatic cancer is one of the most hypoxic and low-oxygen cancer tissues because of its pathologically extremely massive desmoplastic stromal compartment. Many of the reviewed reports demonstrate that the magnitude and extent of tumor hypoxia are strongly associated with poor clinical prognosis. Advanced pancreatic cancers are desmoplastic and hypoxic, both of which might be related with poor prognosis.

17.3 Antitumor Drugs and Hypoxia

Chemotherapy failure comes from the three basic categories; inadequate pharmacokinetic properties of the drug tumor cell internal factors, expressed as drug efflux pumps and the extrinsic condition of the tumor cell microenvironment, including hypoxia, acidosis, nutrient starvation, and increased interstitial pressure. It is known that tumor hypoxia affects therapy outcome negatively. Hypoxia decreases tumor cell proliferation and promotes cell cycle arrest. Ultimately, hypoxia is derived from chemoresistance, because anticancer drugs predominantly target rapidly proliferating cells. When screening antiproliferative substances in vitro, this knowledge has been ignored, resulting in the failure of developing novel anticancer drugs in hypoxia condition in vivo. In tumors, large areas of hypoxic microenvironment often exist, and these are related to a poor prognosis. These regions of massive hypoxia in tumor are thought to be resistant to the treatment of chemotherapy and radiotherapy. Regarding traditional older types of chemotherapy, poor tissue penetration and targeting were due to a more rapid wash-out from regions of tumors, that are located to the tumor vascularity.

The critical unmet medical needs that exist with focus on hypoxic tumors and novel therapeutics, that selectively target hypoxic tumor cells, have to be developed clinically. Aggressive efforts of prodrugs, which are highly and selectively activated in hypoxic regions, began with the nitrobenzyl systems over a quarter century ago [16]. Recently, the hypoxia region activated prodrug, tirapazamine, is in a clinically advanced stage. Many different solid tumors have been investigated in phase III clinical trials of tirapazamine; however, the results have been disappointing due to poor tumor penetration and low in vivo potency at tolerated doses [17]. Hypoxia-activated phosphoramidate DNA cross-linking mustards were introduced by Borch et al. Among the most successful prodrugs were 5-nitrothiophene- and 5-nitrofuran-triggered prodrugs of phosphoramidate toxins. This active form was based on cyclophosphamide, a commonly used antitumor drug. Isophosphoramide mustard is the prodrug of ifosfamide, a clinically useful anticancer agent, and it is the cytotoxin generated from the cytochrome P450 activation. Its clinical efficacy has been proven in trials [18].

17.4   A Promising Prodrug

TH-302 (Threshold Pharmaceuticals, San Francisco) (1-methyl-2-nitro-1H-imidazole-5-yl) N, N0-bis (2-bromoethyl) diaminophosphate is defined as a 2-nitro-imidazole-linked prodrug of a brominated version of isophosphoramide mustard (Br-IPM) [19]. Bioreductive enzymes reduce one-electron from TH-302, thereby generating a free radical anion. Under aerobic conditions, these anions are reported to be restored to their original state, and are induced to the production of superoxide via redox cycling. TH-302 has shown almost no cytotoxic activity under normoxic conditions, and massively augmented cytotoxic activity under hypoxic conditions in terms of in vitro cytotoxicity and clonogenic assays using human cancer cell lines [16, 20]. Both nondividing and dividing cells are killed by a bis-alkylator, acting as a DNA cross-linking agent. "S139 phosphorylation of histone H2AX is thought to ultimately kill tumor cells, when the Br-IPM moiety is efficiently activated and induces intramolecular cross-linkage of DNA" [21–23]. TH-302 exhibited antitumor activity in a dose-dependent fashion and strongly correlated with total drug exposure. Association between its antitumor activity and tumor hypoxic conditions was found across 11 xenograft models. Animals with tumor breathing 95% O_2 showed a decrease of TH-302 efficacy, while on the other hand those breathing 10% O_2 showed significantly enhanced TH-302 efficacy, both compared with breathing of air (21% O_2). Treatment with TH-302 resulted in reduction in accordnace with the tumor hypoxic conditions and a related increase in the necrotic region. Interestingly, DNA damage introduced by TH-302 as measured by gH2AX was initially only observed in the hypoxic regions, and then expanded to the entire tumor in a time-dependent fashion. This evidence from preclinical experiments has strongly demonstrated a bystander effect of TH-302, which may be related to the diffusion of the active form to adjacent normoxic regions of tumor, and strongly indicated an additional and significant antitumor activity. Since TH-302 is preferentially activated in hypoxic tissues and does not have the same toxic metabolites as ifosfamide following hepatic metabolism, it is considered that TH-302 may show fewer drug-related adverse effects than ifosfamide. This hypothesis might be supported by the reversible skin and mucosal toxicities observed to be dose-limiting factors in a phase I clinical trial of HT-302 [24].

17.5 Clinical Development

Several clinical trials have been performed during last decades, in which the target molecule against hypoxia was HIF-1. A phase I clinical trial of topotecan, an FDA-approved semisynthetic camptothecin analogue, has been opened to patient enrollment. Topotecan is thus supposed to be the first HIF-1 inhibitor to be tried in humans. The second HIF-1 inhibitor likely to enter the clinic might be PX-478, from ProlX Pharmaceuticals in Tucson, Ariz; however, excellent clinical effect targeting hypoxia has not yet obtained for this drug. On the other hand, clinical trials of several prodrugs activated in hypoxia tissue have also been performed.

In particular, TH-302 has shown preclinically and clinically strong antitumor activity in a variety of solid tumors, including pancreatic cancer [22, 25, 26]. In a phase I/II clinical study against solid tumors, investigating TH-302 doses of 240–575 mg/m² on days 1, 8, and 15 of a 28-day cycle, the recommended phase II dose of the combination of gemcitabine with TH-302 was established as 340 mg/m². Dose-limiting hematologic and mucosal toxicities were more frequent at 340 than 240 mg/m². The overall response rate was 21%, and median PFS time was 5.9 months when observed in 46 patients with advanced pancreatic cancer [26]. To evaluate the benefit of combination TH-302 to gemcitabine, an open-label, multicenter, randomized phase II clinical trial was designed and conducted, as systemic therapy in patients with previously untreated advanced pancreatic cancer, as the standard of care at the time, namely first-line chemotherapy against advanced pancreatic cancer.

The randomized phase II study was performed at the 45 sites. A total of 214 subjects with advanced pancreatic cancer were enrolled and randomized to three groups: Gemcitabine (1000 mg/m²) alone, Gemcitabine + TH-302 (240 mg/m²), and Gemcitabine + TH-302 (340 mg/m²) group. Crossover was permitted from 240 to 340 mg/m² of TH-302 plus Gemcitabine. The primary end points were PFS and Safety. Secondary end points were response rate by RECIST 1.1; change in CA19-9

Table 17.2 Clinical response

Response	Gemcitabine alone No. of patients	%	G + T240 No. of patients	%	G + T340 No. of patients	%
Overall RR	8	12	12	17	19	26*
CR	0	0	0	0	2	3
PR	8	12	12	17	17	23
SD	38	55	41	58	37	50
DCR	46	67	53	75	56	76
PFS						
Median, months	3.6		5.6		6.9	
HR (vs G alone)			0.655		0.589	
OS						
Median, months	6.9		8.7		9.2	
6-month OS, %	577		69*		73**	
95% CI	44–67		57–78		61–82	
12-month OS, %	26		37*		38*	
95% CI	16–37		26–48		27–49	

$*p < 0.05$, $**p < 0.2$

including CA19-9 response (>50% decrease); and overall survival. Table 17.2 shows the clinical effect of this phase II trial [11]. Median of PFS values in this trail were as follows: Gemcitabine alone group, 3.6 months ($N = 69$); Gemcitabine + TH-302 240 mg/m^2 group, 5.6 months ($N = 71$); and Gemcitabine + TH-302 340 mg/m^2 group, 6.9 months ($N = 74$). Hazard ratio (HR) vs Gemcitabine alone group was 0.655 (95% CI: 0.46–1.02) and $p = 0.060$ (Log-rank test) in Gemcitabine + TH302 240 mg/m^2 group, and 0.589 (95% CI: 0.4–0.88), $p = 0.008$ (Log-rank test) in Gemcitabine + TH302 340 mg/m^2 group, respectively. RECIST best response was as follows: CR and PR in Gemcitabine alone group were 0% and 12% in Gemcitabine + TH-302 240 mg/m^2 group were 0% and 17% and in Gemcitabine + TH-302 340 mg/m^2 group were 3% and 23%, respectively. P-value of Gemcitabine + TH302 240 mg/m^2 vs Gemcitabine alone was 0.22, and that of Gemcitabine + TH302 340 mg/m^2 vs Gemcitabine alone was 0.021. Maximum decrease and response of CA19–9 was as follows: mean nadir change (U/L) in CA19–9, Gemcitabine alone group, −523; Gemcitabine + TH302 240 mg/m^2 group, −3909; and Gemcitabine + TH302 340 mg/m^2 group, −5385. Percent CA 19–9 Decrease >90% was as follows: Gemcitabine alone group, 16%; Gemcitabine + TH302 240 mg/m^2 group, 24%; and Gemcitabine + TH302 340 mg/m^2 group, 32%. Median OS was as follows: Gemcitabine alone group, 6.9 months; Gemcitabine + TH302 240 mg/m^2 group, 8.7 months; and Gemcitabine + TH302 340 mg/m^2 group, 9.2 months. HR of TH302 240 mg/m^2 group vs Gemcitabine alone group was 0.960 (95% CI: 0.67–1.38) and $p = 0.827$ (Log-rank test), and that of TH302 340 mg/m^2 group vs Gemcitabine alone group was 0.955 (95% CI: 0.67–01.37) and $p = 0.800$ (Log-rank test). Survival at 6 and 12 months by treatment arm was as follows: 6-month survival of Gemcitabine alone group, Gemcitabine + TH302 240 mg/m^2 group, and

Gemcitabine + TH302 340 mg/m^2 group were 57%, 69%, and 73%, respectively. P-value of Gemcitabine + TH302 240 mg/m^2 group vs Gemcitabine alone group was 0.123, and that of Gemcitabine + TH302 340 mg/m^2 group vs Gemcitabine alone group was 0.037. Moreover, 12-month survival of Gemcitabine alone group, Gemcitabine + TH302 240 mg/m^2 group, and Gemcitabine + TH302 340 mg/m^2 group were 26%, 37%, and 38%, respectively. P-value of Gemcitabine + TH302 240 mg/m^2 group vs Gemcitabine alone group was 0.178, and that of Gemcitabine + TH302 340 mg/m^2 group vs Gemcitabine alone group was 0.130. Longer survival after crossover randomization was achieved from 2.6 months to 13.4 months [11]. In terms of safety, there was a decrease in study discontinuations due to AEs from 16% to 12%, in Gemcitabine alone group as compared with Gemcitabine + TH302 340 mg/m^2 group, respectively. In summary it was strongly expected that clinical efficacy would be promising and it showed strong signals for clinical benefits [11].

17.6   Pivotal Clinical Trial Against Pancreatic Cancer

After this randomized phase II clinical trial, a pivotal phase III clinical trial (MAESTRO Trial) was performed. However, despite encouraging signals regarding evofosfamide (TH-302) activity from prior studies, the hypoxia-activated prodrug failed to significantly improve overall survival (OS) when combined with gemcitabine in previously untreated patients with unresectable locally advanced or metastatic pancreatic cancer in the randomized phase III MAESTRO trial when announced in January, 2016.

To closely evaluate this study, the international, randomized, double-blind, placebo-controlled MAESTRO trial was conducted in 693 patients with unresectable locally advanced or metastatic pancreatic cancer to compare evofosfamide (TH-302)/gemcitabine with a control arm of placebo/gemcitabine. Patients could not enter the trial if they had received prior chemotherapy or systemic therapy (other than radiosensitizing doses of 5-fluorouracil or gemcitabine) within 6 months of study entry. At the end of the trial, OS—the primary endpoint—revealed a negative result, meaning that there was no statistically significantly increase (Table 17.3). Median OS was statistically similar between the two arms at 8.7 months with evofosfamide (TH-302)/gemcitabine and 7.6 months with placebo/gemcitabine (hazard ratio [HR] 0.84, 95% CI [0.71, 1.01]; $p = 0.059$), narrowly and closely missing the mark of significance. No difference in OS between the two arms was evident across any patient subgroups, except for Asian patients. Among this group of 123 individuals, median OS reached 12.0 months with evofosfamide (HT-302)/gemcitabine versus 8.5 months with placebo/gemcitabine (HR 0.58, 95% CI [0.36, 0.93]). Dr. Van Cutsem, the Principal Investigator of this trial, suggested that the disappointing OS results may have occurred becuase (1) placebo arm performed better than the initial assumptions, and (2) second-line therapy following disease progression was also slightly increased in the control arm compared with the experimental arm, particularly for FOLFIRINOX, FOLFOX, and gemcitabine/nab-paclitaxel regimens

Table 17.3 MAESTRO trial

	Pla/Gem	Evo (340 mg/m^2)/Gem
ITT Population	($n = 347$)	($n = 346$)
Median OS, months (95% CI)	7.6 (6.7, 8.3)	8.7 (7.6, 9.9)
	HR: 0.84 (95% CI 0.71, 1.01)	
	$P = 0.0589$	
Median OS, months (95% CI)	12	8.5
(Asian population, $n = 123$)	0.58, 95% CI (0.36, 0.93)	
Median PFS, months (95% CI)	3.7 (3.6, 3.8)	5.5 (4.8, 5.6)
	HR: 0.77 (95% CI 0.65, 0.92)	
	$p = 0.004$	
ORR, %	8.6	15.2
	OR: 1.90 (95% CI 1.16, 3.12)	
	$p = 0.0086$	

Refs. [27, 28]

(23.1% vs. 16.4%). Despite the lack of a survival benefit, there were promising signals for antitumor activity for combination of evofosfamide (TH-302)/gemcitabine in regard to PFS and objective response rate (ORR). Median PFS was significantly improved with the combination of gemcitabine and evofosfamide (TH-302) compared with gemcitabine alone (5.5 months vs. 3.7 months; HR 0.77, 95% CI [0.65, 0.92]; $p = 0.004$), and a significant improvement was noted in objective response rate (15.2% vs. 8.6%; odds ratio 1.90, 95% CI [1.16, 3.12]; $p = 0.0086$). There was not a big difference in safety profile of evofosfamide (TH-302) in MAESTRO when compared to other evofosfamide (TH-302) clinical trials. The combination of evofosfamide (TH-302) with gemcitabine, as compared with gemcitabine alone, was noted to have more treatment-related adverse effect [27].

Bertram Wiedenmann, M.D, Ph.D., of the Charité University Hospital, in Berlin, mentioned that despite the disappointing results from MAESTRO, "evofosfamide (TH-302) might have some potential for future development", and there might be potential to use evofosfamide (TH-302) "in the adjuvant setting or even as an induction therapy prior to radiation therapy" [28]. Some meaningful signal of hypoxia-activated drug against advanced pancreatic cancer has been seen from this clinical trial. It may not be far from obtaining the efficacy drug against hypoxic cancer like pancreatic cancer.

References

1. Krock BL, Skuli N, Simon MC. Hypoxia-induced angiogenesis: good and evil. Genes Cancer. 2011;2:1117–33.
2. Bertout JA, Patel SA, Simon MC. The impact of O2 availability on human cancer. Nat Rev Cancer. 2008;8:967–75.
3. Muz B, de la Puente P, Azab F, Luderer M, Azab AK. The role of hypoxia and exploitation of the hypoxic environment in hematologic malignancies. Mol Cancer Res. 2014;12:1347–54.

4. Semenza GL, Wang GL. A nuclear factor induced by hypoxia via denovo protein synthesis binds to the human erythropoietin gene enhancer at a site required for transcriptional activation. Mol Cell Biol. 1992;12:5447–54.

5. Bruick RK, McKnight SL. A conserved family of prolyl-4-hydroxylases that modify HIF. Science. 2001;294:1337–40.

6. Wouters BG, Koritzinsky M. Hypoxia signaling through mTOR and the unfolded protein response in cancer. Nat Rev Cancer. 2008;8:851–64.

7. Sanchez A, Tripathy D, Yin X, Desobry K, Martinez J, Riley J, et al. p38 MAPK: a mediator of hypoxia-induced cerebrovascular inflammation. J Alzheimers Dis. 2012;32:587–97.

8. Cummins EP, Berra E, Comerford KM, Ginouves A, Fitzgerald KT, Seeballuck F, et al. Prolyl hydroxylase-1 negatively regulates IkappaB kinase-beta, giving insight into hypoxia-induced NFkappaB activity. Proc Natl Acad Sci U S A. 2006;103:18154–9.

9. Tafani M, Schito L, Pellegrini L, Villanova L, Marfe G, Anwar T, et al. Hypoxia-increased RAGE and P2x7R expression regulates tumor cell invasion through phosphorylation of Erk1/2 and Akt and nuclear translocation of NF-{kappa}B. Carcinogenesis. 2011;32:1167–75.

10. Sun JD, Liu Q, Ahluwalia D, Li W, Meng F, Wang Y, Bhupathi D, Ruprell AS, Hart CP. Efficacy and safety of the hypoxia-activated prodrug TH-302 in combination with gemcitabine and nab-paclitaxel in human tumor xenograft models of pancreatic cancer. Cancer Biol Ther. 2015;16:438–49.

11. Borad MJ, Reddy SG, Bahary N, Uronis HE, Sigal D, Cohn AL, Schelman WR, Stephenson Jr J, Chiorean EG, Rosen PJ, Ulrich B, Dragovich T, Del Prete SA, Rarick M, Eng C, Kroll S, Ryan DP. Randomized phase II trial of gemcitabine plus TH-302 versus gemcitabine in patients with advanced pancreatic cancer. J Clin Oncol. 2015;33:1475–81.

12. Moore MJ, Goldstein D, Hamm J, et al. Erlotinib plus gemcitabine compared with gemcitabine alone in patients with advanced pancreatic cancer: a phase III trial of the National cancer institute of Canada clinical trials group. J Clin Oncol. 2007;25:1960–6.

13. Conroy T, Desseigne F, Ychou M, et al. FOLFIRINOX versus gemcitabine for metastatic pancreatic cancer. N Engl J Med. 2011;364:1817–25.

14. Von Hoff DD, Ervin T, Arena FP, et al. Increased survival in pancreatic cancer with nabpaclitaxel plus gemcitabine. N Engl J Med. 2013;369:1691–703.

15. Vaupel P, Höckel M, Mayer A. Detection and characterization of tumor hypoxia using pO2 histography. Antioxid Redox Signal. 2007;9:1221–35.

16. Duan J-X, Jiao H, Kaizerman J, Stanton T, Evans JW, Lan L, Lorente G, Banica M, Jung D, Wang J, Ma H, Li X, Yang Z, Hoffman RM, Ammons WS, Hart CP, Matteucci M. Potent and highly selective hypoxia-activated achiral phosphoramidate mustards as anticancer drugs. J Med Chem. 2008;51:2412–20.

17. Gandara DR, Lara Jr PN, Goldberg Z, Le QT, Mack PC, Lau DH, Gumerlock PH. Tirapazamine: prototype for a novel class of therapeutic agents targeting tumor hypoxia. Semin Oncol. 2002;29:102–9.

18. Zhang J, Tian Q, Yung Chan S, Chuen Li S, Zhou S, Duan W, Zhu YZ. Metabolism and transport of oxazaphosphorines and the clinical implications. Drug Metab Rev. 2005;37:611–703.

19. Sun JD, Liu Q, Wang J, Ahluwalia D, Ferraro D, Wang Y, Duan J-X, Ammons WS, Curd JG, Matteucci MD, Hart CP. Selective tumor hypoxia targeting by hypoxia-activated Prodrug TH-302 inhibits tumor growth in preclinical models of cancer. Clin Cancer Res. 2014;18:758–70.

20. Hu J, Handisides DR, Van Valckenborgh E, De Raeve H, Menu E, Vande Broek I, et al. Targeting the multiple myeloma hypoxic niche with TH-302, a hypoxia-activated prodrug. Blood. 2010;116:1524–7.

21. Takakusagi Y, Matsumoto S, Saito K, Matsuo M, Kishimoto S, Wojtkowiak JW, DeGraff W, Kesarwala AH, Choudhuri R, Devasahayam N, Subramanian S, Munasinghe JP, Gillies RJ, Mitchell JB, Hart CP, Krishna MC. Pyruvate induces transient tumor hypoxia by enhancing mitochondrial oxygen consumption and potentiates the anti-tumor effect of a hypoxia-activated prodrug TH-302. PLoS One. 2014;9(9):e107995.

22. Sun JD, Liu Q, Wang J, Ahluwalia D, Ferraro D, et al. Selective tumor hypoxia targeting by hypoxia-activated prodrug TH-302 inhibits tumor growth in preclinical models of cancer. Clin Cancer Res. 2012;18:758–70.
23. Meng F, Evans JW, Bhupathi D, Banica M, Lan L, et al. Molecular and cellular pharmacology of the hypoxia-activated prodrug TH-302. Mol Cancer Ther. 2012;11:740–51.
24. Weiss GJ, Infante JR, Chiorean EG, Borad MJ, Bendell JC, Molina JR, Tibes R, Ramanathan RK, Lewandowski K, Jones SF, Lacouture ME, Langmuir VK, Lee H, Kroll S, Burris III HA. Phase 1 study of the safety, tolerability, and pharmacokinetics of TH-302, a hypoxia-activated prodrug, in patients with advanced solid malignancies. Clin Cancer Res. 2011;17:2997–3004.
25. Liu Q, Sun JD, Wang J, et al. TH-302, a hypoxia-activated prodrug with broad in vivo preclinical combination therapy efficacy: optimization of dosing regimens and schedules. Cancer Chemother Pharmacol. 2012;69:1487–98.
26. Borad MJ, Chiorean EG, Molina JR, et al. Clinical benefits TH-302, a tumor-selective, hypoxiaactivated prodrug, and gemcitabine in first-line pancreatic cancer (PanC). J Clin Oncol. 2011;29 (suppl 4; abstr 265).
27. Van Cutsem E, Lenz H-J, et al. MAESTRO: a randomized, double-blind phase III study of evofosfamide (Evo) in combination with gemcitabine (Gem) in previously untreated patients (pts) with metastatic or locally advanced unresectable pancreatic ductal adenocarcinoma (PDAC). J Clin Oncol. 2016;34:(suppl; abstr 4007).
28. ASCO-GI 2016, San Francisco.

The Potential of Oncolytic Virus Therapy for Pancreatic Cancer

Hideki Kasuya

18.1 Introduction

Oncolytic viruses belong to a new category of biological anticancer drugs. Oncolytic viruses infect and replicate in cancer cells, which results in direct tumor lysis and viral spread to neighboring cancer cells without any severe adverse damage to normal tissue. Besides this direct cell-killing effect, it is also a type of cancer immune therapy, in situ vaccination. In October 2015, an oncolytic herpes simplex virus type-1 (HSV-1), talimogene laherparepvec (T-VEC, IMLYGIC™), was approved as a new therapy in the United States by the Food and Drug Administration (FDA). An oncolytic viral therapy is not just a dream of a few physician-scientists. It has become a real new biological therapy. We have studied the oncolytic HSV-1 for treating pancreatic cancer for over 20 years, starting in 1996. Now, we will look at the current state of development of oncolytic viruses for the treatment of pancreatic cancer based on our clinical experiences.

18.2 Biological Properties of Viruses and Selectivity for Cancer Cells

In general, each virus has tropism for a specific type of organ or tissue. For example, adenoviruses prefer to infect respiratory cells, and herpes viruses prefer to infect neurons. HF10 is an attenuated spontaneous mutant of HSV-1, which was originally established at Nagoya University. HF10 differs from wild-type HSV-1 by a 3832 base pair (bp) deletion of the *UL56* gene, which is associated with a lack of neuro-invasiveness and is believed to result in attenuation of its pathogenicity and

H. Kasuya
Cancer Immune Therapy Research Center, Nagoya University Graduate School of Medicine, 65 Tsurumai-cho, Showa-ku, Nagoya, Aichi 466-8550, Japan
e-mail: Kasuya@med.nagoya-u.ac.jp

© Springer Science+Business Media Singapore 2017
H. Yamaue (ed.), *Innovation of Diagnosis and Treatment for Pancreatic Cancer*,
DOI 10.1007/978-981-10-2486-3_18

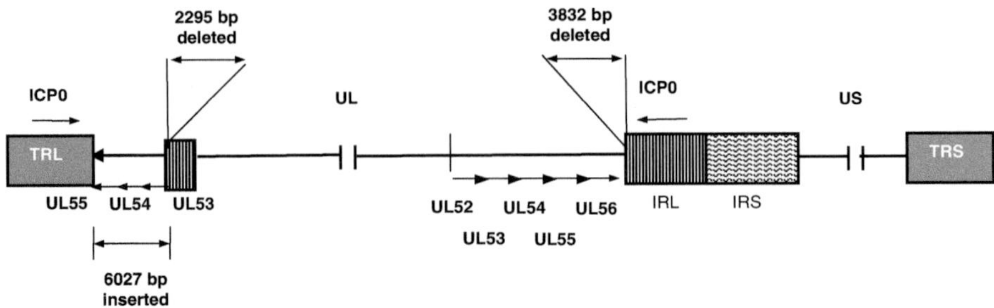

Fig. 18.1 HF10 structure

neurovirulence compared with wild-type HSV-1. It also has an additional 2295 bp deletion and genetic rearrangement. It has not been modified by genetic engineering technique and contains no external genes (Fig. 18.1). It is well known that normal cells produce interferon which activates protective antiviral signalling in surrounding cells, and replication pathway is inhibited, and then surrounding normal cells survive. On the other hand, cancer cells support viral replication due to weak response of interferon and overexpression of replication pathways such as Ras at antiviral signalling pathways including PKR. Therefore, surrounding cancer cells are susceptible to cell death after viral infection. HF10 can show the tumor selectivity by using this difference between normal cells and cancer cells.

Gene deletion and insertion of promoters are techniques for modifying viral characteristics in order to increase their selectivity for cancer cells. ONXY-015, a replication-competent oncolytic adenovirus, was used in the first clinical trial for pancreatic cancer [1, 2]. It has been engineered to lack the *E1B* gene that codes for a 55 kDa protein that binds to tumor suppressor p53 in normal cells and causes progression of the cell cycle and viral replication [3, 4]. *E1B*-deleted viruses do not generally replicate in normal cells. Since approximately 50–75% of pancreatic tumors lack normal p53, *E1B*-deleted viruses can replicate in pancreatic cancer cells.

There is another way to enhance replication and oncolysis of tumor cells. A gene that is regulated by tumor-specific promoters is affected in the case of double or triple mutation viruses that complement the gene and activate mutated gene, similar to single-mutation viruses, but only in target tumors. The mutated HSV-1 virus Myb34.5 has a double-mutation locus that comprises both ICP34.5 and ICP6. The *β*-Myb promoter regulates ICP34.5 (*γ*34.5) at the ICP6 locus. Thus, the *β*-Myb promoter complements the deficient *γ*34.5 gene only in tumor cells [5]. Studies of carcinoembryonic antigen (CEA) [6], Muc-1 [7], ERBB2, amylase, and insulin show that they might be suitable as promoters of an oncolytic virus for the treatment of pancreatic cancer. An upcoming study of a mutated virus using a suitable promoter for pancreatic cancer will show that it resembles the albumin promoter-regulated replication-competent herpes virus against hepatoma 80, or the Muc1 promoter-regulated replication-competent herpes virus against pancreatic cancer [8].

18.3 Dual Mechanism of Action: Local and Systemic Immune Effects

Oncolytic viruses can induce T cell-mediated tumor immunity and cause regression of distant metastases [9–11]. For tumor regression, CD8-positive T cells and NK cells are required because depletion of these cell types has been shown to abolish the antitumor ability of oncolytic viruses. Thus, in addition to their proven efficacy against a variety of tumors through a direct cytotoxic effect, these viruses can activate innate or adaptive tumor immunity, or both [12–15]. In particular, fusion type virus is a strong stimulus for host immunity against tumor antigens. These types of viruses make tumor cell membranes fuse and strongly express tumor cell antigens to antigen-presenting cells. Their effect might be due to changing cell surface characteristics of receptors and ligands, including immune suppressor such as PD-L1.

18.4 HF10 Monotherapy in Eight Patients with Pancreatic Cancer

In 2005, we started a phase I clinical trial of HF10 in patients with pancreatic cancer. The study consists of two stages. The first stage is for three intratumoral injections of HF10, and the second one is for six injections. (Fig. 18.2) The objectives were to evaluate the safety and tolerability in patients with pancreatic cancer. We also examined the tumor response as well as the extent of lymphocyte infiltration induced by viral infection.

In the first stage, six patients with unresectable pancreatic cancer were enrolled. The first two patients received the intratumoral injections of 1×10^5 pfu on three consecutive days (once intraoperatively and twice postoperatively), followed by the next four patients with the dose escalation up to 1×10^6 pfu. All patients were monitored

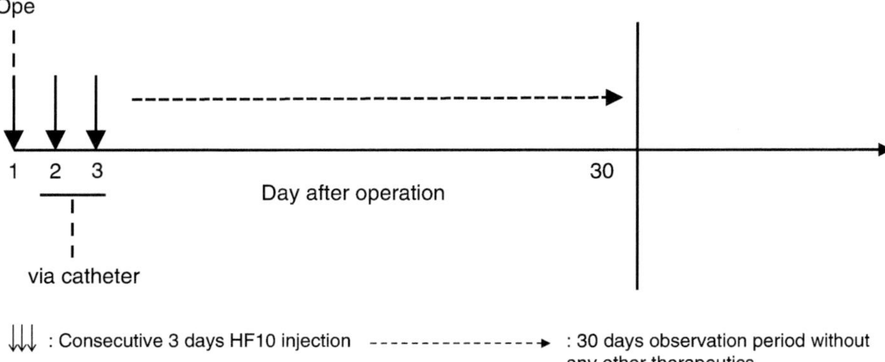

Fig. 18.2 Design of clinical trial for pancreatic cancer. *Three down arrows* consecutive 3 days HF10 injection, *long dashed right arrow* 30 days observation period without any other therapeutics

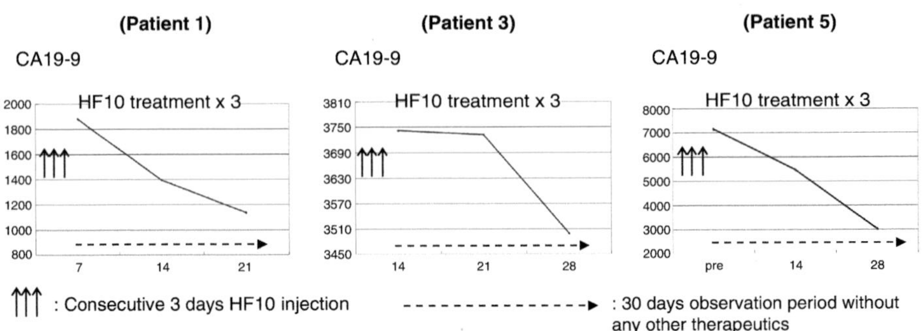

Fig. 18.3 Pancreatic cancer tumor marker movement. *Three up arrows* consecutive 3 days HF10 injection, *long dashed right arrow* 30 days observation period without any other therapeutics

for adverse effects and efficacy without other additional therapy for 30 days. No treatment-related adverse event was observed in the six patients. The tumor responses were classified as SD in three patients, PR in one patient, and PD in two patients. We also examined the infiltration of CD4 and CD8 cells into tumors with immunostaining. Tumors injected with HF10 had much greater infiltration of CD8 cells than resected tumor specimens that did not receive intraoperative HF10 injection with statistically significant differences. There was more CD4 cells infiltration into treated specimens than in control specimens, but this difference was not statistically significant [16]. The number of NK cells in the peripheral blood increased after injection of virus. Antigen-presenting cells and macrophages were also examined by immunostaining. Macrophages infiltrated the tumor site to a greater extent than in resected specimens that served as control tissue. After only three injections against pancreatic cancer, the CA19-9 levels of Patients 1, 3, and 8 were controlled, and decreased without any other therapy during the 30-day observation period (Fig. 18.3).

During the first stage, we learned that there were some difficulties in the continuous injections through a catheter. Therefore, we developed a new methodology using endoscopy to reach to the pancreatic tumor through the duodenum or gastric wall. It is generally accepted that endoscopic ultrasound (EUS) is useful modality for directly reaching pancreatic tumors with minimal invasiveness. By using the EUS under ultrasound guidance, we were able to directly inject HF10 to the tumor site located in pancreas. In the second stage, two patients were enrolled (Patients 7 and 8). The patients received the three injections by the same route as the first stage + additional three injections via EUS, in a total of six injections. The dose of two patients was 10^6 pfu/1.0 mL weekly for 3 weeks. The treatment period was thus 4 weeks. None of two showed any treatment-related adverse event. The tumor responses of both patients were PD. Despite the progression, the levels of CA19-9 of the patients were stabilized during the treatment without any other therapy although CA19-9 levels increased again after the treatment (Fig. 18.4).

According to the Choi criteria (modified RECIST criteria), the tumors in Patients 1, 4, 7, and 8 were classified as PD; those in Patients 2, 3, and 6 as SD; and that in Patient 5 as PR. The disease stability (PR + SD) was 50%. In Patient 6, tumor size did not change for more than 80 days after injection therapy, as determined by

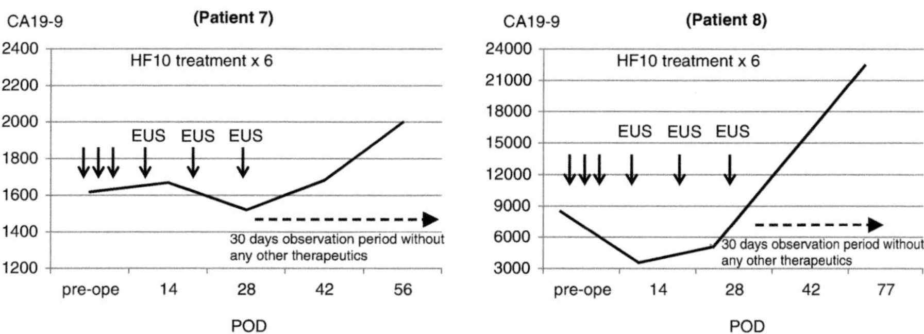

Fig. 18.4 Pancreatic cancer tumor marker movement including EUS method

Table 18.1 Non-resectable pancreatic cancer patient profiles

Patient no.	Age	CHOI	Gender	Contents (pfu) × Time	Histopathology	Toxicity	Non-resectable cause	Survival	Chemo 1 M later
1	68	PD	Male	$1 \times 10^5 \times 3$	Invasive ductal carcinoma	(−)	P, S	200 days	Gem
2	61	SD	Male	$1 \times 10^5 \times 3$	Invasive ductal carcinoma	(−)	P	166 days	Gem
3	60	SD	Male	$5 \times 10^5 \times 3$	Invasive ductal carcinoma	(−)	L	318 days	Gem
4	52	PD	Male	$1 \times 10^6 \times 3$	Invasive ductal carcinoma	(−)	L	98 days	−
5	73	PR	Male	$1 \times 10^6 \times 3$	Invasive ductal carcinoma	(−)	L	209 days	TS-1
6	76	SD	Male	$1 \times 10^6 \times 3$	Invasive ductal carcinoma	(−)	P, C	315 days	−
7	49	PD	Male	$1 \times 10^6 \times 6$	Invasive ductal carcinoma	(−)	L	206 days	Gem
8	64	PD	Male	$1 \times 10^6 \times 6$	Invasive ductal carcinoma	(−)	P	113 days	−

P peritoneal dissemination, *S* superior mesenteric artery invasion, *C* common hepatic artery invasion, *L* liver metastasis

radiography; this patient did not receive any treatment other than HF10 injection, due to anorexia. These patients survived longer than those who underwent ordinary bypass surgery (cholangiojejunostomy or gastrojejunostomy) for non-resectable pancreatic cancer at our institution in the period, and the median OS was 203 days (6.8 months). In patients with pancreatic cancer who received six injections of HF10, CA19-9 levels immediately increased after the end of treatment although they were suppressed during treatment. We hypothesize that multiple cytokines related to immune response and inflammation promote tumor angiogenesis after treatment. Several oncolytic HSV-1 researchers have reported a relationship between tumor angiogenesis and oncolytic HSV-1 injection [17, 18]. It might be a cause for rapid increases in CA19-9 during the observation period (Table 18.1).

18.5 HF10 Combination Therapy with Erlotinib and GEM Against Pancreatic Cancer in Nine Patients

Recently, combination therapy that includes an oncolytic virus and conventional chemotherapy has been reported to be a promising treatment strategy for advanced cancers [19–22]. In 2013, we initiated a clinical trial of HF10 in combination with conventional anticancer therapy in Japan.

Prior to the clinical trial, we conducted the nonclinical pharmacology study of HF10 in combination with erlotinib, an epidermal growth factor receptor tyrosine kinase inhibitor, using a mouse model bearing human pancreatic cancer cell lines (BxPC-3 and PANC-1) [23]. HF10 was also evaluated in combination with gemcitabine, using a mouse colon cancer (CT26) model [24]. After we evaluated the effect of erlotinib and gemcitabine plus HF10 in a mouse model, we started a clinical trial of HF10 in combination with erlotinib and gemcitabine against locally advanced unresectable pancreatic cancer, following the approval from the institutional review board/ethics committee of Nagoya University Hospital. In this trial, ten patients were enrolled, and 9 of 10 were evaluable. The acceptable safety and encouraging efficacy data were observed so far. The final results will be presented somewhere in the near future.

On the other hand, abraxane (nab-paclitaxel) was approved as the treatment for late-stage pancreatic cancer and is likely accepted as the standard-of-care. Taking the treatment trend into consideration, we are planning to further investigate the HF10 combination therapy. In any combination therapies, the balance between adverse effects and efficacy might be implicated (Fig. 18.5).

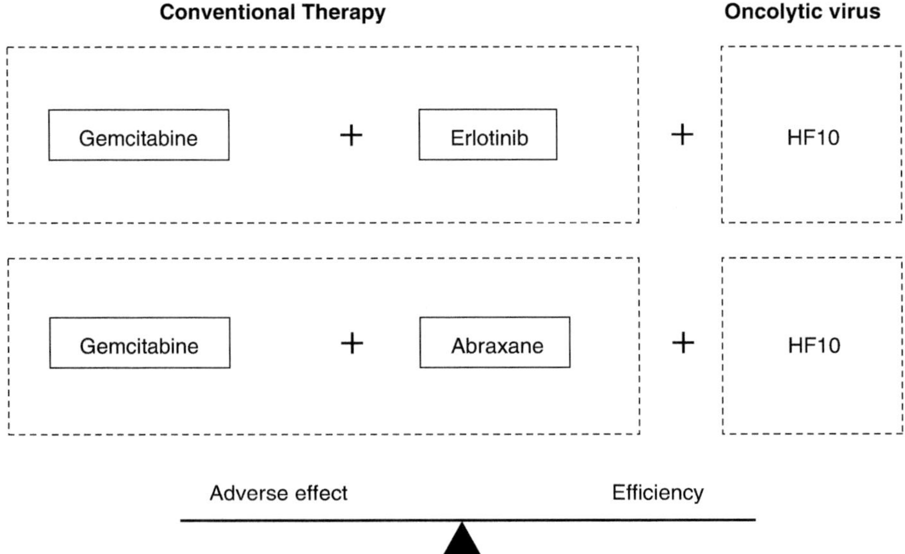

Fig. 18.5 Combination therapy against pancreatic cancer

18.6   Conclusion and Possibilities for Oncolytic Viruses

We are convinced that oncolytic virus therapy including HF10 is a promising new biological drug for solid tumors. Many promising studies have been published in academic journals and commercial news sources. Recently, a large pharmaceutical company has invested big fundamental background to this field. For example, AstraZeneca announced that MedImmune, its global biologics research and development arm, has entered into a licensing agreement with Omnis Pharmaceuticals (Omnis), a privately held biotechnology company focused on the development of oncolytic viruses. This agreement will allow MedImmune to combine key agents from its investigational immunotherapy portfolio with Omnis' lead investigational oncolytic virus, a genetically engineered vesicular stomatitis virus (VSV). The program is currently being studied in a phase I clinical trial as for hepatocellular carcinoma and other cancers with liver metastasis.

In October 2015, Amgen received approval from the FDA for talimogene laherparepvec (IMLYGIC™). In December 2015, the European commission approved talimogene laherparepvec (IMLYGIC™) for the treatment of adults with unresectable melanoma with regional or metastasis (Stage IIIB, IIIC, or IVM1a disease) with no bone, brain, lung, or other visceral organ involvement. Talimogene laherparepvec (IMLYGIC™) has become the first world class of novel agents known as oncolytic immunotherapeutics, and launched in the UK in March 2016. It has been now available to registered users.

Oncolytic viruses will soon be constituted a major type of therapeutic agent in the treatment of solid tumors in the world. Knowledge in this field will continue to grow for many types of tumors, including pancreatic cancer.

References

1. Mulvihill S, Warren R, Venook A, et al. Safety and feasibility of injection with an E1B-55 kDa gene-deleted,replication-selective adenovirus (ONYX-015) into primary carcinomas of the pancreas: a phase I trial. Gene Ther. 2001;8(4):308–15.
2. Hecht JR, Bedford R, Abbruzzese JL, et al. A phase I/II trial of intratumoral endoscopic ultrasound injection of ONYX-015 with intravenous gemcitabine in unresectable pancreatic carcinoma. Clin Cancer Res. 2003;9(2):555–61.
3. Heise C, Lemmon M, Kirn D. Efficacywithareplication- selective adenovirus plus cisplatin-based chemotherapy: dependence on sequencing but not p53 functional status or route of administration. Clin Cancer Res. 2000;6:4908–14.
4. Habib NA, Sarraf CE, Mitry RR, et al. E1B-deleted adenovirus (dl1520) gene therapy for patients with primary and secondary liver tumors. Hum Gene Ther. 2001;12:219–26.
5. Chung RY, Saeki Y, Chiocca EA. B-myb promoter retargeting of herpes simplex virus gamma34.5 gene-mediated virulence toward tumor and cycling cells. J Virol. 1999;73:7556–64.
6. Mullen JT, Kasuya H, Yoon SS, et al. Regulation of herpes simplex virus 1 replication using tumor-associated promoters. Ann Surg. 2002;236:502–12.
7. Kasuya H, Pawlik TM, Mullen JT, et al. Selectivity of an oncolytic herpes simplex virus for cells expressing the DF3/ MUC1 antigen. Cancer Res. 2004;64:2561–7.
8. Kurihara T, Brough DE, Kovesdi I, et al. Selectivity of a replication-competent adenovirus for human breast carcinoma cells expressing the MUC1 antigen. J Clin Invest. 2000;106:763–71.

9. Sahin TT, Kasuya H, Nomura N, et al. Impact of novel oncolytic virus HF10 on cellular components of the tumor microenviroment in patients with recurrent breast cancer. Cancer Gene Ther. 2012;19:229–37.

10. Takakuwa H, Goshima F, Nozawa N, et al. Oncolytic viral therapy using a spontaneously generated herpes simplex virus type 1 variant for disseminated peritoneal tumor in immunocompetent mice. Arch Virol. 2003;148:813–25.

11. Carroll NM, Chiocca EA, Takahashi K, Tanabe KK. Enhancement of gene therapy specificity for diffuse colon carcinoma liver metastases with recombinant herpes simplex virus. Ann Surg. 1996;224:323–9.

12. Nomura N, Kasuya H, Watanabe I, et al. Considerations for intravascular administration of oncolytic herpes virus for the treatment of multiple liver metastases. Cancer Chemother Pharmacol. 2009;63:321–30.

13. Todo T, Rabkin SD, Sundaresan P, et al. Systemic antitumor immunity in experimental brain tumor therapy using a multimutated, replication-competent herpes simplex virus. Hum Gene Ther. 1999;10:2741–55.

14. Miller CG, Fraser NW. Requirement of an integrated immune response for successful neuroattenuated HSV-1 therapy in an intracranial metastatic melanoma model. Mol Ther. 2003;7:741–7.

15. Thomas DL, Fraser NW. HSV-1 therapy of primary tumors reduces the number of metastases in an immune-competent model of metastatic breast cancer. Mol Ther. 2003;8:543–51.

16. Nakao A, Kasuya H, Sahin TT, et al. A phase I dose-escalation clinical trial of intraoperative direct intratumoralinjection of HF10 oncolytic virus in non-resectable patients with advanced pancreatic cancer. Cancer Gene Ther. 2011;18(3):167–75.

17. Kanai R, Rabkin SD. Combinatorial strategies for oncolytic herpes simplex virus therapy of brain tumors. CNS Oncol. 2013;2:129–42.

18. Kaufmann JK, Bossow S, Grossardt C, et al. Chemovirotherapy of malignant melanoma with a targeted and armed oncolytic measles virus. J Invest Dermatol. 2013;133:1034–42.

19. Watanabe I, Kasuya H, Nomura N, et al. Effects of tumor selective replication competent herpes viruses in combination with gemcitabine on pancreatic cancer. Cancer Chemother Pharmacol. 2008;61:875–82.

20. Tysome JR, Lemoine NR, Wang Y. Combination of antiangiogenic therapy and virotherapy: arming oncolytic viruses with antiangiogenic genes. Curr Opin Mol Ther. 2009;11:664–9.

21. Ottolino-Perry K, Diallo JS, Lichty BD, et al. Intelligent design: combination therapy with oncolytic viruses. Mol Ther. 2010;18:251–63.

22. Cheng PH, Lian S, Zhao R, et al. Combination of autophagy inducer rapamycin and oncolytic adenovirus improves antitumor effect in cancer cells. Virol J. 2013;10:293.

23. Yamamura K, Kasuya H, Sahin TT, et al. Combination treatment of human pancreatic cancer xenograft models with the epidermal growth factor receptor tyrosine kinase inhibitor erlotinib and oncolytic herpes simplex virus HF10. Ann Surg Oncol. 2014;21(2):691–8.

24. Esaki S, Goshima F, Kimura H, et al. Enhanced antitumoral activity of oncolytic herpes simplex virus with gemcitabine using colorectal tumor models. Int J Cancer. 2013;132(7):1592–601.